Haynes

# Man
# Manual

*Including extracts from*

Haynes HGV Man Manual (ISBN 978 1 84425 183 4)
Haynes Brain Manual (ISBN 978 1 84425 371 5)
Haynes Cancer Manual (ISBN 978 1 84425 158 2)
Haynes Sex Manual (ISBN 978 1 84425 086 8)

D0190496

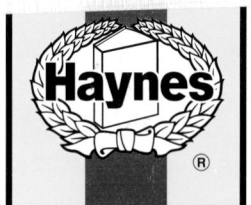

## Ian Banks

Cartoons by Jim Campbell

2199410

6/2199410

© Ian Banks 2007

All rights reserved. No part of this publication may be reproduced or stored in a retrieval system or transmitted, in any form or by any means, electronic, mechanical, photocopying, recording or otherwise, without prior permission in writing from Haynes Publishing.

**Haynes Publishing**
Sparkford, Yeovil, Somerset BA22 7JJ, England

**Haynes North America, Inc**
861 Lawrence Drive, Newbury Park, California 91320, USA

**Haynes Publishing Nordiska AB**
Box 1504, 751 45 Uppsala, Sweden

British Library Cataloguing in Publication Data:
A catalogue record for this book is available from the British Library

ISBN: 978 1 84425 616 7

Printed in Britain by J. H. Haynes & Co. Ltd., Sparkford.

**The Author and the Publisher have taken care to ensure that the advice given in this edition is current at the time of publication. The Reader is advised to read and understand the instructions and information material included with all medicines recommended, and to consider carefully the appropriateness of any treatments. The Author and the Publisher will have no liability for adverse results, inappropriate or excessive use of the remedies offered in this book or their level of effectiveness in individual cases. The Author and the Publisher do not intend that this book be used as a substitute for medical advice. Advice from a medical practitioner should always be sought for any symptom or illness.**

**Illegal Copying**
*It is the policy of Haynes Publishing to actively protect its Copyrights and Trade Marks. Legal action will be taken against anyone who unlawfully copies the cover or contents of this Manual. This includes all forms of unauthorised copying including digital, mechanical, and electronic in any form. Authorisation from Haynes Publishing will only be provided expressly and in writing. Illegal copying will also be reported to the appropriate statutory authorities.*

**Illustration and photo credits:**
Front cover photos, clockwise from top right (all iStock): Gloria-Leigh Logan, Leigh Schindler, Andy Hill, François Etienne du Plessis, Ravet007, David Crockett, Wessel Du Plooy, Janine Hannibal

Other iStockphoto images as marked.

Haynes photos courtesy Paul Buckland and Bob Jex.

Illustrations by Jim Campbell, Mark Stevens, Matthew Marke and Roger Healing.

# Contents

# Author's acknowledgements

My thanks are due to the numerous contributors to the series over the last four years; to the staff at Haynes for their miraculous transformation of a bucket of bits into a finished book; to Jim Campbell for his inimitable cartoons; and finally to the late and much missed Ian Mauger of Haynes, without whose enthusiasm the first edition would never have begun.

**Note:** *The similarities between NHS Direct Online and some sections of this book are no coincidence. It is with grateful thanks that the author acknowledges the invaluable contribution from the NHS Healthcare Guide and Encyclopaedia. For more information see NHS Direct Online (www.nhsdirect.nhs.uk).*

# Foreword

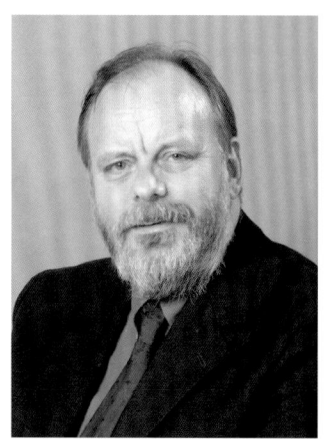

A Man Manual is a pretty obvious idea, but only once someone has thought of it. When the first edition of this book was published in 2002 it rapidly became a best-seller, reprinting three times between October and December and later being translated into German, Russian and Finnish. It was the first title in a series which became known as the Haynes Family Manuals, a range which currently consists of eight titles with more in preparation. This new edition has included material from some of the other manuals in the range to produce a much more comprehensive and up-to-date work than the original, which (it can now be admitted) was a little bit rushed.

Medical science continues to advance, but the use of the health service by men does not. Men do visit their GPs more often than they did 25 years ago, but still nothing like as often as they ought; they are still dying too early from conditions which are largely preventable through lifestyle changes, or treatable if caught in time. Books such as this, and the work of charities such as the Men's Health Forum, will help to reverse that trend.

# How to get the best from your GP

**Write down your symptoms before you see your doctor**

● It is easy to forget the most important things during the examination. Doctors home-in on important clues. When did it start? How did it feel? Did anyone else suffer as well? Did this ever happen before? What have you done about it so far? Are you on any medicines at present?

**Arrive informed**

● Check out the net for information before you go to the surgery. There are thousands of sites on health but many of them are of little real use. Click on NHS Direct as a start, or look in *Contacts* at the back of this book for up-to-date and accurate information.

**Ask questions**

● If a mechanic stuck his head into the bonnet of your car you would most certainly want to know what he intended. This doctor is about to lift the lid on your body. Don't be afraid to

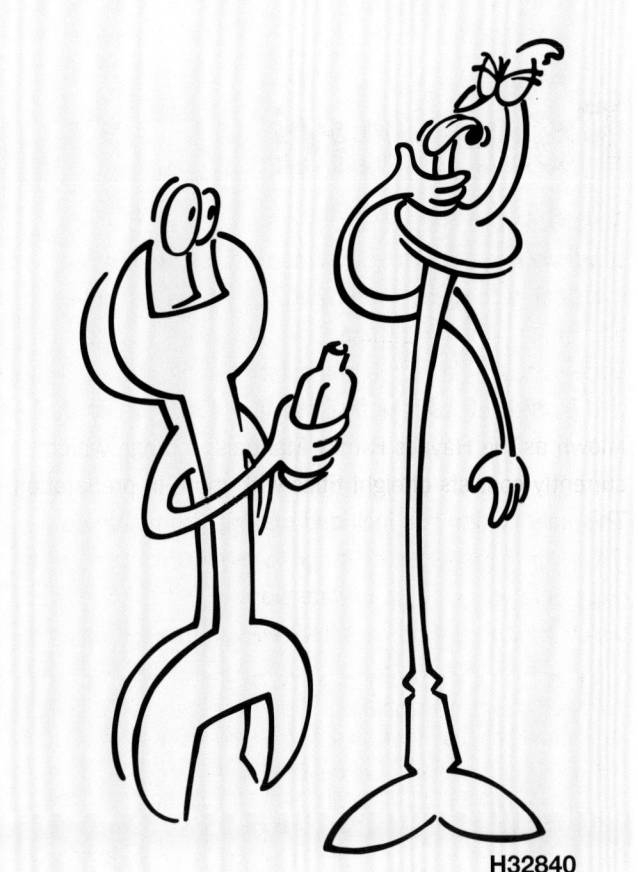

Do your homework with our insider information

H32840

ask questions about what a test will show, how a particular treatment works, and when you should come back. After all, it's your man machine.

## Avoid asking for night visits unless there is a good reason
- Calling your GP after you have 'suffered' all day at work will antagonise a doctor who thinks personal health should come before convenience. If you put money before the quality of family life don't be surprised if you are asked to come to the surgery the following morning.

## Don't beat around the bush
- If you have a lump on your testicles say so. With an average of only seven minutes for each consultation it's important to get to the point. There is a real danger of going to your doctor with erection problems and coming out with a prescription for piles cream.

## Your health is a partnership
- Now is the time to convince your family doctor to take a serious look at men's health, in particular yours. No screening system exists at present but nothing prevents you from asking for a consultation to examine risk factors. A strong family history of conditions such as heart disease, diabetes, cancer or eye problems like glaucoma should prompt some basic tests.

## Listen to what the doctor says
- If you don't understand, say so. It helps if they write down the important points. Most people pick up less than half of what their doctor has told them.

## Have your prescription explained
- Three items on a scrip will cost you as much as a half decent tyre. Ask whether you can buy any of them from the chemist. Make sure you know what they are all for. Some medicines clash badly with alcohol. Even one pint of beer with some popular antibiotics will make you feel very ill. Mixing antidepressants and alcohol can be fatal. Are there any side effects you should look out for? Many prescribed medicines cause erectile dysfunction (impotence).

## If you want a second opinion say so
- Ask for a consultant appointment by all means but remember you are dealing with a person with feelings and not a computer. Compliment him for his attention first but then explain your deep anxiety.

## Flattery will get you anywhere
- Praise is thin on the ground these days. An acknowledgment of a good effort, even if not successful, will be remembered.

## Be courteous with all the staff
- Receptionists are not dragons trying to prevent you seeing a doctor. Practice nurses increasingly influence your treatment. General practice is a team effort and you will get the best out of it by treating all its members with respect.

## Be prepared to complain
- If possible see your doctor first and explain what is annoying you. Family doctors now have an 'in-house' complaints system, and most issues are successfully resolved at this level. If you are still not satisfied you can take it to a formal hearing.

## Trust your doctor
- There is a difference between trust and blind faith. Your health is a partnership between you and your doctor where you are the majority stakeholder.

## Change your GP with caution
- Thousands of people change their doctor each year. Most of them have simply moved house. You do not need to tell your family doctor if you wish to leave their practice. Your new doctor will arrange for all your notes to be transferred. The whole point of general practice is to build up a personal insight into the health of you and your family. A new doctor has to start almost from scratch.

## Don't be afraid to ask to see your notes
- You have the right to see what your doctor writes about you. Unfortunately doctors' language can be difficult to understand. Latin and Greek are still in use although on the decline. Doctors use abbreviations in your notes. Watch out for:

  a) TATT: An abbreviation for Tired All The Time.
  b) TCA SOS: To Call Again if things get worse. Most illnesses are self-limiting. A couple of weeks usually allows nature to sort things out.
  c) RV: Review. Secretaries will automatically arrange a subsequent appointment.
  d) PEARLA: Pupils Equal and Reacting to Light and Accommodation. A standard entry on a casualty sheet to show that your brain is functioning.
  e) RTA: Road Traffic Accident.
  f) FROM: Full Range Of Movement at a joint.
  g) SOB: Short Of Breath. If this comes on after walking in from the waiting room it turns into SOBOE – On Exercise.
  h) AMA/CMA: Against Medical Advice/Contrary Medical Advice: You went home despite medical advice not to do so.
  i) DNA: Did Not Attend. You didn't turn up for your appointment.
  j) SUPRATENTORIAL: If your doctor thinks you are deluding yourself over your symptoms and it's really all in your head, he might think the problem lies above (supra) your tentorium. Rarely used these days.
  k) HYSTERIA: A dangerous diagnosis. In essence your doctor believes you are possibly over-dramatising the situation. Rarely used these days.
  l) $C_2H_5OH$: The chemical formula for alcohol. Your doctor probably believes alcohol plays a role in your problem. Rarely used these days.

# Home medicine chest

Minor illnesses or accidents can happen at any time so it's worth being prepared. It makes sense to keep some first aid and simple remedies in a safe place in the house to cover most minor ailments and accidents. The picture shows an example of a well stocked and maintained kit. Ask your pharmacist for advice on which products are best.

- Painkillers.
- Anti-diarrhoeal, rehydration mixture.
- Indigestion remedy, eg antacids.
- Travel sickness tablets.
- Sunscreen – SPF15 or higher.
- Sunburn treatment.
- Tweezers, sharp scissors.
- Thermometer.
- A selection of plasters, cotton wool, elastic bandages and assorted dressings.

## Remember

- Keep the medicine chest in a secure, locked place, out of reach of small children.
- Do not keep in the bathroom as the damp will soon damage the medicines and bandages.
- Always read the instructions and use the right dose.
- Watch expiry dates – don't keep or use medicines past their sell-by date.

Home medicine kit

Photo: © iStockphoto.com, Dana Bartekoske

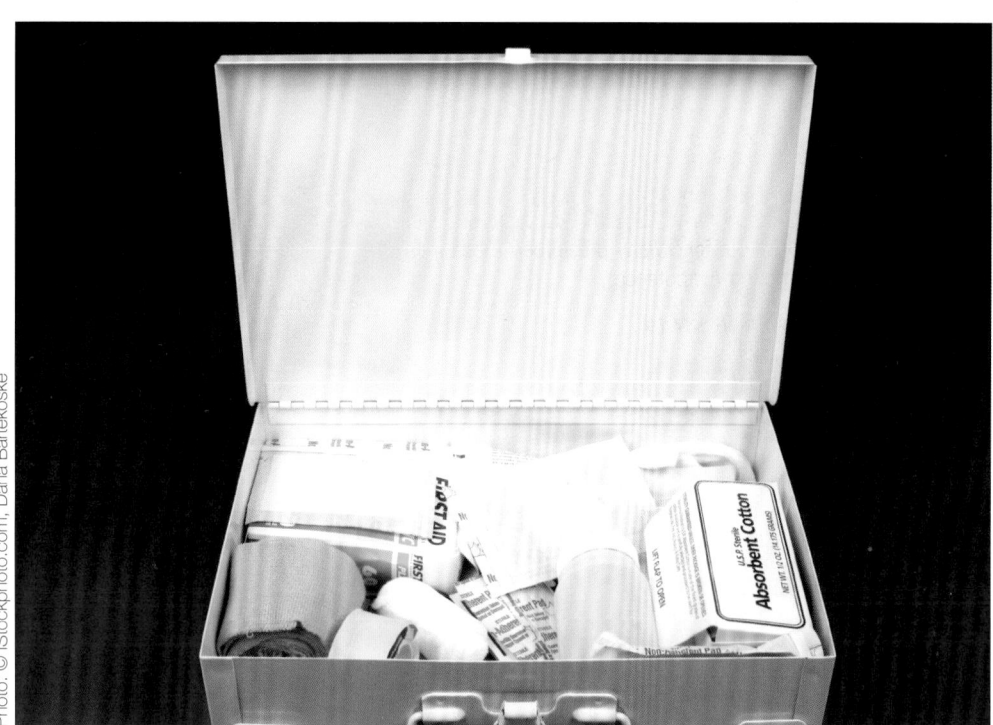

# How your pharmacist can help you lose the pounds but not the £s

Your local pharmacist (chemist) is your health care professional in the high street and is perhaps the most accessible part of the health service. No appointments are needed, advice is free, there are no long waiting lists and you can get a large range of goods and services to help you fight the inch (25 millimetre) war.

Your pharmacist will supply
- Condoms – have more safe sex and burn more calories. 20 minutes of sex burns twice the calories of 20 minutes of mixed doubles tennis.

Sex burns more calories than doubles tennis

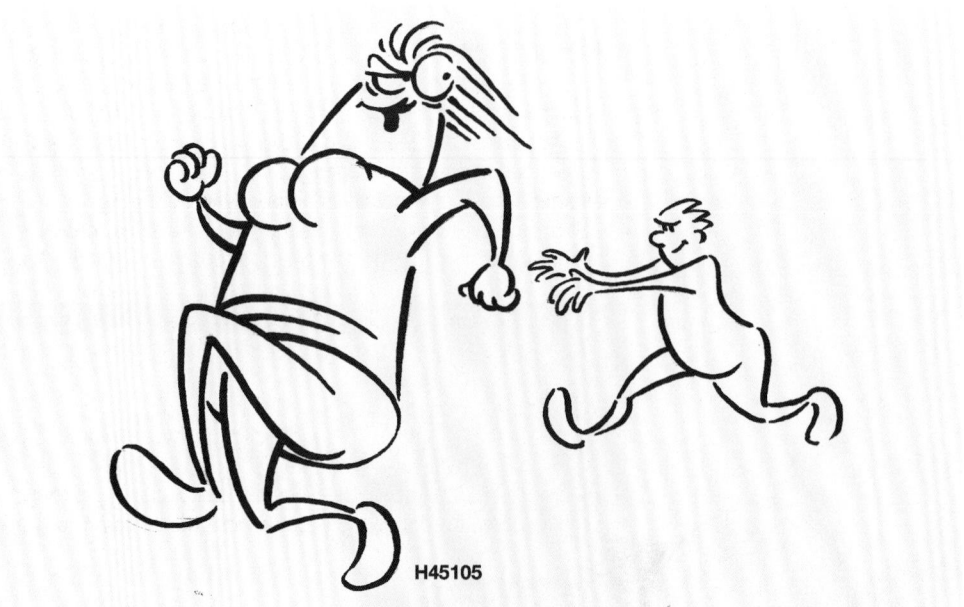

H45105

- Perfume/aftershave – buy some for the wife/girlfriend/partner to increase the likelihood of the above!
- A new toothbrush, floss, mouthwash and sugar free gum – look after your mouth and keep it busy and active so it doesn't miss the full English, Welsh, Scottish or Irish fried breakfasts. Will also increase the likelihood of the above!
- Giving up smoking aids – tobacco and nicotine substitutes – gums, patches, lozenges, micro-tablets, and inhalers to will help you stop raiding the biscuit-tin or hitting the bottle by reducing your cravings for fags (and increasing your desire and performance for the above!).
- Pain-killers for your wife/girlfriend as she is probably developing headaches to *decrease* the likelihood of the above!

The best way to lose those inches for good is exercise and eating healthily

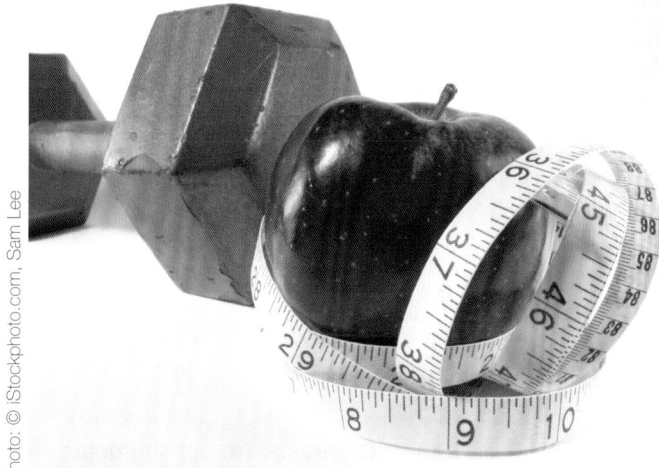

Photo: © iStockphoto.com, Sam Lee

● Tape measures and weighing scales – car or lorry mirrors, the opinion of Doris in the transport café, the views of your workmates or trying to use HGV weighbridges will not be good enough to see if your waistline really is shrinking.
● Sweeteners and sugar substitutes – some things in life can be substituted successfully.

Your pharmacist can also give you free help and advice on
● Figuring out the figures on food labels – understand how 'Low Fat' or 'Diet' food doesn't always 'do what is says on the can'.
● Discussing your prescription and over-the-counter medicines – a few medicines contain lots of sugar, some could cause weight gain as a side effect, and some may not work as well as they should if you have changed your diet, stopped smoking or started drinking grapefruit or cranberry juice, for example.
● Understanding how losing weight will reduce your chances of getting diabetes, high blood pressure or a heart attack. Some pharmacists will be able to measure your blood pressure or cholesterol level for you, so you can see how your health is improving.

Your pharmacist will not supply
● Laxatives – if you take these to try to lose weight you will be as full of sh*t as you were before!
● Quack diet pills and potions – there is no such thing as a magic pill or potion, the only weight you will lose will be from your wallet!

Checking blood pressure

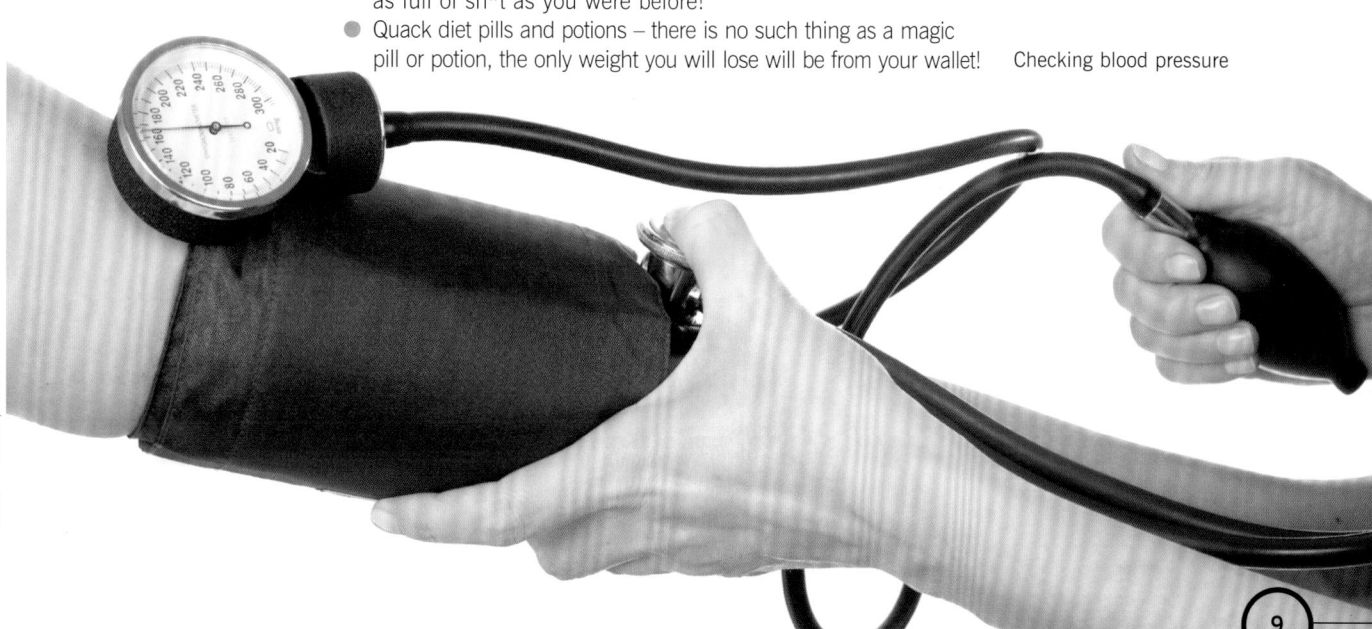

Photo: © iStockphoto.com

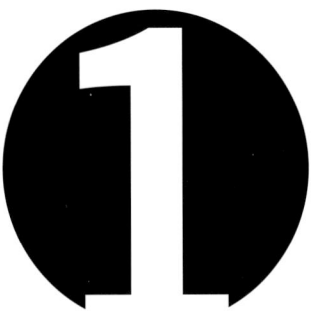

# First aid

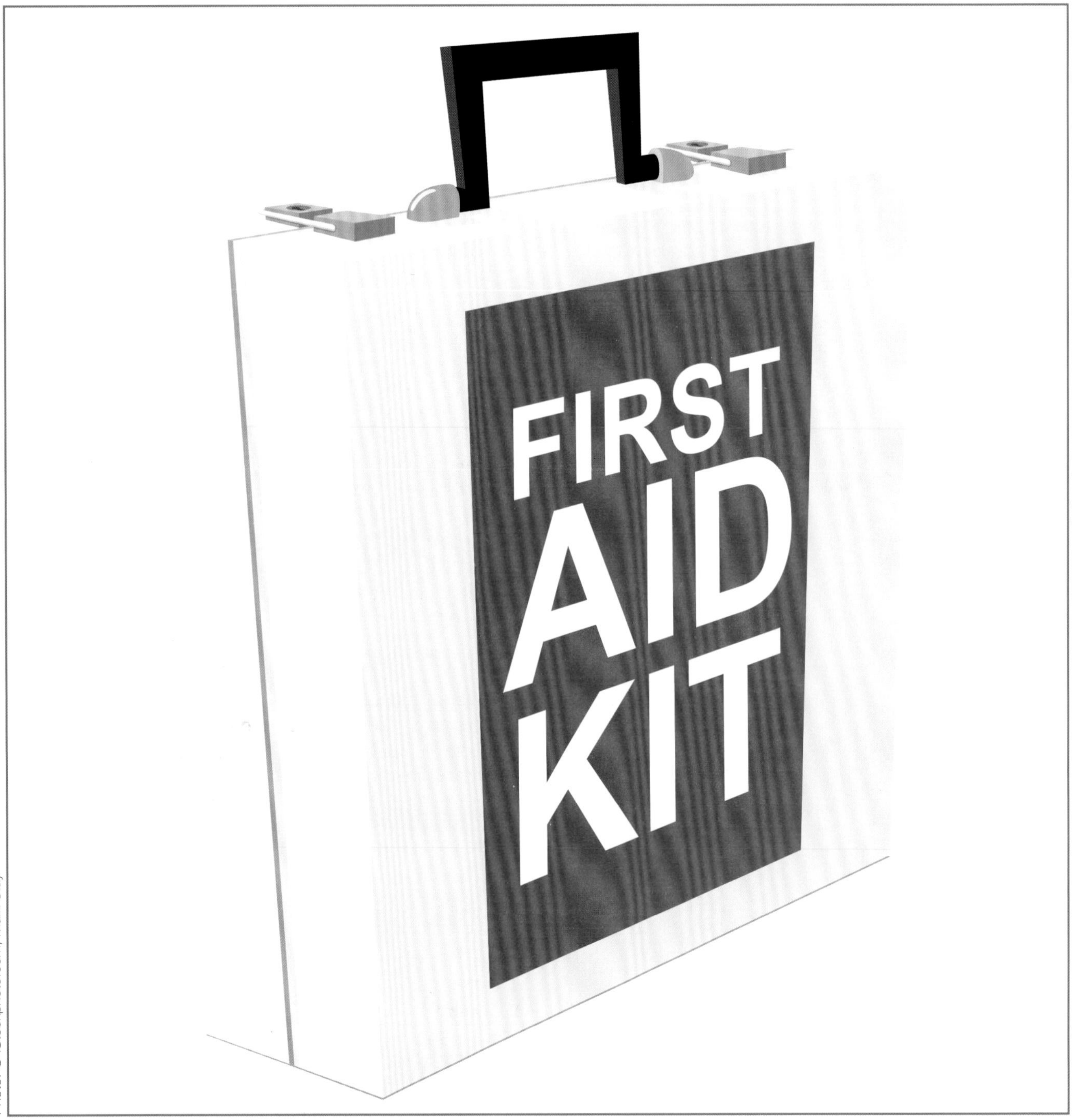

Photo: © iStockphoto.com, Mark Stay

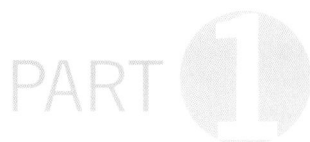

PART **1**

# Introduction

Accidents account for greatest loss of life amongst young men. Car crashes, sports injuries, industrial accidents and dodgy DIY are all major causes of injury and death.

Having someone around with first aid knowledge can make the difference. Anyone can learn these simple but often life saving techniques.

## Myths of first aid

Below are some commonly asked questions and answers:

**You will be successfully sued if you look after someone and they think you were negligent**
- **Wrong:** The Good Samaritan principle should keep you safe from successful litigation in most cases. You are only expected to be able to do what any other non-medically trained person could do.

**Men should not look after injured women in case they are accused of sexual harassment**
- **Wrong:** Common-sense prevails. Do what you need to do to save her life. If another woman is present, use her to chaperone. Explain out loud what you are doing even if she appears unconscious, it also helps to calm onlookers.

**People always faint when they see all the blood**
- **Wrong:** If you know what you need to do and you get on with it you will probably not faint.

**You will catch HIV if you perform mouth to mouth resuscitation on someone with AIDS**
- **Wrong:** Although there is a small theoretical risk, the chances of becoming infected are extremely small.

**First aid makes no difference. Getting them to hospital takes precedence**
- **Wrong:** It is vital to get professional help as soon as possible but ambulance drivers generally like to pick up live people on the way to casualty. A person can lose all their blood from a serious wound in a relatively short space of time. You can save someone's life before the ambulance even arrives. After one hour, the so called 'Golden Hour', a person's fate is more or less sealed. You make the difference in the equation.

**A little knowledge is a dangerous thing**
- **Wrong:** This is usually quoted by people who would rather not bother. So long as you stick to what you know and use common sense it is unlikely you will make the situation any worse.

**Doing something is always better than doing nothing**
- **Wrong:** People with no idea can be a danger to your health. Giving a badly injured person alcohol might bring their colour back but if they're bleeding it could kill them. Get trained.

## It seemed like a good idea (common mistakes)

We all carry ideas on what to do in an emergency. Most of them come from the movies.

**Don't give a casualty anything to eat or drink**
- If a person is unable to swallow properly, for example after a stroke or head injury, you could choke them, and if they need surgery the anaesthetist would not thank you.

**Don't leave an unconscious or drunk person lying on their back**
- Vomit or even their own tongue could block their airway. Stay with them, but shout to attract help or if possible use a mobile telephone.

**Don't be afraid to call the emergency services**
- If you are not sure whether you are out of your depth you probably are. Send two people to phone at the same time. Get one to return and let you know what's happening, and tell one to stay and direct the ambulance.

**Don't use a tourniquet**
- Once a tourniquet is released all the debris in the blood blocks up the kidneys. Instead press firmly on the wound to stop the bleeding.

**Don't put yourself in danger**
- If it goes wrong the emergency services have two casualties to deal with. Check your surroundings first for falling rocks, fumes, cars, live electricity, etc.

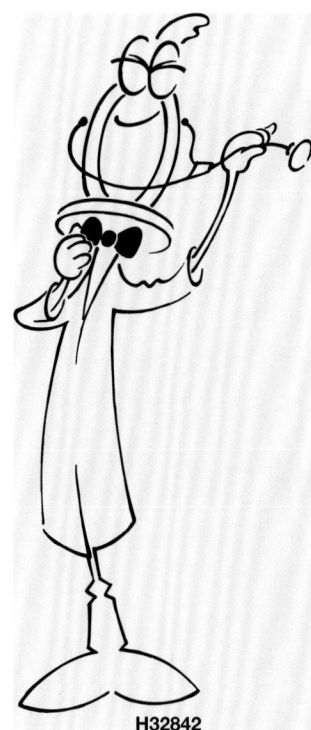

H32842

The best way to gain new skills is from an expert. Do a course and look like Dr Kildare in an emergency. Contact the St John Ambulance or the British Heart Foundation

PART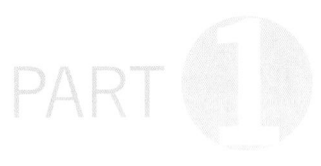

# Cardio-pulmonary resuscitation (kiss of life)

Simply reading how to perform cardio-pulmonary-resuscitation (CPR) is like expecting to be able to drive a Porsche after reading the workshop manual. You need to be trained before having to do it for real.

## Cardio-pulmonary resuscitation (kiss of life)

Check the area for danger, if safe kneel to one side of the casualty. Lean over the casualty and into each ear ask in a loud voice if they can hear you and to open their eyes for you. You can also gently shake the casualty's shoulders while doing so. If there is no response shout for help

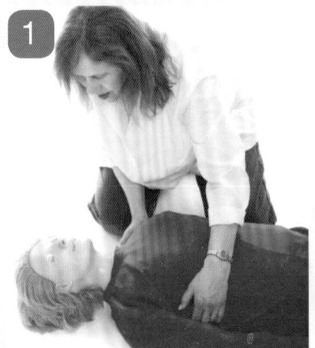

Open the airway by gently placing one hand on the casualty's forehead and two fingers under the chin and gently tilt the head backwards

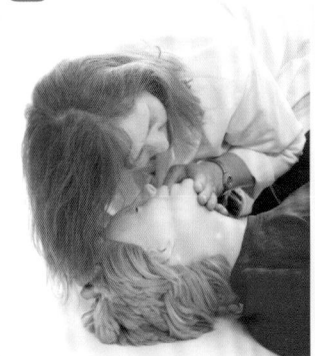

Check for normal breathing by placing your ear close to the casualty's mouth and looking at the chest for a rising and falling motion. Do this for no more than 10 seconds. If there is no response send or call for help. Ensure the rescue service knows that the casualty is unconscious and not breathing normally

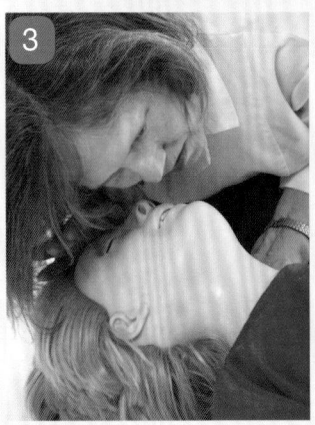

Give 30 chest compressions using two hands in the centre of the chest, at a rate of 100 per minute to a depth of 4 to 5 cms. If you think of the tune 'Nelly the Elephant' this will give you an idea of the pace the compressions need to be

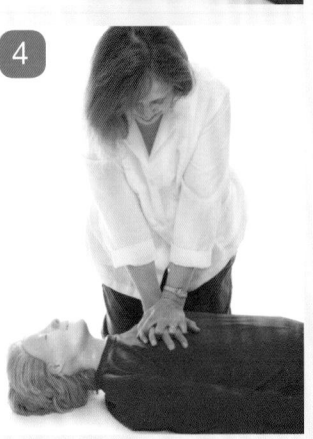

Attempt 2 rescue breaths. Seal your lips over the casualty's mouth and holding their nose deliver the breath over 1 second and remove your mouth then repeat once more. Continue artificial respiration with the correct ratio of 30 chest compressions to 2 rescue breaths. Continue until the rescue services tell you to stop or the patient begins to breathe normally, in which case place them into the recovery position and monitor their responses until help arrives

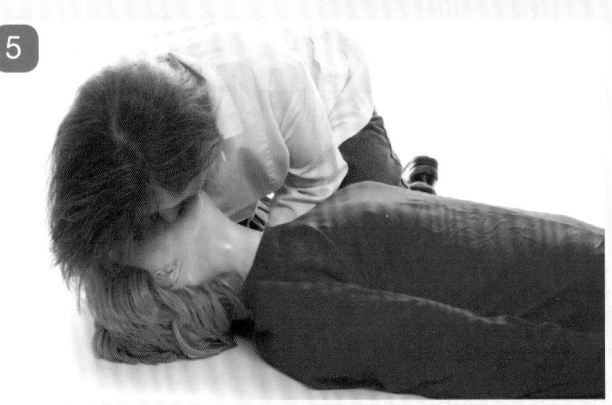

Photos: © iStockphoto.com, Sharon Dominick

## Putting someone in the recovery position

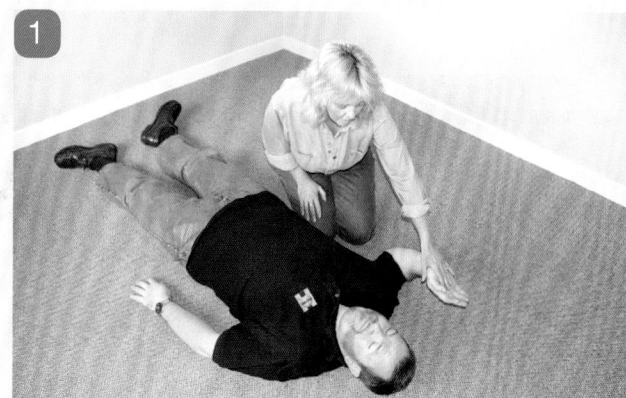

Make sure that the legs are straight and place the nearest arm at right-angles to the body

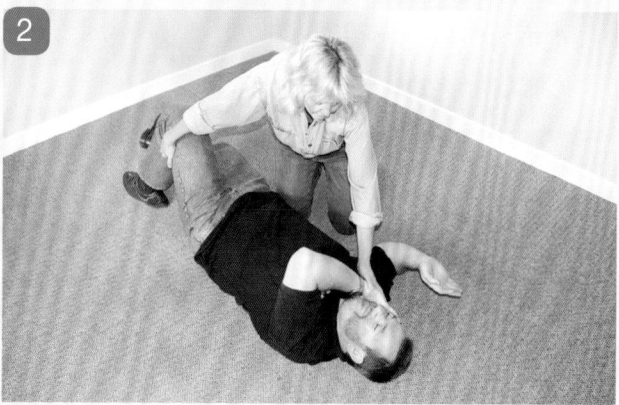

Hold the casualty's hand against the cheek, palm outwards, and raise the furthest leg, keeping the foot on the floor

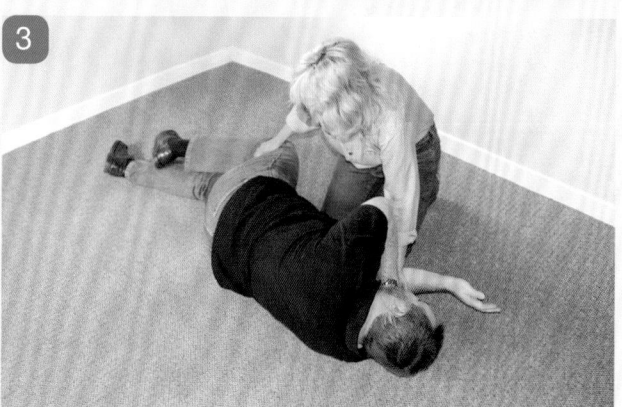

Keeping the hand against the cheek, pull the raised leg and roll the casualty

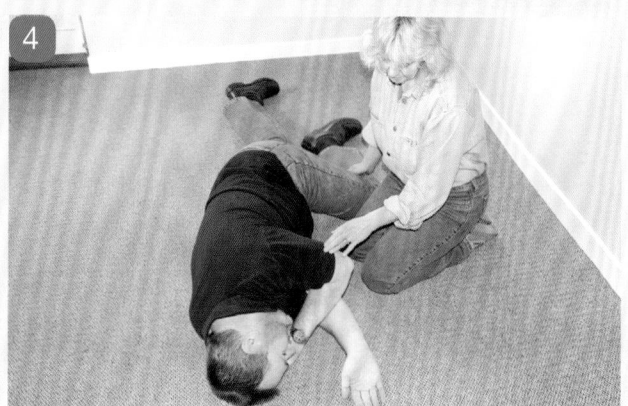

Adjust the upper leg so that both hip and knee are at right-angles, and check that the hand below the cheek helps keep the airway open

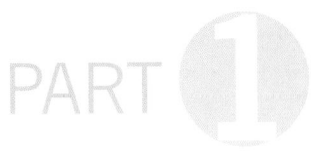

PART **1**

# Common conditions requiring first aid

## Broken bones

Bones contain blood vessels and nerves. A fracture is painful, more so if the broken ends are sticking into flesh. Follow these simple rules:

● Tell the injured person to keep still. Steady and support the limb with your hands.

● Cover any wounds with a dressing or clean non fluffy material, eg shirt. Press as hard as required to stop the bleeding. Bandage the dressing onto the limb.

● If a leg is broken, tie both legs together with a piece of wood or rolled up magazines between them. Tie the knees and ankles together first then closer to the broken bone.

● Suspected broken arms or collar bones should be supported by fastening the arm on the affected side to the body.

● Always check that the hands or feet are warm and colour returns after squeezing a nail. If not, loosen the bandages a little.

● Swelling can tighten bandages so check every fifteen minutes.

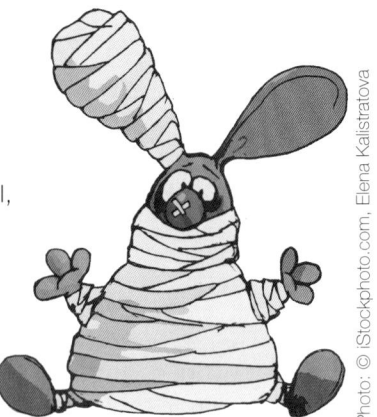

Wrap broken limbs against the body for support, but check for blood circulation regularly

## Broken spine

A broken neck or spine will not necessarily kill or paralyse you, but if you suspect a broken spine it is essential you follow these simple rules.

● Do not move the person unless there is imminent danger within the area. If they must be moved, always support the head on each side with gentle but firm pulling and use a number of people to lift in as many places as possible. If possible use a flat piece of wood to carry him while still supporting his head.

● Reassure the person and tell him not to move. Steady the head with hands on either side of the ears.

● Get helpers to place rolled blankets or coats around the sides to stop him rolling.

● Dial 999 or 112 and explain what has happened.

● Continue to check his breathing while you wait for help.

## Dislocated joints

Dislocating any joint can damage surrounding nerves, blood vessels, and ligaments. Trying to force the joint back into place can make this ten times worse. Dislocated shoulders are common because it is a relatively lax joint. Horrendous damage can be done by well meaning offers to 'pop it back in'.

● Simply support the arm against the front of the body and get him to casualty. Don't give him anything to eat or drink as he may need a general anaesthetic.

## Burns

● Cool the burn area with cold water. This can take 10 minutes. Send someone for the ambulance if the burn is severe (greater in size than the size of their own palm).

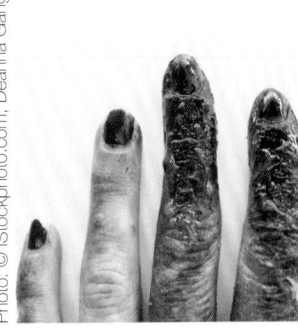

Cool the burn area with cold water

- Remove watches, bracelets or anything which will cause constriction once the flesh begins to swell. This includes shoes and necklaces.
- Don't remove clothes if they are sticking to the skin.
- Cover the burn area with light non-fluffy material.
- Don't apply creams or burst any blisters.
- With severe burns there will be a rapid loss of fluid from the blood system with a loss of blood pressure. Lay him down and raise his legs. This helps keep blood available for the vital organs as well as the heart, brain, kidney and lungs.

## Choking

It takes surprisingly little to choke a person. Here's what to do if you see someone choking:
- Check inside his mouth. If you can see the offending obstruction pull it out. If you can't see it, bend him over and use the flat of your hand to slap him firmly on the back between his shoulder blades five times.
- If all this fails, go for the Heimlich manoeuvre (the abdominal thrust).
- Stand behind the person. Put both arms around his waist and interlock your hands.
- Pull sharply upwards below the ribs. Try five times and go back to checking inside the mouth.

## Eye injury

Eyes are amazingly tough. Blows from blunt instruments, such as a squash ball, cause extensive damage to the surrounding bone but the eye usually remains intact. Penetrating injuries are a different matter. Flakes of steel from a chisel struck with a hammer travel at the speed of sound. That's significantly faster than the blink of an eye.
- Lay him on his back and examine the eye. Only wash the eye if there is no obvious foreign body stuck to the eye and it has no open wound.
- Place a loose pad over the eye and bandage.
- Take him to hospital.

## Heart attacks

Heart disease is the single biggest killer of men so you are likely to see it happen at some time. Modern treatment can significantly improve chances of survival if you can get him to hospital quickly. Recognise what's going on. Central chest pain can move upwards to the throat or arms, usually the left arm.
- Fear causes the release of adrenaline which makes the heart beat faster, increasing the pain, so talk calmly and reassure.
- Call for an ambulance.
- If they normally take a tablet or oral spray for chest pain, let them do so.
- Sit them down but don't force them to lie down if they don't want to.

## Heavy bleeding

- Lay them down. Bleeding from a vein is generally slow and simply pressing a cloth against the wound and raising the affected limb above the level of the heart will stop the bleeding. Get him to hospital.
- Arterial bleeds can be seriously different. It's hard to miss when it happens. The blood is bright red and comes out in spurts with each heart beat.
- Press a cloth against the wound and hold it down firmly. If you have to leave them, secure it to the wound with a shirt or towel.
- Raise their arms and legs to keep the blood pressure up. Some seepage will occur but you may save their life. Get them to hospital.

## Do the knowledge

The principles of First Aid are easy when explained by an expert on a training course. Whether you end up reassuring an elderly relative after a fall, or saving a choking child, the sense of reward is amazing. The British Heart Foundation and St John Ambulance charities offer courses, why not give them a call today? See *Contacts* for details.

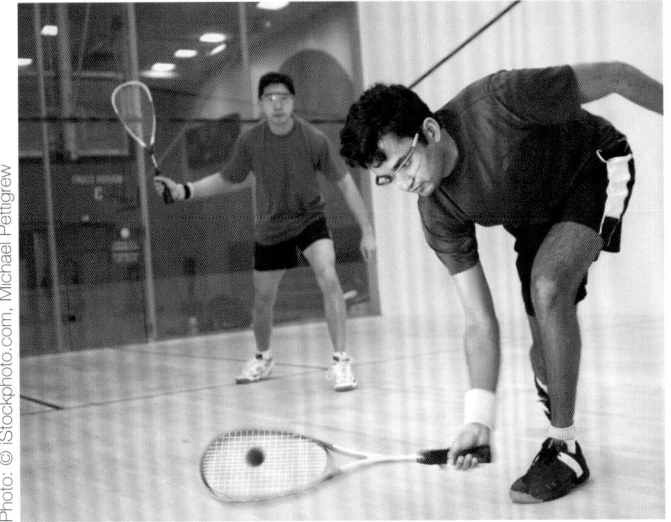

Photo: © iStockphoto.com, Michael Pettigrew

No matter how tough the eye is, it always makes sense to wear some sort of protection

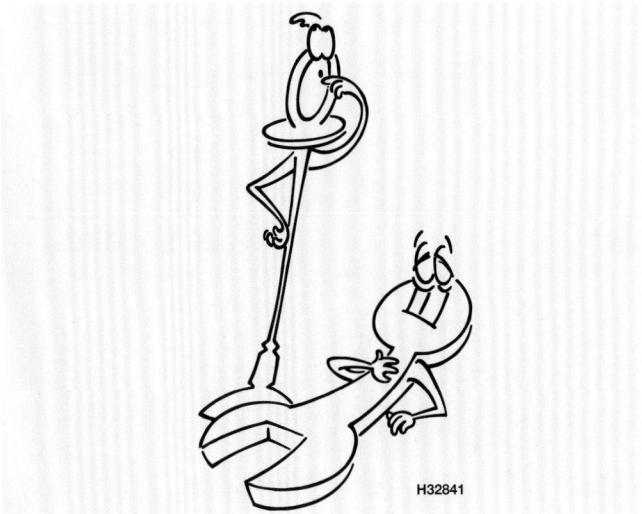

H32841

Don't be a Dipstick, get trained

# Routine maintenance (staying healthy)

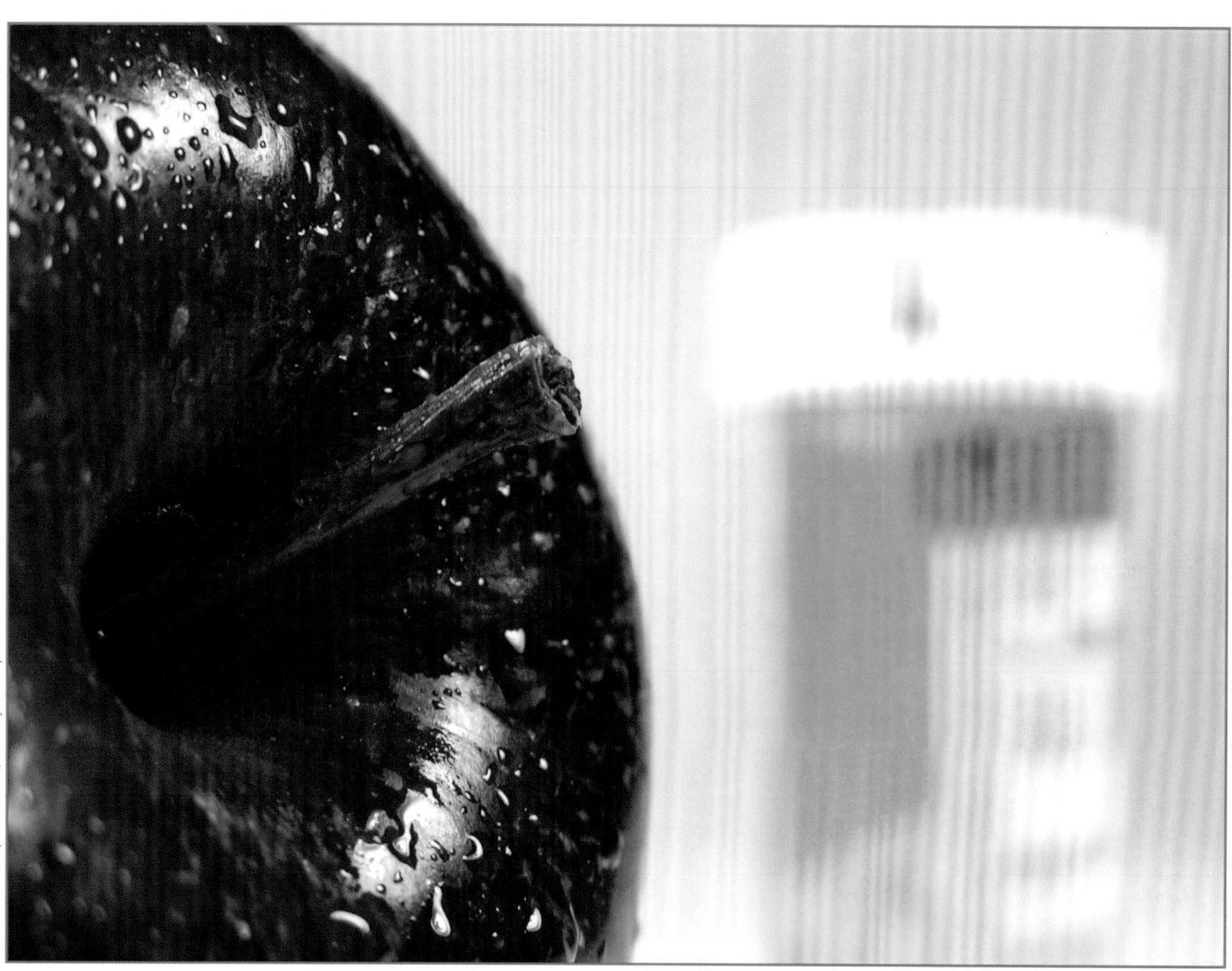

Photo: © iStockphoto.com, Christy Thompson

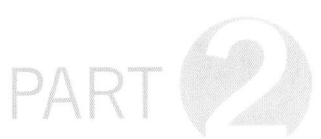

# PART 2

# Ageing

The natural human life-span appears to be about 100 years although this can vary enormously across the globe. Even within Europe men live different lengths of time depending on their country and environment.

The bodily and mental changes that occur with ageing usually cause a general improvement and increasing power, both of body and mind, up to about the mid-20s. After that, in most men, there is a gradual decline.

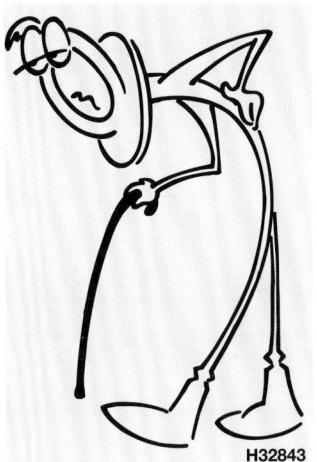

Ageing is one thing that comes to us all, although a regular body service will help keep you running like a Rolls Royce

## Symptoms

There are some generally common facets to the ageing process which include:
- Loss of muscle power.
- Deterioration in efficiency of the nervous system.
- Loss of hair colour.
- Decreased skin elasticity with wrinkling and sagging of the skin.
- Thinning of the skin.
- Brittleness of the bones.
- Hardening and narrowing of the arteries.
- Damage to the lenses of the eyes (cataract).
- Poorer recall of memorised facts.

## Causes

A number of things make ageing worse, including:
- Unhealthy diet.
- Reduced or lack of exercise for body and mind.
- Smoking.
- Substance abuse, including alcohol.
- Excessive exposure to sunlight.

All of these can be modified. The earlier the better.

It's also worth keeping an eye out for warning signs. Even as we get older the best way to stay healthy is to catch problems early. Warning signs of dangerous changes include:
- A new, changed or persisting cough.
- Blood in your sputum.
- Black or blood stained stools (motions).
- Any persistent change in your bowel habit.
- Indigestion coming on for the first time in later life.
- Difficulty in swallowing possibly with food returning to your mouth undigested.
- Blood in your vomit.
- Urine or semen with blood stains.
- Any obvious change in a coloured skin spot, mole or wart.
- Any wound or sore that fails to heal in a month.
- Hoarseness or loss of voice, without obvious cause.
- Unexplained weight loss.

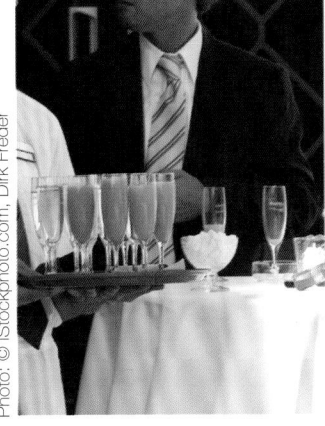

Photo: © iStockphoto.com, Dirk Freder

Take alcohol in moderation

## Action

- Eat less to maintain a normal, low-end-of-range body weight. Avoid saturated fats.
- Exercise to the point of breathlessness at least three times a week.
- Stop smoking.
- Take alcohol in moderation. Aim for no more than 3-4 units of alcohol per day, hopefully less.
- Have regular blood pressure checks.
- Take your hobbies seriously, involve others.
- Make an appointment to see your GP.

PART 2

# Allergies

Allergies are caused by the body producing antibodies to specific substances (allergens). The reactions can range from a mild flush to a serious and life threatening condition. Coming into contact with products containing normally innocent foodstuffs such as peanuts can actually kill susceptible people. Thankfully this is rare. Many people will suffer from allergies for years without realising they are the victim of their own body's defence system.

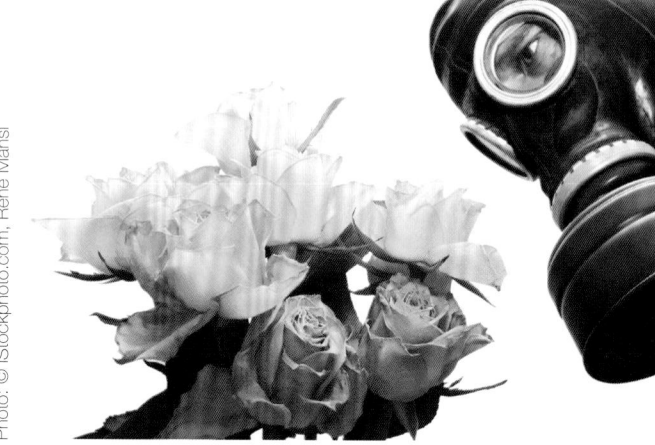

Photo: © iStockphoto.com, René Mansi

Allergic reactions include hayfever . . .

Allergic conditions include:

- Hay fever and allergic asthma. Pollen, house mites, pets and mouldy dust can all cause respiratory and nasal problems.
- Eczema. Contact dermatitis is easily recognised. Cement dust is particularly bad.
- Urticaria (itchy hives). This tends to be harmless, though it can be very annoying. Nettles will produce it in most people but foods like strawberries or seafood can also be causes.
- Drug reactions (eg, to penicillin).

. . . and eczema

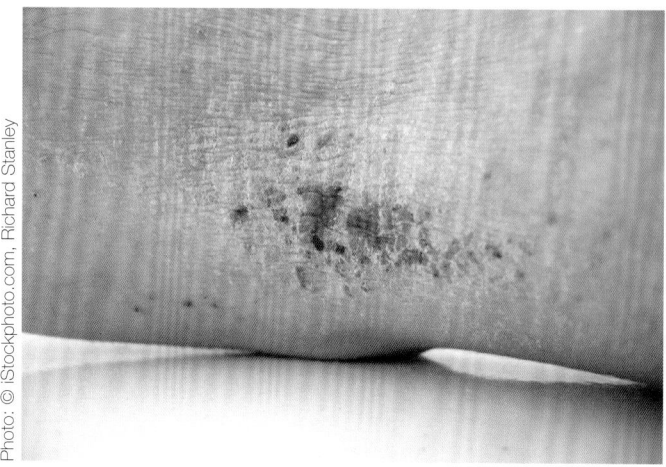

Photo: © iStockphoto.com, Richard Stanley

## Symptoms

Immediate reactions can affect the whole body or just around the contact area. For some people, the skin becomes sore and broken with even the slightest exposure to the allergen. Symptoms include:

- Itchiness.
- A blotchy red rash over the body.
- Blocked or running nose.
- Eye irritation.
- Fluid retention.
 More serious reactions can lead to:
- Chest tightness.
- Shortness of breath.
- Swollen lips and tongue.
- Fatigue.

## Causes

There is a wide range of possible allergens and a great deal depends on your own particular allergy state. You are more likely to suffer from strong allergic reactions if you have hay fever, asthma or have had a reaction to a particular substance in the past. Subsequent contact, for instance the second time you are stung by a bee, can be worse than the first time.

## Possible allergens include

- Drugs (both over the counter and prescribed).
- Foods, particularly, in susceptible people, peanuts, seafood and strawberries.
- Dairy and grain produce (associated with longer term allergies).
- Soap powders.
- Latex (eg, rubber gloves, condoms), plasters.
- Nickel jewellery or watches.
- Hair dye.
- Cement dust.

## Prevention

Once the allergy is established, its cause must be either removed or avoided. Other substances, foods or material are often available which do not provoke an allergic response.

- Wear hypoallergenic gloves.
- Use a filter in the vacuum cleaner to remove dust mite droppings.
- Use the correct protective clothing when handling material such as cement.
- Use a filter face mask when in dusty areas.
- Check food labels for potentially allergenic ingredients, such as peanut products.
- Use a barrier cream.
- Check with your pharmacist/doctor before taking any new medicines.

## Complications

Serious allergic reactions can be fatal. Long term reactions can cause debilitation even after there is no further contact with the allergenic substance. Anaphylactic shock is an extreme allergic reaction. Immediately after contact there is difficulty breathing, itchiness, swelling of the lips and throat, drop in blood pressure, and finally collapse. Dial 999 or 112.

## Self care

- Wash off any of the suspected allergen if it is on the skin.
- Bathe in a cool bath with a large spoonful of baking soda.
- Ask your pharmacist for something to treat the allergy.
- Susceptible people should carry antihistamine tablets in case of a reaction.
- If you have ever had anaphylactic shock, you should also carry injectable adrenaline available from your doctor.

You should make an appointment to see your doctor if:
- There are any serious allergic reactions (see above).
- There are any new and unexpected reactions.

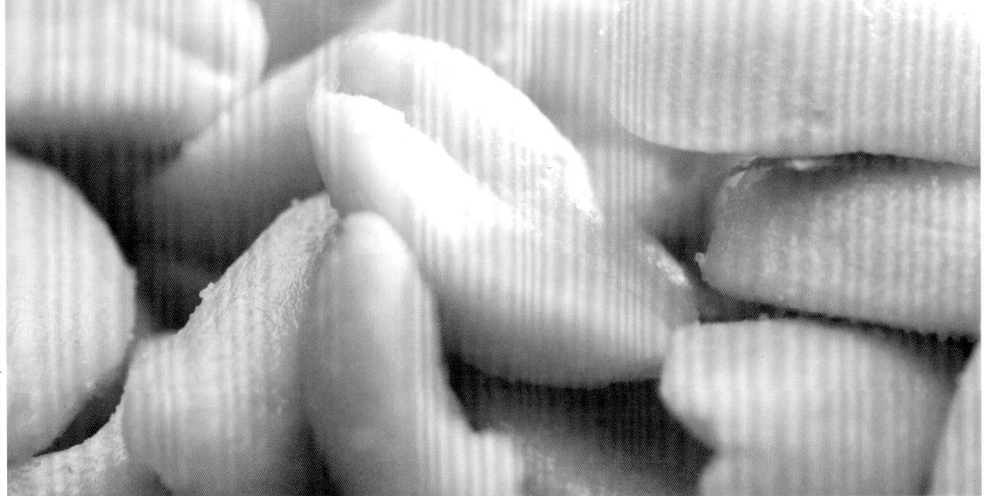

Photo: © iStockphoto.com, Paul Reid

Peanuts are a common allergen

PART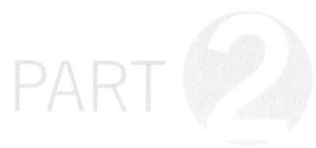

# Eating disorders

Everyone has different eating habits and there are a large number of 'eating styles' which can allow us to stay healthy. However, some eating habits can actually damage our health. These are called 'eating disorders', and the most common are Anorexia Nervosa and Bulimia Nervosa.

Although girls and women are 10 times more likely to suffer from anorexia and bulimia, boys and men seem to be getting eating disorders more often. Anorexia is a serious illness which can damage your heart, lungs and bones. It has the highest death rate of any psychological disorder.

Anorexia usually starts in the teenage years and affects around one 15 year-old boy in every 1,000. Bulimia often starts in the mid-teens, but people don't usually seek help for it until their early to mid-twenties because, unlike anorexia, they are able to hide it.

Symptoms can include not eating and taking exercising to extremes

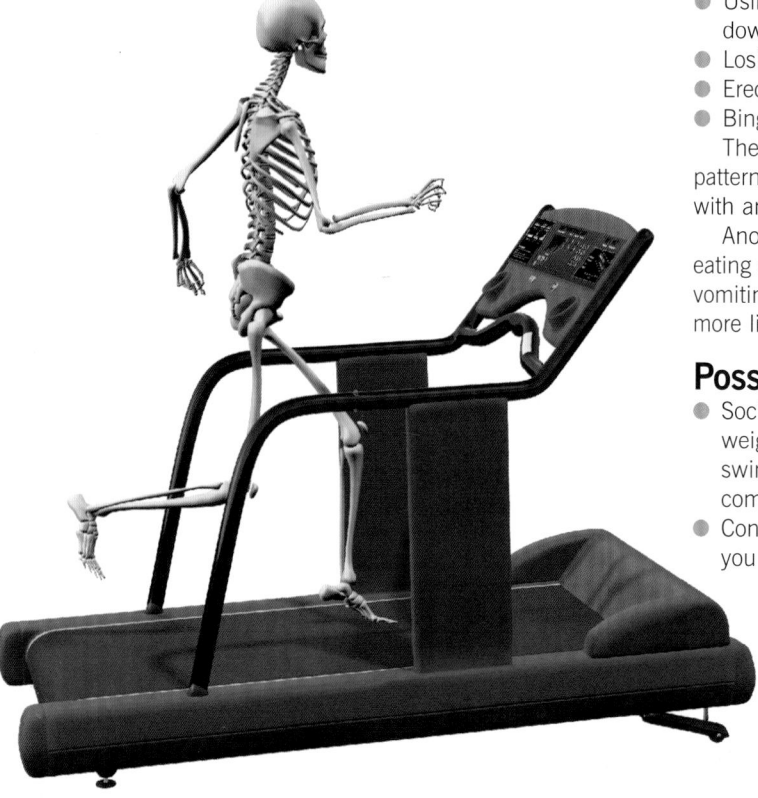

## Symptoms (for men in particular)
- Eating less and less.
- Worrying more and more about your weight.
- Using harmful ways to get rid of calories, such as vomiting and using laxatives.
- Exercising more and more to burn off calories.
- Using slimming pills, or smoking more to keep your weight down.
- Losing interest in sex.
- Erections and wet dreams stop, your testicles shrink.
- Binge eating.

The symptoms of anorexia and bulimia are often mixed. The pattern of symptoms can change over time – someone may start with anorexic symptoms, but later develop those of bulimia.

Another eating disorder has recently been recognised – binge eating disorder. It involves dieting and binge eating, but not vomiting. It is much less harmful than bulimia and sufferers are more likely to become overweight.

## Possible causes
- Social pressure – occupations which demand a low body weight (or low body fat) – body building, wrestling, ballet, swimming and athletics – seem to make eating disorders more common.
- Control – your weight may be the only part of your life that you feel you can control.
  - Puberty – anorexia can reverse some of the physical changes of becoming an adult – pubic and facial hair for example. This may help you put off the demands of getting older, particularly sexual ones.
  - Family – saying 'no' to food may be the only way you can express your feelings or have a say in family affairs.

Photo: © iStockphoto.com, Linda Bucklin

- Depression – people with bulimia are often depressed. Bingeing may start as a way of coping with feelings of unhappiness.
- Self-esteem – people with anorexia and bulimia often don't think much of themselves and compare themselves unfavourably with other people.
- Emotional distress – anorexia and bulimia can develop as a result of sexual abuse, physical illness, and important life events.

## Treatment

Most people with a serious eating disorder will end up having some sort of treatment, as the condition does not appear to get better on its own. Bulimia can sometimes be tackled using a self-help manual and some guidance from a therapist. However, anorexia usually needs more organised help from a clinic or therapist. Although half of people with anorexia make a recovery, on average they will be ill for five to six years. A full recovery can happen even after 20 years. About 1 in 5 of the most seriously ill may die.

Although Cognitive Behaviour Therapy and Interpersonal Therapy have been found to be beneficial for bulimia, many patients have responded to other therapy approaches, particularly forms of family therapy. In the case of anorexia, no particular therapy has advantages over others.

What you see in the mirror isn't how the world sees you

Photo: © iStockphoto.com, Gary Milner

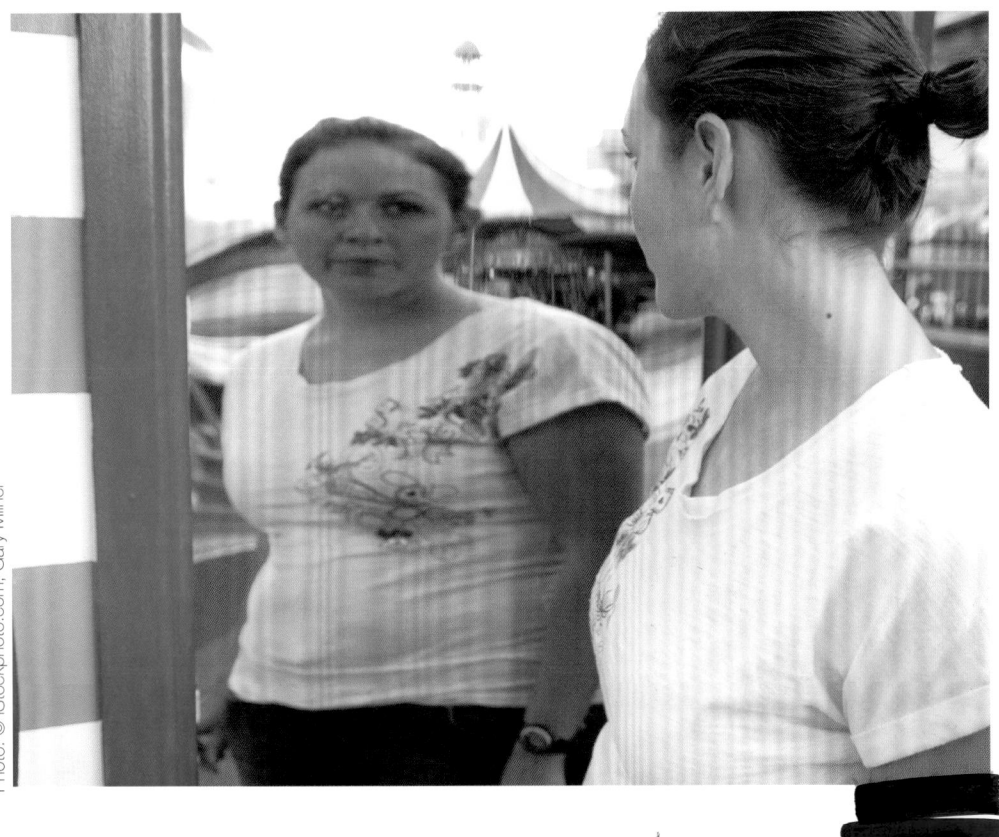

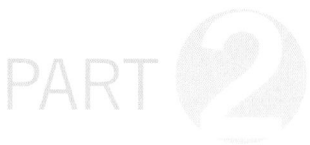 PART **2**

# Exercise

Exercise is not just good for the heart, it is also good for the mind. Just as pumping iron makes you stronger and able to lift heavier loads, taking regular exercise enables your brain to cope better when things get stressful. The fitter your body, the more reserves you have to draw on when under pressure. The same applies for the brain.

Scientists have shown that people who take regular physical activity are less likely to suffer from depression and anxiety, and are better able to cope with stress. Studies have found that exercise can be as effective as anti-depressant drugs in cases of mild or moderate depression. More evidence on just how exercise affects the brain is emerging all the time. The latest research suggests that fitter people have better cognitive functioning. This means they are better at remembering things, planning, organising and juggling different tasks. Also, regular physical activity can help some of the mental decline that is associated with ageing. Being physically active is part of the routine maintenance for a healthy brain.

Both exercise and physical activity are good for mental health. Just going out for a stroll can improve mental well-being, so you don't have to be a fitness fanatic to benefit. Generally, the more exercise you do, the better it is for preventing depression. A few people become addicted to exercise, but cases of this are rare and, for most of us, just getting enough exercise is a challenge! If you haven't done much exercise in the past or if you are very unfit, then start slowly with something like walking and build up gradually.

> Walking is man's best medicine
>
> Hippocrates, Ancient Greek Physician

## Definitions

**Exercise**
This usually refers to a structured session of physical activity taken at a specific time and performed to enhance health and well-being.

**Physical activity**
This could be any activity, at work, during leisure time or in the home, which uses large muscle groups (such as the leg muscles) and contributes to energy expenditure. It can include structured exercise sessions.

## Operating systems – how exercise improves mental health

There are probably many reasons why physical activity improves mental health and several theories about the mechanisms involved. Some theories relate to the biochemical effects of exercise and others to the psychological effects. Proponents of the biochemical theories believe that, during exercise, our brains release chemicals similar to morphine called endorphins. These are sometimes called feel-good hormones and are important

> Moderate intensity activity is described as any exercise that uses the large muscle groups (such as walking, dancing, sport, gardening, cycling) and makes you breathe slightly deeper and feel slightly warmer.

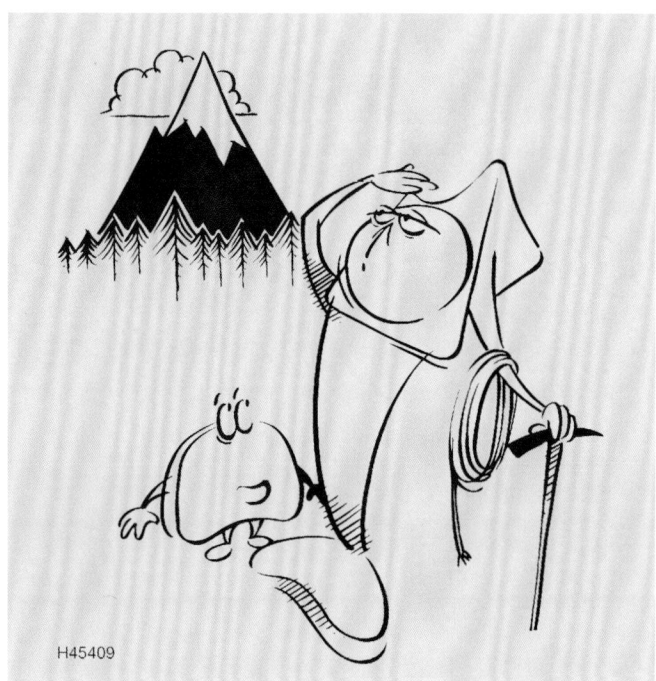

H45409

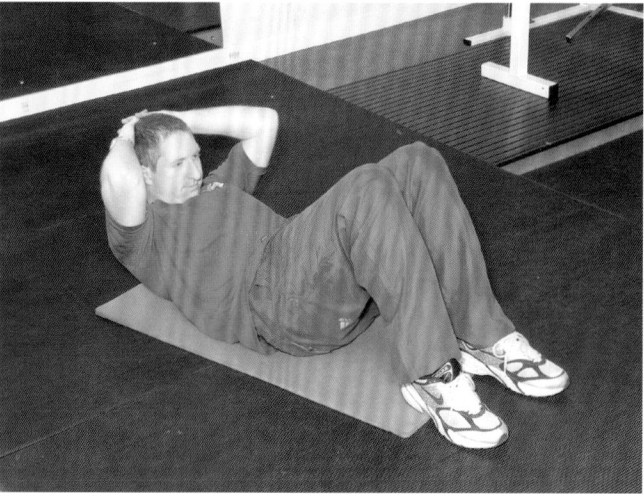

Left: Exercise can also boost our self-esteem by making us feel more confident by completing an activity, whether it is a marathon or simply a walk to the top of a hill

Below: If you are struggling for breath, or unable to hold a conversation while you exercise, you are probably working too hard! This chap's technique is not perfect either. . .

in regulating emotion and pain perception. Anti-depressants produced by drug companies are designed to improve the balance of these brain chemicals. It is likely that exercise does this naturally and therefore leads to improved mood and feelings of well-being.

Another theory is referred to as the thermogenic hypothesis. Exercise increases the body temperature, which in turn leads to reduced muscle tension and feelings of relaxation and well-being. The Scandinavians obviously think this is true judging by their love of saunas!

As well as these biochemical reasons, there are also psychological reasons why physical activity and exercise may help improve mental health. One psychological reason is the 'distraction theory'. This simply means that exercise provides us with 'time out' and takes our mind off anxious or stressful thoughts. But exercise can also boost our self-esteem by making us feel more confident by completing an activity, doing something worthwhile or accomplishing a challenge, whether it is marathon or simply a walk to the top of a hill.

It is likely that these theories all have an element of truth and they probably all work together to bring about the benefits to the brain. Physical activity gives us something positive to focus on and aim for and provides opportunities to meet new people. This stops us from feeling isolated and unsupported. Although more research is needed to fully understand why exercise is so good for mental health, what we do know for sure is that being more active makes us feel better and that should be reason enough to get started!

## Rebooting the system

Have you ever watched a toddler at play? They stand up, sit down, run around, gyrate and contort their little bodies into all sorts of positions. This activity is vital for their development and their health. As we get older, we lose much of that natural physical activity as life's demands get the better of us. By the time we reach our teens, very few of us actually still do enough

exercise to benefit our health. We need to make a special effort to build activity back into our lives, especially as technology seems hell-bent on removing every opportunity to be active by giving us cars, computers, escalators, power tools and remote controls.

The Government has come up with guidelines, based on years of research, about the minimum amount of physical activity we should be doing. These guidelines state that, to maintain good health, we should aim to be active at a moderate intensity for thirty minutes, at least five times a week. Only about 30% of the UK population meet the current Government guidelines and 6 out of 10 men currently don't do enough physical activity to benefit their health. Most people believe that they are active enough and describe themselves as 'fit', but the statistics tell a different story.

Researchers are unclear about the amount of activity needed to maintain a healthy mind, but the evidence suggests that 30 minutes, five times a week at a moderate intensity is also the level of physical activity needed to improve mental health.

## Are you getting enough?

The chief Medical Officer says that we should aim to be physically active on at least five days of the week for at least 30 minutes. If you are very unfit, you can break this down into 3 x 10 minutes or 2 x 15 minutes. Brisk walking, dancing, gardening, football and cycling are all examples of suitable exercise for improving health. But any activity is better than none, and for maximum benefit you should try to limit the time you spend on non-active pursuits like TV watching or sitting at a desk. Get up and move around whenever you can, take the stairs instead of the lift or park the car further away from the shops.

Visit Sport England's Everyday Sport website to see how you can build more physical activity into your life (see *Contacts*).

By feeling and gradually looking fitter and healthier, physical activity leads to a more positive body image and boosts self-confidence and self-esteem.

# Where do I start?

Exercise is good for you whatever your mental state. It is the oil that lubricates a healthy mind and keeps it healthy. It can also help as a remedy when things aren't so good. If you're feeling down, then exercise may be the last thing on your mind and starting an exercise programme can be challenging. That's why it is important to start gently and build-up gradually and choose something that is manageable and fun.

It is a good idea to check with your doctor before you increase the amount of physical activity that you do or before starting an exercise programme. Take a look at the questions below. If you have answered 'yes' to one or more of them, then discuss your plans with your doctor before you start.

This questionnaire is designed to help you decide whether you are physically ready to take up more exercise. Answering 'yes' to any of these questions does not necessarily mean that you cannot become more active, but you may need to check with your doctor so that he or she can help you structure a safe and effective programme.

❑ Has your doctor ever said that you have a heart condition or have you ever experienced a stroke or blood clot?

❑ Do you ever experience pain in your chest when you are physically active or at any other time?

❑ Do you ever feel faint, lose your balance or lose consciousness?

❑ Do you have a bone or joint condition such as rheumatoid arthritis?

❑ Is your doctor currently prescribing medication for high blood pressure or a heart condition?

❑ Have you had surgery in the last three months?

❑ Do you suffer from epilepsy that is hard to control?

❑ Do you suffer from diabetes?

It is very unlikely that your doctor will tell you that you cannot increase your activity level. Very few conditions are made worse with exercise. In fact most physical and mental conditions are improved with regular physical activity. The main thing is to choose the right exercise for your level of fitness and ability and build-up gradually.

Physical activity makes you sleep better. Lack of sleep (or poor quality sleep) is a problem that is commonly associated with depression. Becoming more active can therefore help with this condition.

# Is it safe?

Very few conditions do not benefit from regular physical activity or exercise. In fact, not becoming more active is likely to be much more detrimental to your health. Choose gentle activities such as walking to get you started and seek out professional help if you are trying something new like a gym or a new sport.

Many GPs can 'prescribe' exercise for patients, referring them to schemes where they will be helped to develop their own personal exercise programme under the supervision of a qualified trainer. Not every doctor's surgery can offer this service, but it is worth finding out from your doctor whether such a scheme is available in your area and whether it is suitable for you.

## STOP SIGNS

**Pain or discomfort**
Expect to feel a little discomfort at first, especially if you are unused to physical activity, but any pain in the chest or upper body, particularly the left arm, is a sign to stop exercising and seek your doctor's advice.

**Breathlessness**
If you are finding it hard to control your breathing or gasping for breath and this does not subside as you decrease the intensity of your physical activity, stop and consult your doctor.

**Fainting**
If you faint during or just after exercise, seek your doctor's advice before continuing. If you experience dizzyness or nausea during exercise, slow down and wait to see if it subsides. If it does not, then stop the activity.

It is quite natural to feel hot and sweaty during exercise and to be breathing much more heavily. This is usually a sign that you are working at the correct intensity. However, experiencing any of the 'Stop Signs' should act as a warning that you may be overdoing things.

**Palpitations**
A fast or irregular heartbeat is a danger signal.

## What physical activity should I choose?

If you don't fancy the idea of joining a gym, there are plenty of other ways of becoming more active and getting more exercise. Many people who start on a physical activity or exercise programme give up within a matter of months. Usually this is because they have chosen activities that are unmanageable, either because they make too many demands on their time, or because they are too strenuous. Physical activity shouldn't feel like hard work, it should be fun and enjoyable. Aim to include lots of variety in your exercise programme, combining daily walks or cycle rides with weekly sporting activities like football or fencing. You could also try more adventurous activities like kayaking or orienteering.

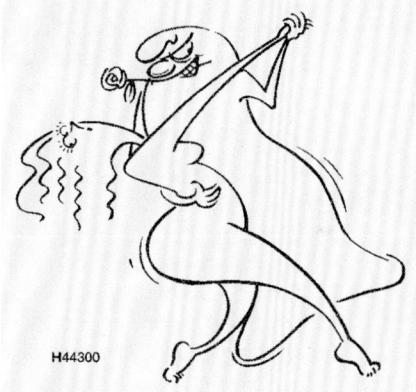

Physical activity shouldn't feel like hard work, it should be fun and enjoyable

## Tips for fitting exercise into your day

Write your exercise sessions into your diary as you would any other appointment. Remember that this time spent on physical activity is just as important as other commitments.

**Get up earlier**
Go for a walk or an early gym session. Research has shown that people who exercise in the morning are more likely to stick with it. It is often easy to find excuses not to exercise as the day progresses and fills with unforseen demands on your time.

**Do the housework and make it count**
Vigorous sweeping, mopping or scrubbing are all excellent form of exercise. You'll also get the pleasure of a clean home and a happy family.

**Take the kids out for a walk or a game of football**
Kids need exercise too!

**Get off the train or bus a stop earlier and walk the last part of your journey to work**
If there is a lot of traffic, it may even prove to be quicker than the motorised option.

**Take the stairs insead of the lift or escalator**
Remember every little bit counts and it all adds up.

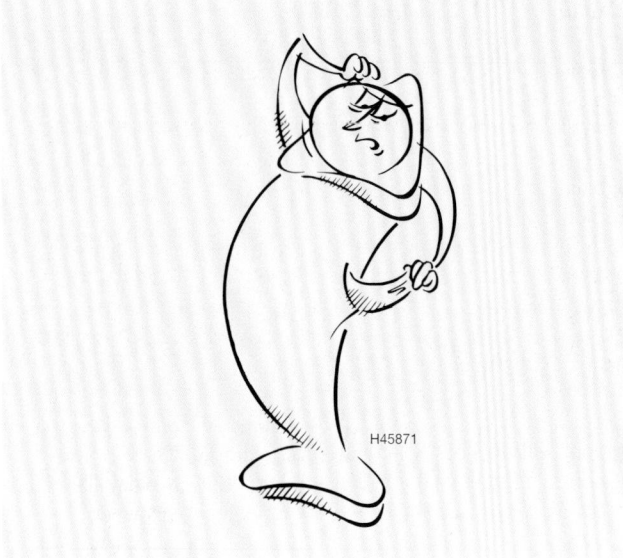

When choosing which activities to take up, it is a good idea to consider the following:

### Am I fit enough?
Some sports require a basic level of fitness before you can take part. If you are very unfit or have a disability or injury you may be best to chose an activity like walking or swimming. Remember: any activity is good for you and you don't have to be fit or be 'sporty' to benefit.

### Where does the activity take place?
If the activity is too far from where you live or work, it will give you another excuse not to go when the sofa and TV beckon.

### What are the costs of the activity?
Is the activity something you can realistically afford to do on a regular basis? Skiing and horse riding may be appealing and excellent for improving your fitness, but how often can you realistically afford to go? Make your daily activities ones that are free or affordable. Walking, cycling, swimming, and an exercise class at your local leisure centre are more likely to be sustainable.

### Do I need supervision?
Some people find it hard to get motivated to exercise on their own or without supervision. If you are unsure of how to get started then go along to your local gym and discuss how they can help you become more active. Alternatively, try joining a local group such as a walking group. You will meet new people and you will get the encouragement you need to keep going. Exercising with a friend is a great way of ensuring you stick with your programme and the social side of exercising in this way will boost your mental health.

Walking the Way to Health is a Countryside Agency and British Heart Foundation initiative that organises regular led walks across the UK. To find out about walks in your area see *Contacts* for details.

Sport England is the strategic lead for sport in England. It aims to encourage people of all ages to start, stay and succeed in sport and increase participation in physical activity. It is at the heart of developing sports policy and infrastructure and works in partnership with health, education and local agencies to boost

Is the activity something you can realistically afford to do on a regular basis?

participation and performance. Sport England distributes funding and invests in a range of sporting projects including the Active England fund. It is responsible for delivering the Government's sporting objectives. To find out more about Sport England, and for information about activities that you could join in your area, see *Contacts*.

### How often should I exercise?
Try to get some physical activity every day, even if it is a short, brisk walk to or from work or the shops. As you become fitter, you can start to include more strenuous activities into your exercise programme.

### How hard should I work?
Research has shown that aerobic exercise such as brisk walking, dancing, running and sports like tennis are best for counteracting depression and anxiety. Resistance exercise such as lifting weights has also been shown to have an effect on mental health if performed regularly. Although you are likely to feel less stressed and improve your mood by taking a gentle stroll, the evidence suggests that regular, moderate exercise is likely to have the greatest effect. Moderate intensity exercise is less likely to lead to injury, is often more enjoyable and is more sustainable than very strenuous activities like running. You should be able to sustain the exercise for at least 30 minutes at a time.

### What exercise is best?
The best exercise for you is one you enjoy, can sustain for 30 minutes without pain and can do on a regular basis. Many people find that a walking programme provides them with all the exercise they need. Regular brisk walking can give you all the physical health improvements associated with regular

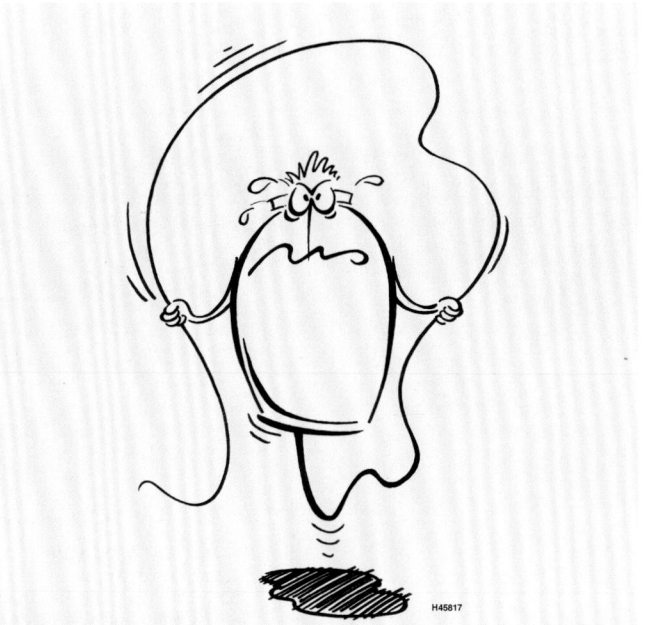

Choose an activity that leaves you glowing and refreshed rather than exhausted exercise: improved heart health, reduced cholesterol, reduced risk of diabetes, weight control, muscle strength and tone, and a stronger immune system. Many people think that walking does not count as 'proper exercise' but research has shown that this is not the case. Walking a mile and jogging a mile burn roughly the same number of calories. If you find that walking does not make you feel warmer and slightly out of breath, try increasing the pace or add some gently hills. But for most people walking is an excellent way to start getting more active as it can easily be built into your daily life. Walking has been described as 'the perfect exercise' as it is something that for most of us is natural and has a very low risk of injury.

You can use your exercise time to help you deal with any stresses that may have built up. While out on a walk think about the things that are troubling you. Many anxieties can be reduced simply by managing your life more effectively. Think about the issues that could be causing you stress and put them into categories. Consider what practical changes you could make to make your life easier. Would outside help be useful, whether it is a financial advisor, a baby-sitter or just the ear of a good friend?

# Motivation troubleshooter

Sometimes it is hard to get motivated to exercise. As many of us know all too well, exercise is a habit that is easily lost. The key is to start gently and build-up gradually.

Even if you don't feel like doing your usual workout, use the time to go out for a gentle walk instead. That way you will still be getting a benefit and you won't fill the time slot you set aside with non-active pursuits.

Set yourself realistic goals and keep a diary of when you exercise. A great way of getting motivated is to use a gadget called a pedometer or step-o-meter to monitor your progress and set yourself goals. Set yourself weekly as well as monthly goals. Keep a diary of your exercise sessions. Set yourself targets for to how much and often you would like to exercise and reward yourself with a small indulgence (like going to the cinema, or a night out with friends) when you reach your goals.

Choose activities that can be built into your everyday life. There are 168 hours in a week, finding 30 minutes a day (3.5 hours a week) is not that difficult. Think about where you could save time to be set aside for exercise. How many hours do

Seasonal Affective Disorder (SAD) is a type of winter depression that affects an estimated 1/2 million people every winter in the UK particularly between September and April. Although it can be treated with light therapy and drugs just getting out in the daylight hours can help many people. Exercising outdoors particularly at lunchtime during the winter can help counteract the effects of SAD.

All truly great thoughts are conceived by walking.
*Friedrich Nietzsche*

**Cut Down On**

**If You're Consistent**
(Active most days of the week)
Choose activities from all levels of the pyramid. Change your routine if you start to get bored. Explore new activities.

Sitting
Watching TV
Working or playing
on a computer

**If You're Sporadic**
(Active some of the time, but not regularly)
Become more consistent with activities in the middle of the pyramid. Plan activity in your day. Set realistic goals.

**3 or more times a week**

*Stretch and strengthen your muscles*

Take stretch breaks   Weight lifting
Yoga or Tai Chi   Push ups or sit ups

**3 to 5 times a week**

*Give your heart and lungs a workout*

Play golf or hike   Brisk walking
Running or jogging   Football
Swimming or water aerobics   Rollerblading

**Everyday**

*Walk often and stay active*

Walk the dog   Go cycling or walk to the shops   Do housework

Park your car further away   Take the stairs instead of the lift

**If You're Inactive**
(Rarely active)
Increase daily activities at the base of the pyramid. Walk whenever you can. Make leisure time as active as possible.

Each week balance your physical activity using the pyramid

H45400

you spend watching TV? Could you go for a walk in your lunch hour? Many employers are happy to encourage their employees to have more active lifestyles. It has been shown that fitter employees are more productive and take less time off sick than unfit colleagues. As you get fitter you will have more energy and be able to accomplish more in less time, freeing up even more time to exercise.

## Exercise and addiction

Most of us have our vices. Some of these, such as enjoying the occasional chocolate bar or a flutter on the lottery are harmless enough. Sometimes, however, vices can turn into addictions. Exercise can help overcome addictions in a variety of ways:

Physical activity helps reduce stress. As anyone who has quit smoking will tell you, stress can be a major problem when you are giving up.

Exercise can help counteract some of the weight gain that people experience when they give up smoking.

Getting out and being active can help take your mind off the addiction and give you something else to focus on.

As you start to become fitter and enjoy your exercise programme, you will find that you no longer want to feel like your lungs are on fire every time you walk up a hill. Smokers who take up exercise tend to cut down naturally as they find they enjoy their exercise more without the symptoms of smoking. Similarly, you will find your morning run much easier if you are not nursing a hangover.

Exercise is, for many, the first step in adopting a healthier lifestyle. As you become fitter you will find that you also are more conscious of what you eat and drink, and start to take more care of your body and mind.

Do the housework with vigour

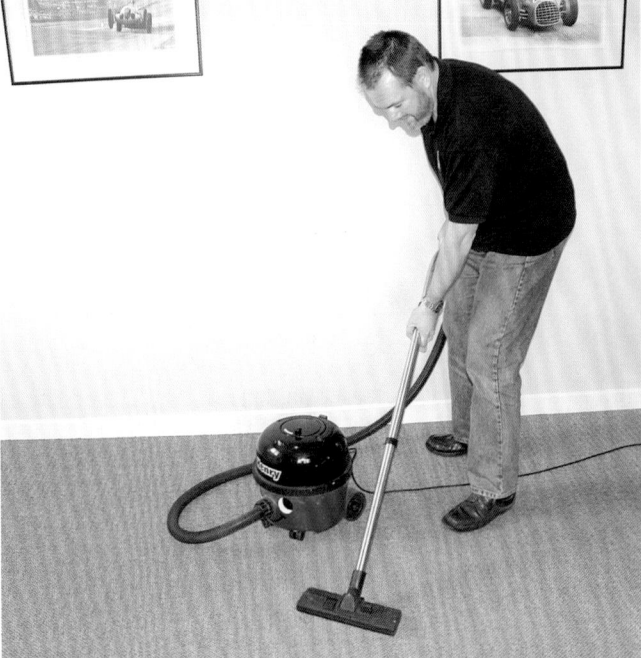

Don't try to change too many things at once. Giving up smoking, alcohol, starting a diet and an exercise programme all at the same time is a recipe for disaster. Take one step at a time and be realistic about your goals.

PART

# Healthy living

Life is for living and it would be much more pleasant if we were all healthier and lived longer to enjoy it. Simple things can make a big difference and don't mean a complete change in the way you live. Here are some tips on how to stay healthy and live longer, without worrying about it.

## Eating for pleasure and health

Being overweight is on the increase, particularly in men. We know this can increase your risk from heart disease so cutting down on fatty food, especially animal fats, makes sense. Simply grilling food rather than frying will significantly reduce the amount of fat you are eating.

Some foods are known to reduce your risk from many illness and possibly even cancer yet are cheap and taste good. Fruit supplies both vitamins and fibre and can replace sweets for children, especially as a 'treat' or reward. Aim for around five servings of fruit or vegetables each day. (One serving is roughly 1 piece of fruit, 1 dessert bowl of salad, 1 glass of fruit juice or 2 tablespoonfuls of vegetables.)

Try gradually cutting down on salt with your food. You'll be surprised how little you need after getting used to less. It will protect you from high blood pressure.

Fish, especially the oily varieties such as mackerel or sardines are loaded with special oils which actually protect your heart.

Bread, especially wholemeal types, potatoes and pasta are all great forms of carbohydrate which provide energy and should be the main part of the meal. Enjoy your food and go for as wide variety as possible.

## In a puff of smoke

The more we look at smoking and health the more we know that cigarettes are the single greatest killer in our society. Over 300 people die every day from smoking related diseases. Smoking 25 cigarettes a day increases your risk of lung cancer by 25 times and doubles your chances of heart disease.

- Get someone to give up with you and name the day to start.
- One day at a time is the best plan, but reward yourself each day by putting the money normally spent on cigarettes in a jar.
- Tell people in the pub or at work that you are trying to stop. These days they will understand and support you.
- Get rid of all the tobacco stuff in the house like ashtrays, lighters and matches.
- See your pharmacist, GP or practice nurse about nicotine replacement which will help ease the cravings.

Go for it. You've only your cough to lose in the long run!

## Are you active?

Most people think they are more active than they actually are. Even a small amount of moderate activity will help protect you from heart disease, still the greatest single cause of death in the

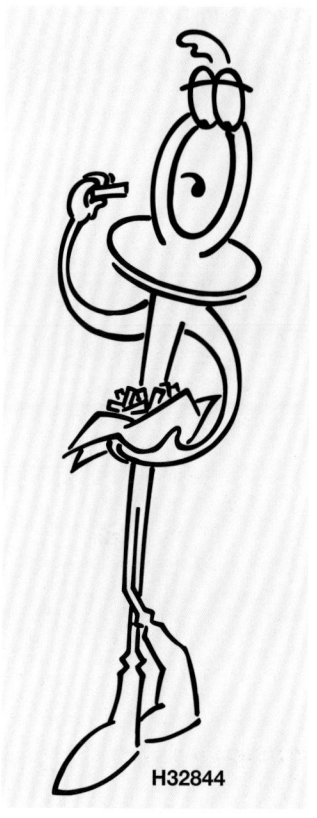

H32844

Ever tried running a diesel engine on petrol? Men need the right fuel too

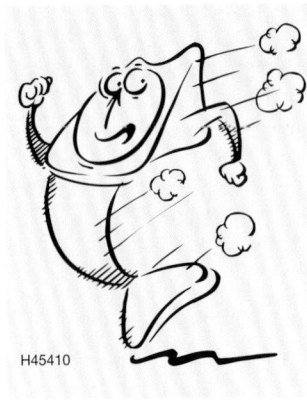

H45410

Exercise to the point of breathlessness at least 3 times a week

UK. Aim to exercise until the point of breathlessness at least three times a week. You don't need to buy expensive machines or even go to gyms or leisure centres.

- Take the stairs instead of the lift.
- Get off the bus one stop early and walk briskly.
- Play with the children. Being a 'horse' for them gets your heart pumping.
- Climb briskly up the house stairs.
- If possible cycle rather than take the bus or use the car. Most towns are making special tracks for cyclists.

## Sexual health

The UK has the highest rate of teenage pregnancies in Europe. At the same time sexually transmitted disease is on the increase. Using simple protective contraception like male or female condoms would help protect against both pregnancy and infections such as HIV.

- Don't be a dipstick. Always use a condom. They are on sale in supermarkets and chemists, and free from family planning clinics.

## Alcohol

Relatively recently we found out that moderate drinking for men and women over 40 years can actually help prevent heart disease. The problem is that the message gets confused and there is a temptation to drink too much without realising that this protection is very soon lost as the amount of alcohol consumed rises. Aim for no more than 3-4 units of alcohol per day and preferably less. Alcohol abuse is on the increase and children are drinking heavily at a much earlier age, setting the pattern for later life.

1 unit of alcohol is roughly the same as:

- An English measure (25ml) of spirit. Scotland and Northern Ireland use larger measures.
- Half a pint of normal strength beer.
- One measure of sherry (50ml).
- One small glass of wine (100ml).

Some beers are very strong and we all pour out more generous measures at home.

Always use a condom

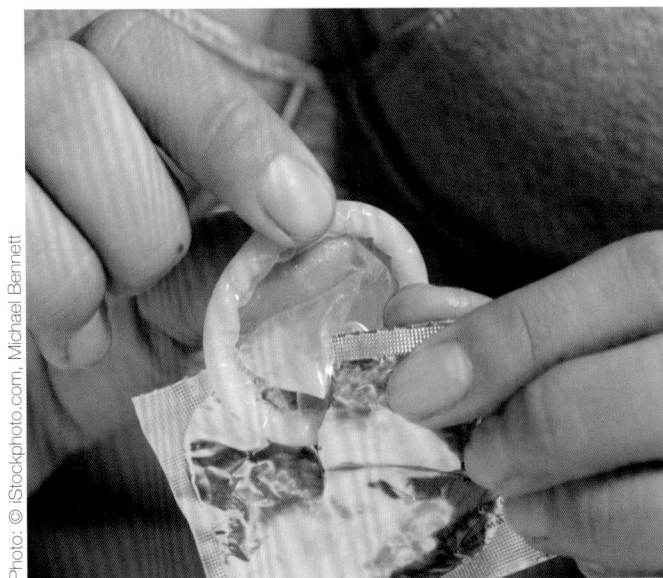

Photo: © iStockphoto.com, Michael Bennett

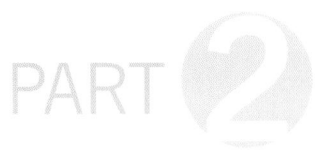

PART

# Are you ready to lose weight for life?

*By Dr David Haslam*

## Choosing your vehicle

You may have a multitude of reasons for wanting to lose weight. For example, you may have suddenly noticed your reflection in the mirror and decided to change your appearance, or you may have recently suffered a clinical warning signal such as shortness of breath or frequent tiredness.

Whatever your incentive, a weight-loss manoeuvre is usually an extremely sensible option.

This is because obesity (defined as having a body mass index (BMI) over 30), is closely linked to a number of serious, life-threatening diseases. For example, compared to thin people, people who are obese are four times more likely to contract heart disease. They are also more likely to suffer a fatal course of cancer[1].

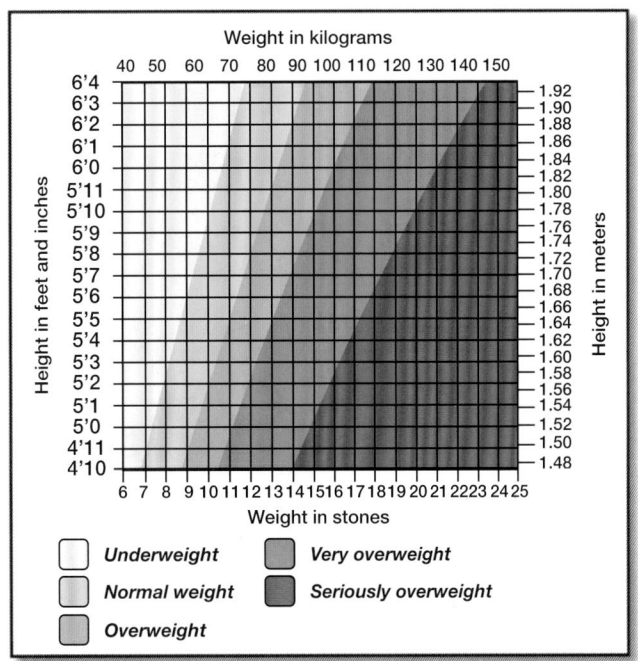

H45398

## Understanding what's under your bonnet

If you want to lose weight, it is important that you have realistic expectations.

If you feel that you have a lot of weight to lose, it is not a good idea to try to lose it all in one go. A much better idea is to

## Fat facts

Being obese increases your chances of developing one or more of these serious medical conditions[2]:

- Arthritis.
- Asthma.
- Back pain.
- Cancer.
- Cirrhosis.
- Depression.
- Diabetes.
- Gallstones.
- Gout.
- Haemorrhoids.
- Heart disease.
- Heart failure.
- Heartburn.
- High blood pressure.
- Increased surgical risk.
- Infertility.
- Stress urinary incontinence.
- Varicose veins.
- Wound infections.

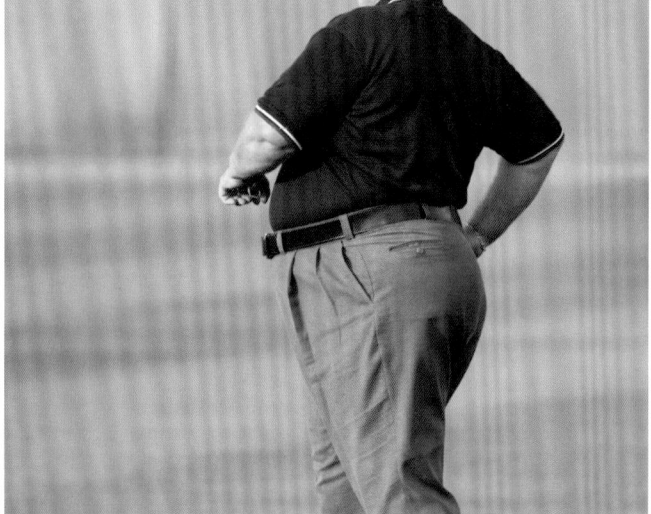

Photo: © iStockphoto.com, Rob Friedman

Any weight loss is best achieved
in small chunks

break your overall target into smaller chunks and then aim to lose
a small amount at a time. For example, if you would eventually
like to lose 25 kg (4 stone), it would be sensible to set an initial
target of losing 10 kg (22 lbs).

This is an excellent initial target to set yourself because
research shows that this amount of weight loss can result in a
substantial number of health benefits. Losing 10% of your body
weight (eg, 10 kg in a 100 kg man) decreases your chances of
dying from an obesity-related cause by around 20%[3].

You should also aim to lose weight gradually, so that your
metabolism remains high. If you try to lose weight too quickly (ie,
by starving yourself), your metabolism may slow right down and
go into 'starvation mode'. This means that your body needs fewer
calories to function, so although you have cut down your calorific
intake, some calories will still be converted into body fat.

A weight reduction of 0.5-1 kg per week is a sensible average
rate. To achieve this, you should reduce your calorific intake by
500-600 kcal per day.

To lose weight healthily, you should also increase your daily
exercise regime, and aim to take 30 minutes of exercise, five
days a week.

Brisk walking, cycling or swimming are good examples of
suitable fat-burning exercises. You should also revert to a low-fat
diet.

## How to improve your diet
- Do not shop for food when hungry.
- Store healthy foods where you can see them.
- Use smaller plates and utensils.
- Eat more slowly.
- Chew food thoroughly before swallowing.

## Your weight-loss journey
Your willpower also plays an important part in your weight-loss
attempts. If you want to lose weight successfully, you must be
mentally ready for the challenge. Put simply, you must be totally
dedicated to making the necessary changes to your lifestyle.

Making any major change involves six key stages. These
stages closely resemble a car journey. Using the list below, at
what stage would you currently place yourself?

### Leaving the car in the garage (the pre-contemplation stage)
At this stage, you have not yet decided that you want to lose any
weight.

### Getting in the driver's seat (the contemplation stage)
At this stage, you have thought about losing weight, but are not yet
ready to start.

### Starting the engine (the preparation stage)
You have decided that you want to lose weight, and are prepared
to make the necessary lifestyle changes within the next few
weeks. You may already have set a date to start dieting. You may
also feel that you need some additional guidance and support to
help with your weight loss attempts.

Your reasons for wanting to lose weight may be:
- To be able to walk upstairs without panting.
- To look better.
- To be able to wear off-the-peg clothes.
- To lower the strain on your knees.
- To put on shoes and socks more easily.
- To lower your blood pressure.
- To achieve long-term health benefits.

### Releasing the handbrake (the action stage)
Well done. You have got over the first hurdle and have started
to make the lifestyle changes which will help you to lose your
excess weight.

### Reaching your destination (the maintenance stage)
Congratulations, you have reached your target weight. You must
now concentrate on maintaining your new reduced weight.

### The return journey (the relapse stage)
For whatever reason, you have gone back to your old ways of
eating too much and not exercising regularly. The weight that
you initially lost has started to return. You must find the inner
strength to turn your behaviour back around.

For a fat-burning exercise, try
cycling

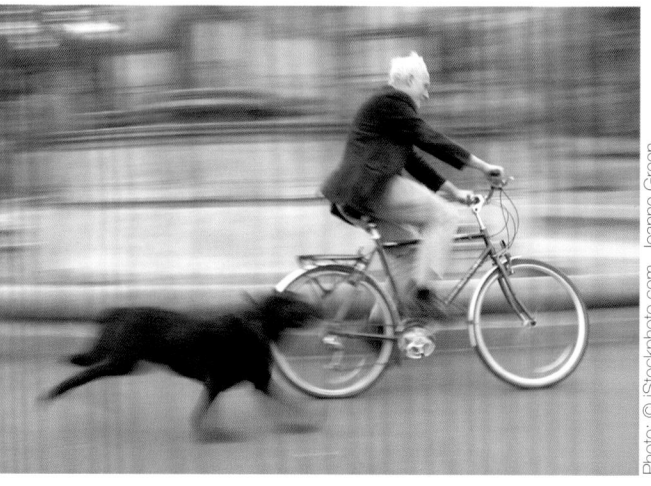

Photo: © iStockphoto.com, Joanne Green

Whatever stage you find yourself at, your doctor can provide additional help and support. Some of the ways that he can help are listed in the following table.

| Stage of your weight-loss journey | How your doctor can help |
|---|---|
| Pre-contemplation | At this stage, you will not yet have decided to visit your doctor because you have not yet accepted that your weight is a problem. However, if you are visiting your doctor for another ailment, he or she may proactively mention that you should lose some weight. |
| Contemplation | At this stage, your doctor may be able to help you develop a list of pros and cons associated with your weight loss. For example, you could discuss:<br>● What you will gain from losing weight.<br>● The likely difficulties you will face.<br>● The barriers that are stopping you from losing weight right now. |
| Preparation | At this stage, your doctor can help you develop a sensible weight loss plan. This could include:<br>● The number of calories to aim for each day.<br>● The types of foods to avoid.<br>● A suitable exercise regime.<br>● A valid start date. |
| Action | At this stage, your doctor can help you overcome any cravings to ensure that you do not lose sight of your weight-loss goals. In addition, if you are finding it increasingly difficult to stick to your original weight-loss plan, he or she may be able to help you regain your motivation and make the necessary modifications to put you back on track. |
| Maintenance | At this stage, you are unlikely to need any additional support, as you are managing quite nicely on your own. However, your doctor is always there if needed, and may be able to offer medications to complement your diet and exercise programme. |
| Relapse | At this stage, you are not likely to visit your doctor as a result of your weight problem because you have lost interest in maintaining your new, reduced weight. However, if you are visiting your doctor for another ailment, he or she will almost certainly ask about your weight, and may try to pursue the triggers that made you revert to your old behaviour. This may help to put you back on track with your weight-loss attempts. |

One type of weight-loss aid that you can only get from your doctor is medication (eg, sibutramine and orlistat).

These two medications can help to boost your weight loss attempts. Both of these medications must be taken alongside a sensible diet and exercise programme, and are only suitable if your BMI is more than 27 and if you have other obesity-related conditions, or if your BMI is greater than 30.

## References

1  Haslam DW. *Obesity - the scale of the problem.* General Practitioner July 2001; p31-32.
2  Haslam DW. *Time to tackle obesity.* Family Medicine February 2000; p25-31.
3  Colditz GA, Willett WC, Rotnitzky A et al. *Weight gain as a risk factor for clinical diabetes mellitus in women.* Annals of Internal Medicine 1995; 122: 481-486.

PART 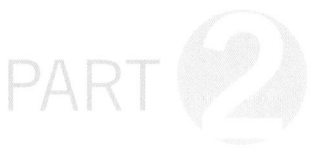 

# Slow down – the lazy man's way to lose weight

## The body mass index

There are two ways to calculate your body mass index (BMI):

a) *Using pounds and inches. Multiply your weight in pounds by 700 and divide that figure by the square of your height in inches. For example, if you're 68 inches tall and weigh 185 lb, your BMI = 185 x 700 ÷ (68 x 68 = 4624) = 28.*

b) *Using kilograms and metres. Dividing your weight by the square of your height. This means that if you're 1.78 metres tall and weigh 78kg, your BMI = 78 ÷ (1.78 x 1.78 = 3.2) = 24.4.*

**Men know Diets with a capital D don't work. So how do you build weight-loss into your daily routine?**

A survey published by Mintel in 2004 claimed that record numbers of men are attempting to lose weight. Apparently one in four of us would like to shift a kilo or two – up from one in six in 1980.

Perhaps we've all been inspired by the recent Danish research showing that being overweight lowers your sperm count and makes you less fertile. The University of Southern Denmark found that, compared with men of normal weight, overweight men – defined as men with a body mass index over 25 – had a 24% lower sperm count.

Anyway, regardless of its impact on your fertility, the general tone of the media coverage of the Mintel report was that men trying to lose weight must be a good thing at a time when two-thirds of the male population is overweight or obese. Maybe. But the trouble is that diets don't work. And the whole weight-loss obsession can be very damaging to the self-image. Fortunately, many men already know this. Twice as many men as women told the researchers that they would never diet and only 3% would even consider joining a slimming club.

The report found that men tend to want to lose weight for health reasons rather than to get into smaller clothes sizes. As a result we are more likely to cut out the booze or take more exercise than to resort to meal replacements or faddy diets.

So what do you do? If you want to lose weight without actually changing what you eat it comes down to two things: slower and fresher.

## Go slow

To start, don't even think about what you eat. Think about how you eat it. Lots of us stuff our faces in front of the telly hardly noticing what we're shovelling in. No good.

Take it easy. Drink some water. Look at your food. Chew it. Savour the flavour. Drink some more water. You'll enjoy your food more and your body will know that it's actually eating. This is vital because when it comes to food your brain's a bit slow. It takes it a good 20 minutes to wise up that your stomach is full. This means that if you've been stuffing yourself, you'll have eaten tons more than you wanted. Good rule of thumb? The first belch. It's dear old mother nature's way of telling you've had enough. (And, of course, like all mothers she does it in the most publicly embarrassing way possible.)

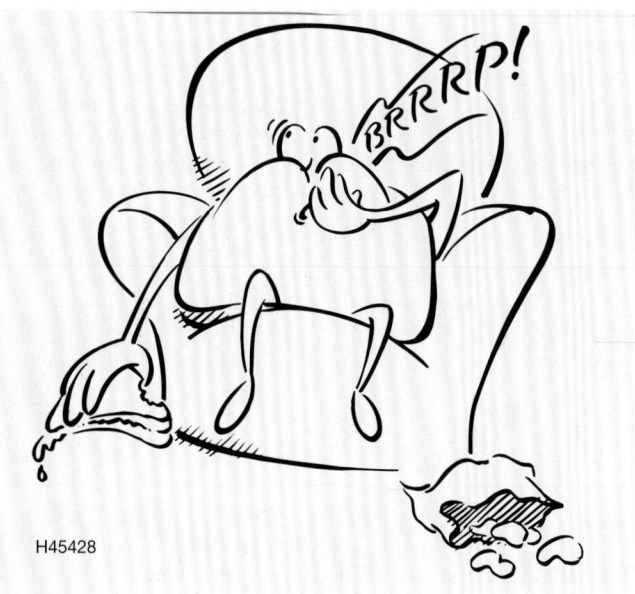

H45428

The first belch is Mother Nature's way of saying you've had enough

## Be a thin couch potato

Don't just sit there. Think thin. Fidget. Sit up violently. Burn more energy by stretching while you yawn. Get up and walk to the TV.

What sorts the bone-idle thin from the most languid obese people? The answer is Neat or non-exercise activity thermogenesis. Neat is more powerful than pumping iron or running on the spot.

Low Neat means obese people sit down on average 150 more minutes each day than even the laziest lean people. Patients with low Neat have a biological need to sit more. The study shows that the calories people burn in their everyday activities – their Neat – are more important in obesity than previously imagined.

The decade-long study required volunteers to wear special underwear that recorded their every movement. They were also given special meals and gave up all unauthorised snacks. Then the scientists tried another regime. They made the thin volunteers consume an extra 1,000 calories a day, and underfed the larger ones by 1,000 calories. Even when they lost weight, the naturally obese moved less, while the naturally thin walked and fidgeted more.

*US journal Science Today*

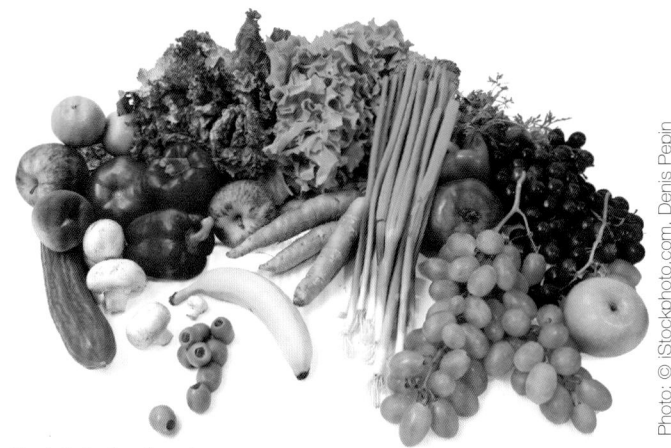

Fresh is better than frozen

## Get fresh

Once you're eating more slowly you'll taste your food better so the smart next step is to choose the tastiest version of it. Now, I'm no farmer but it's clear that the carrot that tastes most like a carrot will be the one you've pulled out of the ground yourself rather than the one that was picked weeks ago and has since been flown round the world, sliced up, salted, sugared and tinned. The good news is that this fresher version is also the most nutritional version with the most vitamins.

So don't change what you eat but choose the least-processed version of it. The more factories and other places your food has been through, the more likely it is to have had sugars, salts and fats added. Avoid ready-meals and convenience pre-packed options. Don't buy a chicken meal, buy a chicken. When it comes to fruit and veg, frozen is better than tinned. Fresh is better than frozen. Organic is better than supermarket.

Not that all fresh food is that fresh. If the item has been flown from the other side of the world it's likely to be less fresh than something produced down the road. Check out the country of origin on fruit and veg and buy local.

It's hardly brain surgery is it? Baked beans are a good example of the problem with processing. The beans themselves are pretty good for you but in the tins we buy they're pumped up with salt and sugar. Nobody's suggesting you bake your own beans – though you could chose a reduced salt and sugar version – but you see the point.

Apart from the reduction in nutrients, processed foods – and fast foods like burgers and fries too by the way – have a high energy density. That means that each mouthful contains a lot of calories. More calories than your body is expecting. Human beings have evolved over thousand of years to guess how much we need to eat by the size of a portion but just an ordinary looking portion of a high-density food can contain double the calories your body expects. If you also have the habit of putting it away like a wolf in a meat factory, you can see how the calories can mount very quickly.

Worst of all, you can become dependent on the sweet, salty, fatty tastes because they give you an instant sugar hit. In tests, rats who are used to this sort of food get the shakes when they're deprived of it. Trouble is that the hit soon wears off and you're back starving again. Now, if only you'd eaten more slowly in the first place. Just like mamma used to say.

## Get fresher

Talking of evolution, you can take that idea a little further and think about what food we've evolved to eat rather than what we actually do eat. Humans have been on Earth for hundreds of thousands of years. In terms of our evolution, the cultivation of crops only began yesterday and the processing of food even more recently.

That's why you hear people going on about the raw food diet or the caveman diet. Sure, they're trying to sell diet books but the basic theory is sound. For most of our time on this planet, we would have been eating what we could hunt and what we could gather from the landscape around us. That means a diet of mainly fruit, nuts, vegetables and meat. Not that the meat would be much like today's meat. The meat on a hunted animal is different to the flab on a factory-farmed one that has never seen daylight and never walked more than a yard or two. Lean meat, free-range, organic or game gets a little nearer to what you're after.

This is not say you shouldn't eat cereals but that you should try to get the version that's closest to nature. That means whole grain or wild rice. Fresh, wholemeal bread rather than factory white. If you're having trouble eating the government's recommended five portions of fruit and vegetable a day, you'll find it a lot easier if you replace one serving of cereals, bread, pasta or rice with one of vegetables.

But sorry, as usual, chips don't count. Why not? Well, since potatoes are pretty disgusting raw (most of their plant relatives are poisonous), we didn't start eating them in quantities until we learned to cook food. Again this happened relatively recently. There's that and the 50g of fat in a portion of fries!

Photo: © iStockphoto.com, Denis Pepin

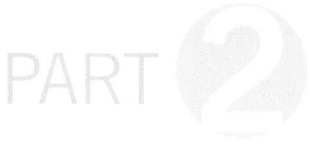

PART **2**

# Nutrition

Traditionally, meals are often planned around meat. Vegetables and other foods that come from plants (such as rice, pasta, bread or beans) are then often added as an accompaniment. But did you know that changing the focus of your meals is actually one of the best ways to improve your health? Swap it around. Instead of focusing on the meat you'll have, make plant foods the main part of your meal. Aim to fill two thirds or more of your plate with these nutritious foods. And try to think of animal foods (that is, the meat, fish or low fat dairy products) as the accompaniment to your meal. These foods should fill the remaining part of your plate – that is, one third or less.

## What's the easy way?
- Aim to have a colourful salad with lunch or dinner – or a side salad when eating out.
- Add beans or lentils to salads, stews, soups or pasta/rice dishes. Try different kinds, such as yellow lentils, chick peas, cannellini, kidney, pinto or black beans.
- Make salads and soups into tasty main dishes by adding some reduced fat cheese, beans or a handful of seeds such as pumpkin or sesame seeds sprinkled on top.
- Make a huge bowl of fruit salad for a healthy start to the day. Keep it in the fridge, ready for breakfast (have with yoghurt and cereal), as a healthy dessert or even just to snack on during the day.
- Buy fresh vegetable soup to have handy when you want something quick and tasty, but healthy at the same time.

Plant foods are foods that come from plants – such as vegetables fruits or grains – rather than from animals. These include: cereals such as grains, bread, rice, and pasta; tubers such as potatoes, sweet potatoes and yams; vegetables and fruits such as fresh or frozen green vegetables, root vegetables, salad vegetables vegetable/fruit juice and canned, dried or fresh fruit; pulses such as beans, peas and lentils; nuts and seeds such as brazil, nuts, cashew nuts, pumpkin seeds and sesame seeds.

Aim to fill two thirds or more of your plate with plant-based foods

Animal foods are those foods that come from animals such as chickens, lambs, pigs or cows. These foods include: meat, game, eggs, cheese, milk, poultry and fish.

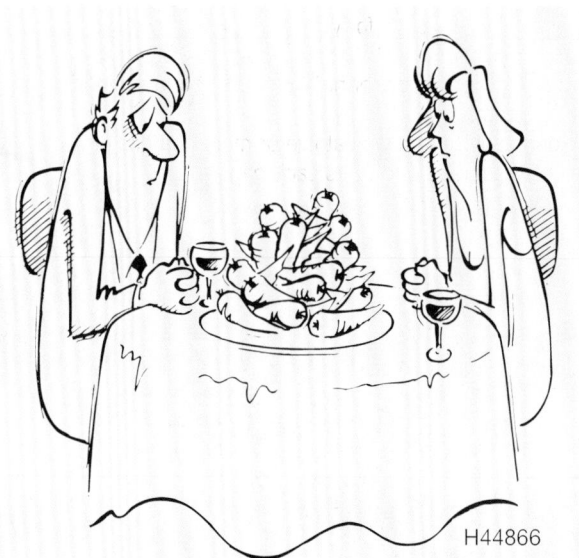

H44866

## Meal makeover

Below is a good example of how changing the proportions of foods on your plate can make a big difference. The healthier version is much lower in fat and salt, and higher in vitamins, so it would definitely be the better option for your health. It will get you well on your way to achieving the recommended five or more portions of vegetables and fruits each day.

| Traditional breakfast brunch | Healthier version |
| --- | --- |
| 2 rashers back bacon, grilled | 2 rashers of reduced salt back bacon, fat trimmed and grilled |
| 2 fried eggs | 1 poached egg |
| 2 grilled sausages | small tin baked beans |
| 1 slice fried white bread | grilled mushrooms |
| Tomato ketchup | grilled tomatoes with chopped basil |
| | 1 slice wholemeal toast with scraping of low fat spread |
| | 1 glass fresh orange juice |
| This breakfast provides 850 calories, 60 grams fat, 2.63 grams sodium and just a trace of fibre and vitamin C. | This healthier version provides 488 calories, 15 grams fat, 1.62 grams sodium, 11 grams fibre and 80mg vitamin C. |

## Natural or pill form?

Would you consider taking vitamin pills in the hope that they'd offset unhealthy living or a poor diet? Although there is no harm in taking a 'regular' multi-vitamin or mineral tablet – one which does not exceed the daily reference nutrient intake – there is a real lack of evidence to show that many of these pills are actually beneficial for health at all. And so far there is little or no evidence to show they help reduce cancer risk.

There are cases where taking vitamin pills may be necessary. For instance, some people can't get all the necessary nutrients from their diet, perhaps because they are not eating enough. Others, such as the elderly, may not be able to absorb vitamins or minerals from their diet so well. If you suspect that you may fall into one or more of these groups, talk to your GP or a qualified dietician.

So, before you reach for your usual stash of dietary supplements, stop and think. If you are relatively healthy, with access to a wide variety of healthy foods, there should be no need for them.

Experts advise that we eat five or more portions of different vegetables and fruits each day. But surveys show that,

Don't overdo the vitamin pills

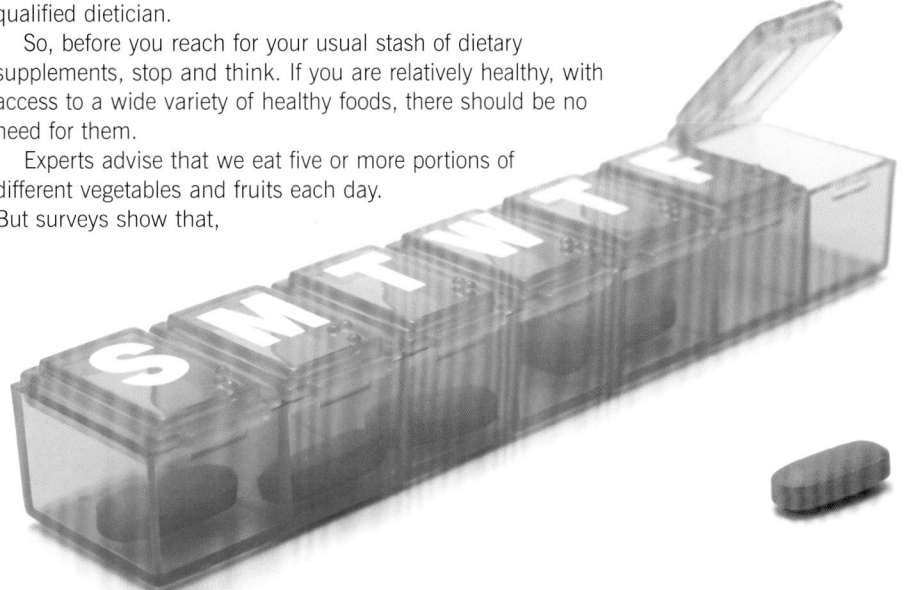

Photo: © iStockphoto.com, Jim Jurica

unfortunately, most of us aren't reaching that target. So, instead of relying on vitamin pills, just aim to double your intake of vegetables and fruits – this is the best way of getting the nutrients your body needs. These nutrients include vitamins, minerals, fibre and 'phytochemicals', substances that have been proven to help prevent cancer.

## How much again?

Below are some examples of what a portion of vegetables and fruits looks like. But this is just a guide. Try not to get too hung up on measurements – you just need to eat a 'decent' sized serving. The overall aim is to double your daily intake – everybody has a different starting point.

**One portion of vegetables is equal to**
- 2-3 heaped tablespoons of most vegetables (like spinach, carrots, peas or sweetcorn).
- 2 heaped tablespoons of beans (like baked beans or kidney beans).
- 1 cereal bowlful of salad (like lettuce, tomato and onion).

**One portion of fruit is equal to**
- 1 large slice of large melon or pineapple.
- 1 whole apple or banana.
- 2 whole plums or satsumas.
- 1 handful of raspberries or grapes.
- 1 glass (150ml) of fresh fruit juice like orange or tomato.
  Fruit juice and beans each count only once towards your 5+ a day total – no matter how much of them you drink or eat. And remember, although potatoes are a healthy component of a balanced diet, they cannot be counted in your 5+ total.

## Tips to fit in 5+ a day

Many people ask 'how can I fit in 5+ portions of vegetables and fruits each day?' Here's how it can be done (choose a few each day to make up 5 or more):

**Breakfast**
- Glass of fruit juice.
- Fruit salad with yoghurt.
- Chopped fresh or dried fruit on cereal.

**Snack**
- Handful of dried fruit.
- Piece of fresh fruit.
- Vegetable crudités with salsa or hummus.

**Lunch**
- Baked beans on toast.
- Home-made vegetable soup.
- Large green/side salad.
- Sandwich with extra salad.

**Dinner**
- Vegetable stir-fry or curry.
- Ratatouille with poultry, fish or lean meat.
- Extra vegetables with your main course.
- Fresh fruit with dessert.

Research shows that if we all ate the recommended five or more portions of vegetables and fruits every day, overall cancer rates could be reduced by about 20%. Despite this, 53% of UK people we asked were not aware that their diet could influence their risk of cancer.

Fit in 5+ portions of vegetables and fruits each day

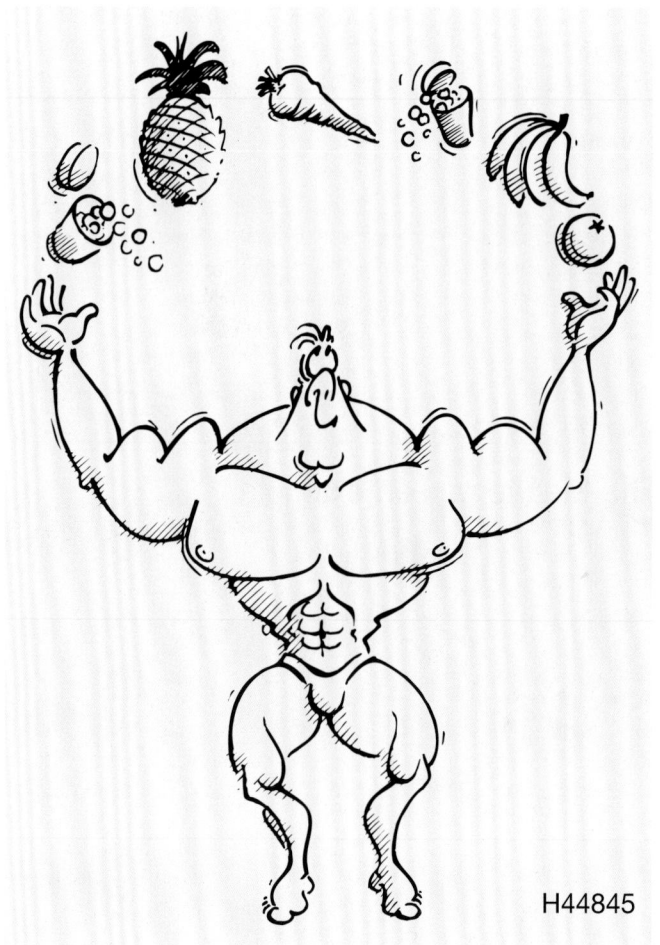

H44845

The Mediterranean diet contains plenty of vegetables and fruits, herbs, fish, small amounts of lean meat, pasta beans, nuts and seeds

## Fat facts

In the UK, many people eat too much fat – probably due to the fact that we're always rushing about and eating 'on the go'. But there is a cost to this: our health. We know that by cutting down on fat we could improve our overall health – so why don't we? The fact is that many of the foods we find most appealing are high in fat. It gives food a certain flavour and a smooth texture as well as giving us a feeling of fullness.

Diets high in fat, particularly when combined with a lack of exercise, can cause you to become overweight – a major cause of cancer. But eating too much fat, in itself, might also increase our risk of certain cancers – particularly those of the lung, bowel and prostate – as well as heart disease.

As a general rule, saturated fat – found in animal foods like red meat and cheese – is the worst type. Unsaturated fats are the healthier option – these are found in plant foods like vegetables, nuts, seeds and cereals.

## Easy ways to cut the fat

| Instead of | Try |
| --- | --- |
| Whole milk | Semi-skimmed or skimmed milk |
| Biscuits | Dried fruit |
| Butter | Low fat spread |
| Fatty meats | Lean meats |
| Processed meat | Fish or chicken |
| Chips | Baked potatoes |
| Cake | Fruit loaf |
| Ice cream | Frozen yoghurt |
| Full fat salad dressings | Low fat dressings |
| Creamy sauces | Tomato-based sauces |
| Crisps | Home-made popcorn |
| Tortillas and cream dip | Vegetable crudités with low fat dip |
| Croissant | Breakfast muffin or crumpet |
| Mayonnaise | Mustard or chutney |

## The Mediterranean example

Many experts believe that the Mediterranean diet is one of the healthiest around. Not only is it rich in fresh vegetables, fruits and cereals, it also provides some of the best sources of 'good' (unsaturated) fats such as olive and rapeseed oils, avocados, nuts and oily fish. Furthermore, levels of physical activity are often higher in Mediterranean countries.

This diet also tends to be low in meat – which can be high in saturated fat. Interestingly, a number of scientific studies have shown that people who regularly eat large portions of red and processed meat have a higher risk of developing cancer, particularly bowel cancer.

A good tip to cut down on saturated fats is to begin eating more plant foods – just like our Mediterranean friends – that way, you'll find that you feel full more quickly and have much less room for foods dripping in saturated fats.

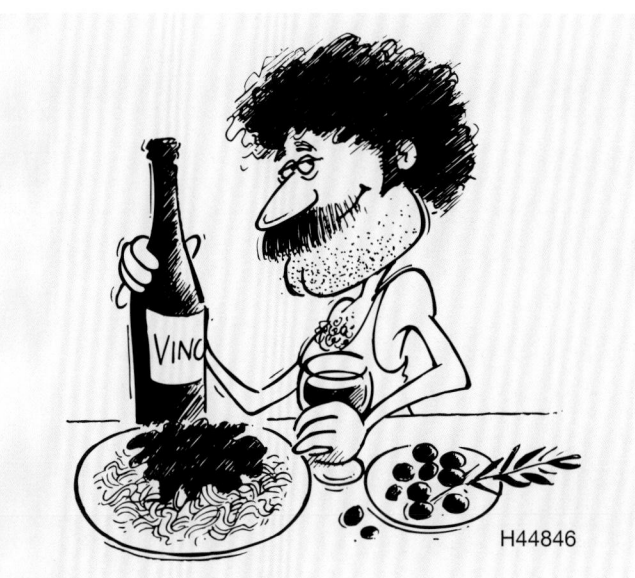

H44846

## Eating out

It's easy to blow all your good intentions in a restaurant or when having a take-away. But you should be able to enjoy your food and still choose the healthier options. That way, you'll save the calories, fat and salt and can feel good about yourself at the same time. So what are the healthiest things to order?

### Chinese

Chinese food can be healthy when meals contain plenty of rice, noodles and vegetables, small meat portions, and tend to have light cooking techniques. Healthy choices:
- Try some of the clear soups with wonton, noodles and vegetables.
- Have steamed rather than fried rice, noodles, dumplings or dim sums.
- Go for dishes with tofu, seafood, poultry or lean meats rather than duck (often served with skin) or pork – both high in fat.

### Indian

Indian meals can be healthy if they are based on grains, vegetables and fruits, are flavoured with spices and contain small amounts of meat and oil, although many Indian dishes are high in fat. Healthy choices:
- Try meat-free dishes such as dhals (lentil dishes) or saag (spicy spinach).
- Go for yoghurt or tomato-based dishes such as rogan josh or dupiaza.
- Have chapattis, rotis, or naan breads without ghee (clarified butter).
- Tandoori or tikka (dry roasted) chicken is healthy without a creamy sauce.

### Italian

The Italian diet is typically healthy as it contains plenty of vegetables and fruits, herbs, fish, small amounts of lean meat, pasta, beans, nuts and seeds. Healthy choices:
- Go for tomato-based sauces like napoletana, marinara, pomodoro or arrabiata.
- Try some of the vegetable or seafood soups such as minestrone or cioppino.

- Use a light sprinkle of parmesan cheese to add flavour to pasta dishes or pizza.
- Choose thin crust pizza with tomato sauce and vegetable toppings (hold the extra cheese).

### Thai

Thai meals based on boiled rice, raw or steamed vegetables and fish flavoured with lemon or garlic are all great choices for healthy eating. Healthy choices:

- Go for low calorie clear soups with noodles, vegetables, lemon grass, herbs or hot and sour soup like tom yum.
- Try spicy Thai salads – often based around seafood and low in fat and calories.
- Order plain boiled rice rather than fried noodles or fried rice, which are high in fat.
- Try dishes with chilli or lemon grass – they add lots of flavour without the fat.

Thai seafood salad

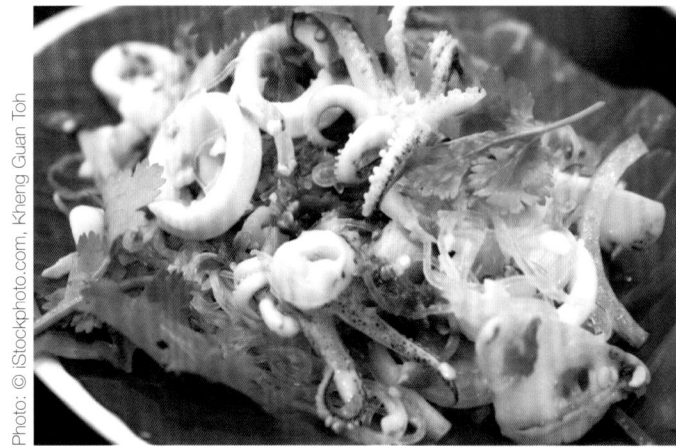

Photo: © iStockphoto.com, Kheng Guan Toh

## Healthy cooking tips from overseas
- Increase the amount of fibre in meals. Include more pulses in meals: for example, try stewed peas/lentils with rice, or yam or sweet potatoes.
- The traditional One Pot Soup (akin to a meat or vegetable casserole) is usually a very healthy option, especially if more peas or pulses are used and less meat.
- If dumplings are prepared, half white flour and half wholemeal or cornmeal should be used.
- Sweet potatoes can be boiled or baked with the skin.
- Reduce fat intake: when and wherever possible cut down on food containing high saturated fats like coconut cream, evaporated milk, etc. Lean meat should be used and remove the skin from chicken.
- Fish, meat and chicken (after being seasoned) should be stewed or baked with little or no fat. Little fat should be used with dishes like 'jollof' rice (recipe with chicken, ham, tomatoes, onion, cabbage and green beans), saltfish (salted cod) and ackee (Caribbean fruit). Plantains (banana-like fruit) can also be baked, rather than fried.
- With soups made with groundnut/peanut or palm oil, allow the soup to cool (after cooking) and then pour off the layer of excess oil.
- Reduce the amount of salt in your diet: gradually cut down on the amount of salt used in preparing food. Many ready-made seasonings contain a fair amount of salt.
- Try using fresh or dried herbs like thyme, coriander, turmeric, paprika, garlic, chilli and black pepper.
- Saltfish, salted mackerel, stockfish (air-cured fish such as cod or haddock) and salted pig-tails are high in salt content and should be soaked overnight in large quantities of water, to remove as much salt as possible before cooking.
- Try to cut down on salty foods/snacks like bacon/ham, packet/tinned soup, crisps and nuts.
- Fresh fruits are a much better option.

## Salt

Just like fat, unfortunately the average adult in the UK eats around 8 times the amount of salt his body needs. The tricky part is that over two-thirds of the salt we consume is found in manufactured foods. Things like ready prepared meals, tinned soups, salad dressings, savoury snacks, cooking sauces and stock cubes, as well as canned meat, fish and meat products and many canned vegetables are high in salt which is added during processing. Bread and cereals can also be guilty of containing too much salt. In fact, salt from bread is responsible for almost a quarter of the salt in our diet.

We now know that diets high in salt can contribute to high blood pressure and may lead to coronary heart disease, kidney disease and stroke. Research also shows that salty diets will probably increase our risk of stomach cancer. While we do need some salt for our bodies to function properly, we don't need too much or we could be putting our health at risk.

To cut down on adding salt to your food, try hiding the salt cellar and using freshly ground pepper or herbs and spices instead – you'll be surprised how easily you get used to this. Also, try to buy low-salt versions of normally high-salt products like stock-cubes, butter, bacon, baked beans, savoury snacks and soy sauce.

## Makes all the difference

The average man, consuming around 2,500 calories a day, should aim to eat less than around 85 grams (3ozs) of total fat and no more than 6 grams of salt (sodium). But it's very easy to notch up too much fat and salt without realising it. Here we show how choosing the right shop-bought lunch makes a big difference to the amount of fat and salt you eat.

| Original choice | Improved choice |
|---|---|
| 1 wholemeal ham and cheese sandwich | 1 wholemeal chicken salad sandwich |
| 1 packet of crisps | 1 slice of malt loaf (28g) |
| 1 chocolate mini roll | 1 medium apple |
| 1 can of cola | 1 glass of pure orange juice (180ml) |
| *Per serving* | *Per serving* |
| 870 calories, 38.8 grams fat and 1.42 grams sodium (salt). Contains zero portions of vegetables and fruits. | 457 calories, 11.3 grams fat and 1.06 grams sodium (salt). Contains 2 portions of vegetables and fruits. |

## Read the label

An easy way to help you keep an eye on the amount of fat and salt you're eating is to know what to look out for on food labels so that you can buy the healthiest choices. Memorise the following and you can impress your friends.

| Find it on the label | A Healthy range (per 100g of product) | But watch out for! (per 100g of product) |
|---|---|---|
| Total fat | 2g – 8g | 14g or more |
| (of which are saturates) | 1g – 3g | 5g or more |
| Sodium (salt) | 0.1g – 0.3g | 0.5g or more |

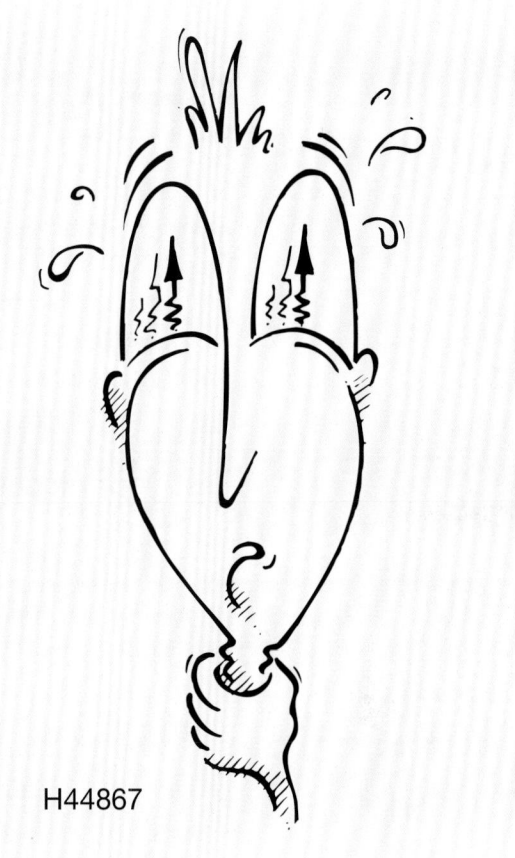

H44867

Diets high in salt can contribute to high blood pressure

## Top 20 superfoods

You're probably already asking yourself 'well, what should I buy?'. Although individual foods cannot yet be linked to specific illnesses, we do know that certain foods contain higher than average amounts of nutrients such as vitamin C, selenium, vitamin E and other 'bioactive compounds' – all of which have been shown to help protect against cancer.

Here is a list of the 'top 20 superfoods for good health'. Try to include as many of these as you can each time you go food shopping. Bear in mind that this is not a definitive list, and that the foods are not ranked in any particular order. Each food has been chosen because it is believed to help boost the body's immune system, thereby keeping it strong and resistant to serious illnesses such as cancer or heart disease.

- Bean sprouts.
- Brazil nuts.
- Broccoli.
- Brussels sprouts.
- Cabbage.
- Garlic.
- Kiwi fruit.
- Mango.
- Onions.
- Orange peppers.
- Oranges.
- Red peppers.
- Spinach.
- Strawberries.
- Sunflower seeds.
- Sweet potatoes.
- Tomatoes.
- Virgin olive oil.
- Watercress.
- Wholegrain bread.

PART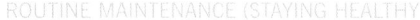

# Smoking and health

Smoking is a major cause of ill health. Every puff of tobacco smoke gives you a very nasty cocktail of over 4,000 chemicals including tar, nicotine, carbon monoxide, arsenic and ammonia. 60 of these chemicals are known to cause cancer. Smoking also increases your risk of heart disease and stroke, and is a major cause of bronchitis, emphysema and impotence.

## Test your nicotine dependence

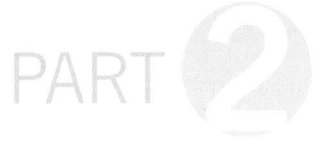

| How many cigarettes do you smoke per day? | | |
|---|---|---|
| 10 or less | ☐ | 0 points |
| 11 to 20 | ☐ | 1 point |
| 21 to 30 | ☐ | 2 points |
| Over 30 | ☐ | 3 points |

| How soon after you wake up do you smoke your first cigarette? | | |
|---|---|---|
| Less than 5 mins | ☐ | 3 points |
| 6 to 30 mins | ☐ | 2 points |
| 31 to 60 mins | ☐ | 1 point |
| Over 60 mins | ☐ | 0 points |

| | Yes (1 point) | No (0 points) |
|---|---|---|
| If you had to refrain from smoking because you were in a public place would it be difficult? | ☐ | ☐ |
| Do you smoke more in the morning than the rest of the day? | ☐ | ☐ |
| Do you smoke if you are ill and have to spend most of the day in bed? | ☐ | ☐ |
| Which would be the hardest cigarette to give up? | The first ☐ | Any other ☐ |

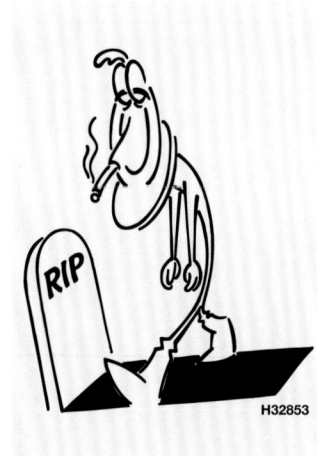

Smoking can lead to all sorts of serious health problems

### Dependence score

0-3 points – low
4-5 points – medium
6-8 points – high
9-10 points – very high

## Tobacco smoking

Despite the bleating from the tobacco industry and their funded 'independent' advocacy groups, the evidence linking cancer of the lung to cigarette smoking is overwhelming. Most people, including governments, now accept this, but what many people don't realise is that smoking can also cause cancer of the tongue and bladder and in various other organs. The cancer-producing substances in cigarette smoke are absorbed into the blood and get everywhere in the body.

Normal cell DNA contains genes called proto-oncogenes. These remain harmless unless acted on by a carcinogen. When this happens, cancer-producing genes (oncogenes) are formed. Mutations in proto-oncogenes can also lead to cancer. One of the arguments is that tobacco doesn't actually cause cancer itself but

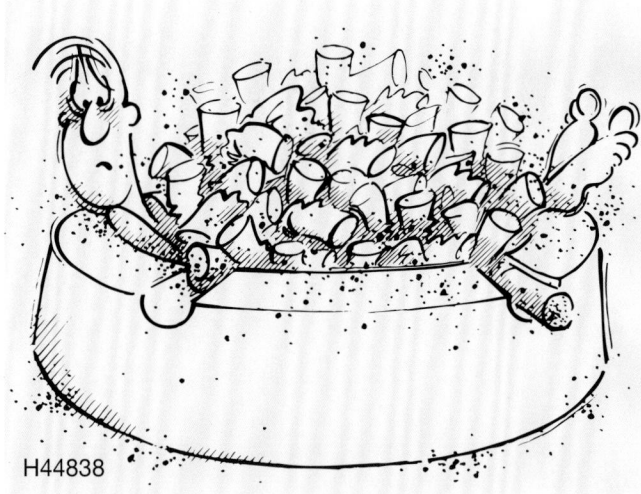

H44838

The cancer-producing substances in cigarette smoke are absorbed into the blood and get everywhere in the body

instead triggers viruses or the oncogenes which then cause all the trouble. Actually it doesn't make much difference. Trying to decide whether it's your finger which pulls the trigger of the gun or the bullet the gun fires that kills you is pretty academic. You still blow your head off.

## No smoke without fire

Okay, so you've heard it all before. But don't turn the page yet. This advice could add years to your life, never mind helping to improve the way you look, feel and smell.

Smoking can lead to all sorts of serious health problems, including heart disease, stroke, various cancers (such as lung, bladder, mouth and throat cancers), bronchitis and emphysema. Our advice is the same as everyone else's. Plain and simple: if you smoke, try to give up. And, if you don't smoke, don't start.

On a more positive note, what you may not know is that the very moment you stop smoking, your health will start to improve. After only 20 minutes of not smoking, your blood pressure and pulse return to normal. In just 48 hours, your body is nicotine free and carbon monoxide is cleared from your system. And, within 2 to 12 weeks, your circulation improves and you'll feel noticeably fitter.

Best of all, within five years your risk of lung cancer will have dropped dramatically. And your risk may be halved by the time you reach your tenth year of being cigarette-free.

## How much could I save?

Because nicotine is highly addictive, many people find it hard to stop smoking. But there are around 12 million ex-smokers in the UK – a living testimony that the habit can be beaten. And these people have since been enjoying the financial – not just physical – benefits of their new tobacco-free lives. If you smoke 20 cigarettes a day, stopping could save you around £1,800 a year. That's a great holiday each year or, over the course of the next five years, a nice new car.

## Smoking habits

After smoking for any length of time, lighting-up becomes a habit and there are probably certain times when you usually have a cigarette. It can be helpful to identify these times and plan ways to handle or avoid the most difficult.

### Lighting-up times

What triggers the 'time for a cigarette' habit? Is it:
- On awakening?
- With the first cup of coffee?
- Talking on the phone?
- Watching TV?
- In the pub?
- After a meal?
- While reading?
- During stressful periods?

These are only examples, and you might have others. Try keeping a diary for a few days to record your smoking patterns; this can help you understand when and why you smoke, and plan what to do instead.

| Time of day | Related event | Alternative activity |
|---|---|---|
|  |  |  |
|  |  |  |
|  |  |  |
|  |  |  |
|  |  |  |
|  |  |  |
|  |  |  |

Some ways of getting through the tricky times are:
- Take one day at a time.
- Get involved in something new.
- Keep busy.
- Go for a walk.
- If you're doing this with someone, tell them how you're feeling.
- Drink a glass of water or juice.
- Change your routine.
- Buy a small 'treat' (not sweets, and definitely not baccy!).

Practise your 'alternative activities' before quitting, and see how they work.

# How do I stop?

There are a few ways to stop smoking:

● Cutting down to a final quit point.
● Cold turkey (stopping all at once).
● Treatments to assist the process.
● Use experienced back-up services and support groups.

Whichever you go for, it will be easier with some sort of structure or quit plan, eg:

---

## Quit plan

● Set a day and date to stop. Tell all your friends and relatives, they will support you.
● Like deep sea diving, always take a buddy. Get someone to give up with you. You will reinforce each other's will power.
● Clear the house and your pockets of any packets, papers or matches.
● One day at a time is better than leaving it open-ended.
● Map out your progress on a chart or calendar. Keep the money saved in a separate container.
● Chew on a carrot. It will help you do something with your mouth and hands.
● Ask your friends not to smoke around you. People accept this far more readily than they used to do.

---

### Cutting down and cold turkey

The problem with tapering off is that the numbers tend to creep up again, so it is better to stop outright. Make sure you are fully prepared to manage without smoking; many fail because they jump into the task before they are ready. Just quitting with no assistance is hard; consider also using other means to help you as well.

### Treatments to assist the process

Things that can help you keep off the weed are:

● Prescription and non-prescription aids.
● Alternative therapies like hypnotherapy and acupuncture.

### Stop-smoking groups

Joining a stop-smoking support group is a good source of professional advice and support from like-minded people. The NHS offers free help and support for people who want to stop smoking.

### One-to-one services

Some people prefer individual help and support, and this is available in many areas.

Some people prefer individual help and support, and this is available in many areas

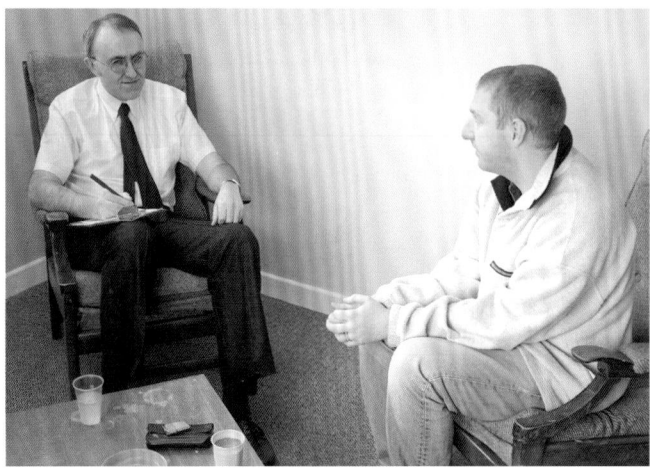

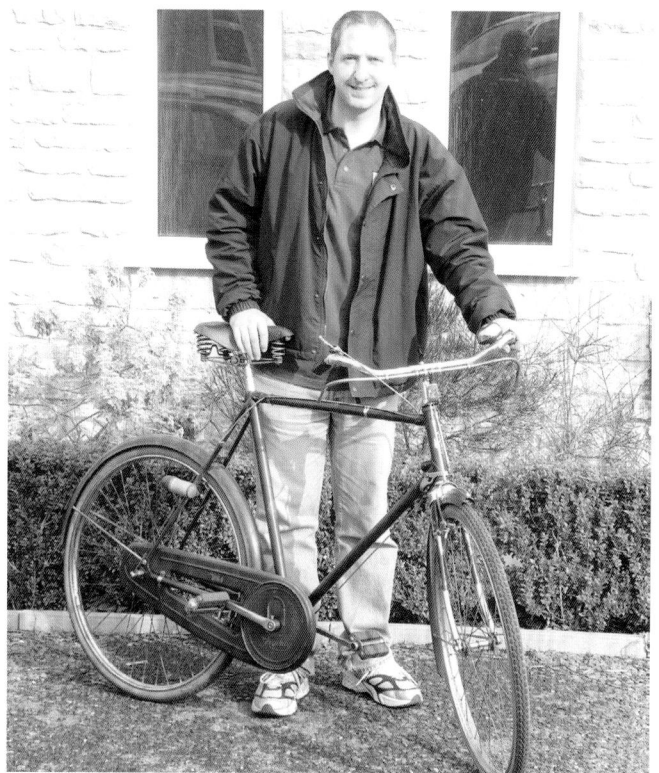

## Managing the cravings of nicotine withdrawal

Lots of people start smoking again very rapidly because of the strong hold both the nicotine and the smoking habit has on them. The first few days really are the worst, and not a lot of fun for anyone, but the symptoms are generally signs that the body is starting to recover. This also gives you the opportunity to start that new sport or hobby – the activity takes your mind off lighting-up, and your body will benefit doubly from the exercise and the nicotine removal.

| Symptom | Coping |
| --- | --- |
| Desire to smoke | This will lessen over a few weeks. In the short-term try: NRT and/or deep breaths or a glass of water. |
| Coughing or a dry mouth | This will be worse initially, as your lungs clear out the tar, but will improve rapidly. Warm drinks can ease the cough, and remember it's the road to recovery. |
| Hunger | Changes to your metabolism, and better-tasting food, can increase hunger. Get a 'survival kit' of fruit and vegetables. Carry chewing gum and drink lots of water. |
| Bowel changes | Constipation or diarrhoea will soon settle down. Drink plenty of water if you are constipated and eat more fibre if suffering from diarrhoea. |
| Trouble sleeping | Nicotine leaving the body can disturb sleep patterns. This should settle down in a few weeks, but consider nicotine patches. Try to get more exercise and fresh air; cut down on tea and coffee. |
| Dizziness | This is the result of more oxygen getting to the brain, rather than carbon monoxide. This will pass after a few days. |
| Mood swings, irritability, poor concentration | These are signs of nicotine withdrawal. All anyone can really do is grin and bear it, though it might be useful to warn family, friends and colleagues! |

## Swap chart for more fibre

| Refined | Unrefined |
| --- | --- |
| Cornflakes | Muesli or prorridge |
| White toast | Wholegrain or wheaten bread |
| Chocolate bar | Nut & seed bar or piece of fruit with a handful of nuts or seeds |
| French bread | Wheaten bread |
| White pasta | Wholewheat pasta |
| Breadsticks | Oatcakes |
| White rice | Brown basmati rice |

## Weight gain worries?

Some people gain weight when they stop smoking. This is because:

- Nicotine suppresses the natural appetite and makes the body burn calories faster.
- Stopping smoking makes food taste better.
- The physical smoking action is often replaced by the consumption of snacks and sweets.

Although some initial weight gain is common, after about a year most people will only have gained a few pounds. To avoid putting on too much weight:

- Get out more – even a walk round the block will help.
- Made a healthy eating program part of your stop-smoking plan.
- Keep an eye on what you eat; steering clear of high calorie and fried foods (see *Fat swaps* on page 69).

Having something to do with your hands breaks the nicotine habit

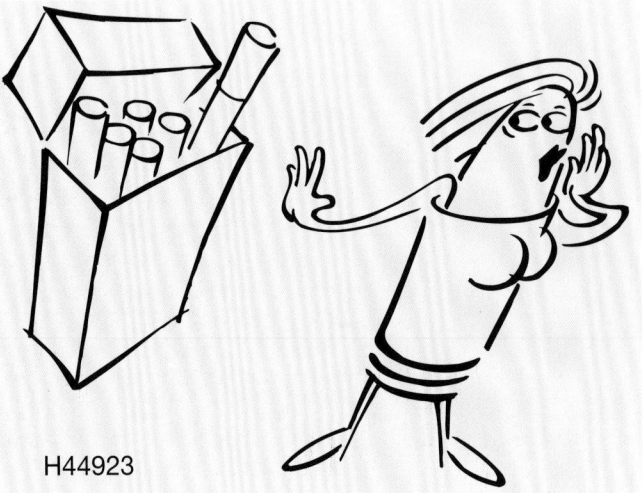

H44923

## Treatments to help during the first few weeks

There are many aids to ease you through the early days of not smoking; they are not all suitable for everyone, so it is worth

checking with your GP or a pharmacist first. You have to bear in mind that these aids cannot:
- Make you **want** to stop.
- Stop you smoking.
- Make the stopping painless and easy.
What they **can** do is:
- Lessen the urge to light-up.
- Ease withdrawal.
- Boost confidence or help relaxation.

## What treatments are available?

There are two main types of product:
- **Unlicensed products** which have not undergone any trials.
- **Licensed product**s which have undergone clinical trials to prove they are effective.
- Also available are **alternative** and **complementary therapies** which have unproven results, but they work for some people. It is important to find a registered practitioner.

### Unlicensed products

These do not need a license under the Medicines Act, and there is no firm evidence of their effectiveness. Be wary of claims of high success rates. In general, the range includes:
- Dummy cigarettes.
- Herbal cigarettes.
- Nicobrevin capsules.
- Tobacco-flavoured gum.

Having something to do with your hands and mouth instead of smoking at least breaks the nicotine habit, although the physical side will have to be addressed at some time.

### Licensed products

The main division in the range of licensed products is with or without nicotine. The nicotine replacement therapies (NRT), which are available on NHS prescription or from a pharmacist, include:
- Gum.
- Patches.
- Lozenges.
- Microtabs.
- Nasal spray.
- Inhalator.

The product which doesn't contain nicotine is only available on prescription:
- Bupropion tablets.

### NRT

Nicotine replacement therapies supply some of the nicotine that you are used to from smoking, but in a different way, so is much less addictive. Although these therapies are available over the counter, it is essential to check with your GP before starting to use them because some affect the action of other drugs. All NRT products are effective, and research shows that it can double your

chances of quitting if you follow the instructions on the packet and use the full 10 to 12 week course. Side-effects can include:
- Feeling sick.
- Indigestion.
- Headache.
- Dizziness.
- Palpitations.

### Nicotine gum

Provides nicotine on demand, by absorption through the lining of the mouth as the gum is chewed. Any nicotine swallowed as you chew is wasted, so a chew-rest-chew technique is best.

### Patches

These provide a continuous supply of nicotine so you cannot respond to a craving for a smoke or a stressful moment. If cravings are a problem, the 24-hour patch is probably the one for you as it provides all-day nicotine, but they can disturb your sleep. There is also a 16-hour patch which is ideal for most smokers. Remember to change the patch site regularly to avoid skin irritation.

### Lozenges

Like the gum, the lozenges can be used to provide a quick 'fix'. They are like sweets and are sucked slowly or allowed to dissolve in the mouth.

### Microtabs

Like the gum, the microtabs can be used to provide a quick 'fix'. They are small tablets which are allowed to dissolve under the tongue.

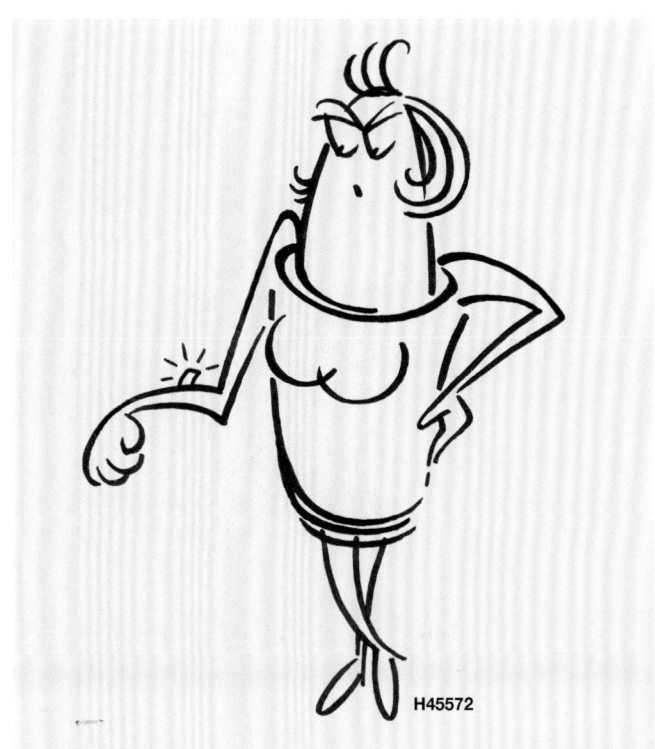

H45572

Patches are one of the NRT products available on the NHS

### Nasal spray

The nasal spray mimics cigarettes most closely by giving a fast effect. The nicotine gets into the body through the linings of the nose, and the sprays are especially suited to people who have high nicotine dependence or are suffering severe withdrawal symptoms. There can be some initial irritation.

### Inhalator

A plastic device shaped like a cigarette with a nicotine cartridge fitted into it. Sucking on the mouthpiece releases nicotine vapour which is absorbed through the linings of the mouth and throat. Most useful to people who miss the hand-to-mouth action of smoking.

### Bupropion tablets

Acts on the pathways in the brain that are responsible for nicotine addiction, so should reduce the desire to smoke and relieve some of the symptoms you get when you stop. Bupropion is only available on prescription and is not suitable for certain people, such as:

- Women who are pregnant or breast-feeding.
- People who have seizures or blackouts (eg, epilepsy).
- People who have had head injury or a brain tumour.
- People with eating disorders (eg, anorexia).
- People with kidney or liver problems.
- People withdrawing from high alcohol intake or tranquilliser/antidepressant-type drugs.
- Care must also be taken when driving and when taking other types of medicine.
- Bupropion should not be taken with NRT.

Bupropion is generally an eight-week course, the first week consisting of one tablet a day while still smoking, and the remainder of the course one tablet twice a day without cigarettes.

Side-effects can include:
- A dry mouth.
- Difficulty sleeping.
- Headache.
- Skin rash.
- Breathlessness.

### Stop-smoking groups

Joining a group of people who are also quitting can be a great help, especially when combined with NRT or bupropion. Working with a trained advisor, either in a group or on a one-to-one basis, has been show to increase quit rates by up to 19 per cent.

Most groups meet for an hour or two a week for six or seven weeks. The first two sessions are usually compiling quit plans, with the third week being the time to stop. After that you get mutual support, a sense of being understood and a sense of competition!

After the main course, many areas offer monthly relapse meetings or regular drop-in sessions.

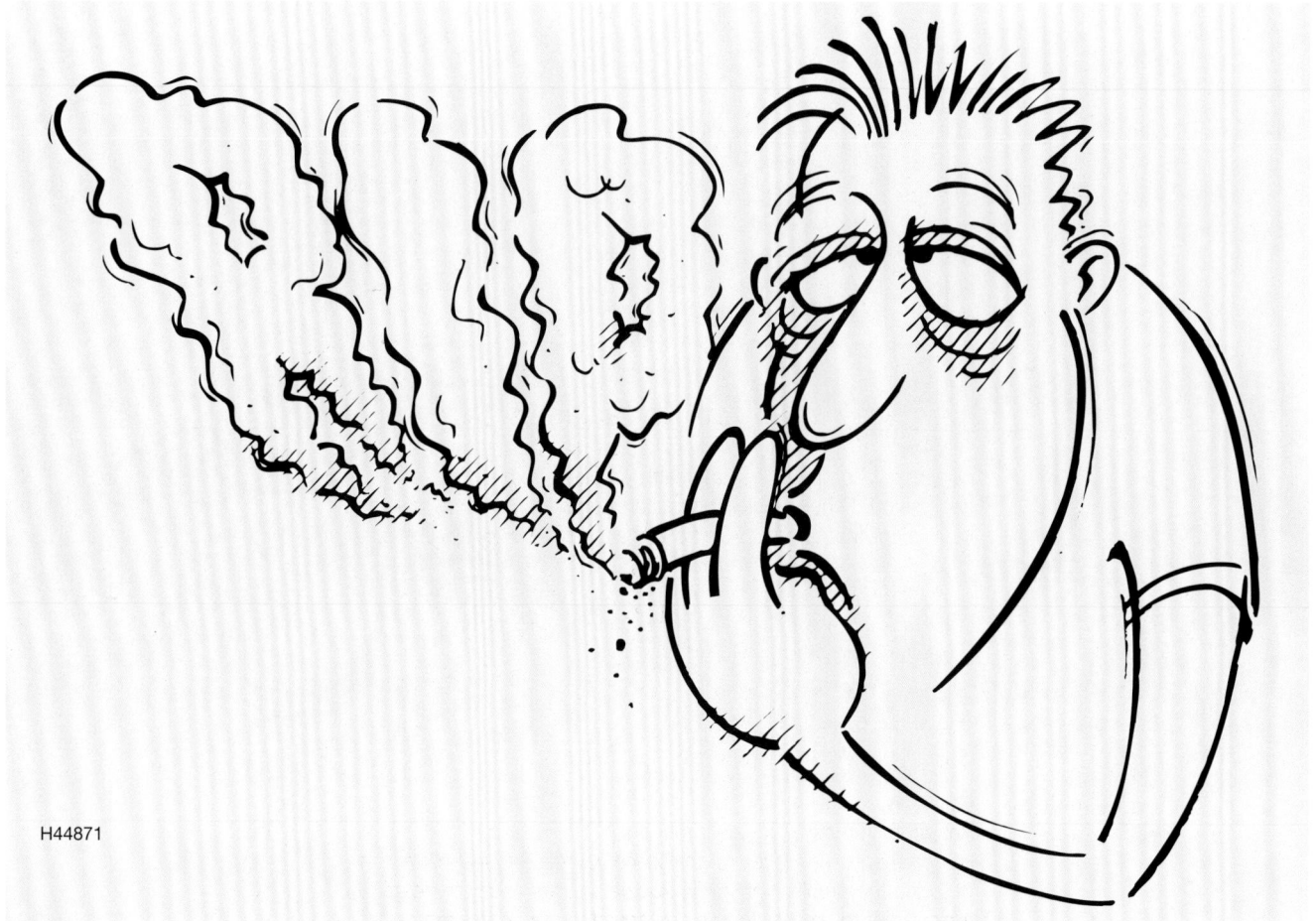

H44871

PART 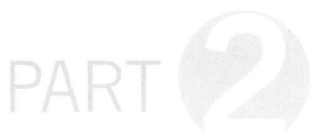 # Stress

## What is stress?

For many people, a certain degree of pressure can have a positive effect, however a build-up of pressure, without the chance to recover, can lead to stress. This can have a negative effect, both physically and emotionally. According to the Health and Safety Executive, stress is 'the adverse reaction that people have to excessive pressure or other types of demand placed on them'.

Most people are familiar with feelings of stress such as being worried or tense and believing that you may be unable to cope. The good news is there are positive steps that you can take to deal with, and manage, stress at home and at work with support from those around you.

## Stress signals

We all deal with some level of stress – however people vary in how much stress they can take before it has an effect on their life. Common stress signals include:

- Eating more/less.
- Mood swings.
- Poor concentration.
- Feeling tense.
- Low self-esteem.
- Anxiety.
- Not sleeping properly.
- Tiredness.
- Poor memory/forgetfulness.

It is useful to know your own stress signals so that you identify the cause and do something about it. This could mean changing your behaviour or how you think about things – sometimes we create our own stress by thinking or expecting too much of ourselves.

## Why is it important to tackle stress?

Too much stress, or stress that goes on for long periods of time, can trigger common mental health problems like anxiety and depression. Other problems that can be related to stress include back pain, indigestion, irritable bowel syndrome, psoriasis, migraine and tension headaches.

There are several things that you can do to help yourself deal with and prevent stress plus improve how you feel both physically and mentally in the long run.

## Time out

It can be hard to be rational when you are feeling very stressed which is why it is important to take time out.

### Quick fix

Physically removing yourself from a stressful situation, even for a few moments, can give you the space you need to feel more able to tackle the problem. If you anticipate a stressful day try to get up a bit earlier to prepare for the day ahead instead of feeling rushed.

### Long term

Taking time out from your everyday routine may help you deal with, and avoid, stress. If you have young children it is important to get a break. Try organising a family member, friend or neighbour to look after them for an evening, or take it in turns with your partner to have time to yourselves. If you work, try to avoid doing long hours, take proper holidays when you can and take breaks away from your work area each day.

## Work out

Exercise has been found to have a positive effect on the common symptoms of stress and it can help to prevent stress related ill-health.

### Quick fix

Go for a quick walk round the block – this can help clear your head and put problems in perspective so you can tackle them with renewed energy. If you work, get some fresh air and get moving during breaks.

### Long term

Aim to do at least 30 minutes of activity a day. This doesn't have to be done all at once and can be done in bouts of 10 minutes. Regular activity may help reduce your stress levels as well as getting you fit and making you feel good. Try building activity into your daily routine like cycling or walking to the shops, taking stairs instead of lifts, going for a walk with friends or family and playing games with the children.

If you work, build activity into your day by doing things like walking or cycling to work or meetings. Perhaps you can take advantage of work-based exercise facilities or corporate deals at local gyms.

## Chill out

Making time for yourself mentally and emotionally, as well as getting enough quality sleep is important so you can focus on relaxing your mind and recharging.

### Quick fix

Learning simple relaxation techniques such as deep breathing can be an effective way of helping you deal with feelings of stress. Try these simple exercises that you can do anywhere if you are hit with stress.

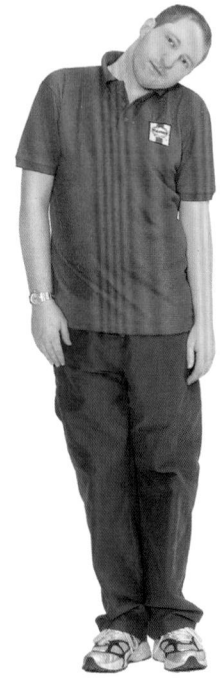

- Deep breathing. Take a long slow breath in then very slowly breathe out. Really concentrate on your breathing – after a few times you should begin to feel more relaxed.
- Tensing and stretching your muscles. Rotate your neck to the side as far as is comfortable, and then relax. Repeat on the other side. Then try fully tensing your shoulder and back muscles for several seconds and relax completely.

### Long term

Plan time to relax even if it's just having a long bath or listening to music. Try and have a good night's sleep – adults usually need, on average, 7 to 8 hours.

This may be difficult for some people, especially if you have children or work shifts. If this is the case aim to have at least 4 hours of sleep at the same time each day as this can help to keep your sleep clock regular.

Research shows that people who are regularly active fall asleep faster and sleep longer and more deeply than people who do less activity. So being active through the day may improve the quality of your sleep.

Relaxation techniques or meditation can also be useful for many people in helping them to feel more able to cope. You can buy relaxation music or there are many types of relaxation classes available like meditation, yoga and pilates. Find information about classes at your local library, gym, health centre, on the internet or look in your phone directory.

## Leave out

Try to avoid taking refuge in smoking, junk food or alcohol! This won't help your stress levels. Avoid too many caffeinated and sugary drinks as they may make you feel more anxious and bursts of sugar can cause mood swings.

### Quick fix

Drink plenty of water. This will help you concentrate better and may stop you getting stress headaches which can be caused by dehydration.

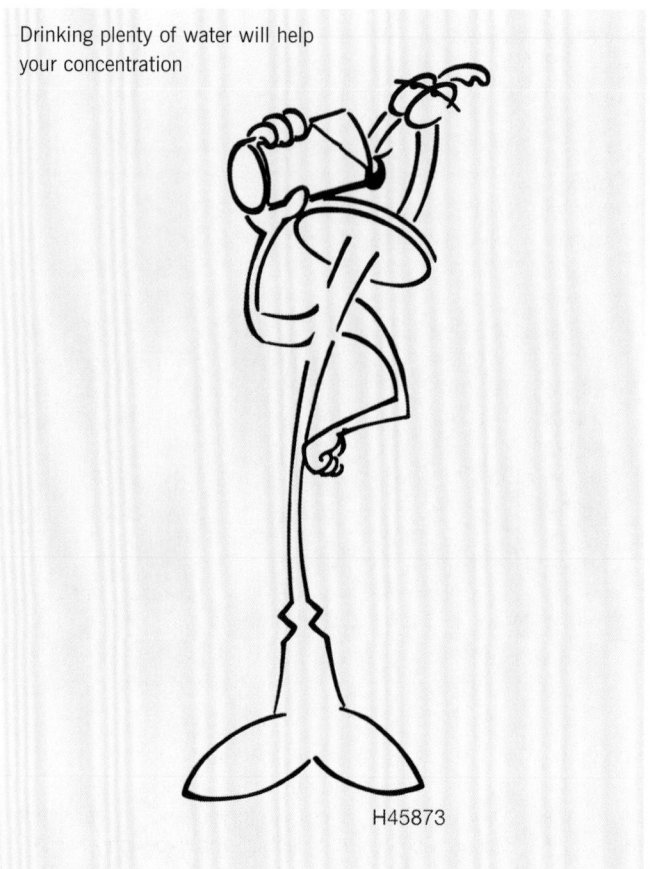

Drinking plenty of water will help your concentration

H45873

### Long term

Improving your diet and drinking plenty of water will increase your body's resistance to stress. Eating fruit and vegetables really boosts your immune system, especially in times of stress. Make small changes to increase your intake like chopping a banana on your cereal or toast and having a glass of fresh fruit juice with your lunch. It's important to make time for proper meals to help you stay energised.

## Talk about stress

Talking about stress may help you see things in a different light and help you find a way forward in tackling practical problems that may be causing you stress.

### Talk with friends or family

Try not to go it alone. A good support network, even if it's just one other person, can help you deal with stress. Talk with family or friends about how you are feeling – they may be able to offer their support. Don't be afraid to ask for their help, even if it's just to lend an ear.

### Talk with colleagues

Work is generally good for our well-being but, at times, it can be stressful. Getting help to improve your work environment or prioritising tasks can help.

Good working relationships are important in dealing with stress. Identifying colleagues who have knowledge of particular areas or who can simply offer a friendly ear can really help to relieve pressure.

### Talk with your boss

If you can't find a solution highlight the problem with your boss – they can support you in finding positive ways to reduce work related stress.

If you find it difficult to broach the subject consider the following tips:
- Book a time with your boss to meet.
- Prepare – think about what is causing you stress and any potential solutions you may have. Make a note of these to discuss.
- Think about positive changes that you would like to make to help you work more effectively.
- Make a list of points and questions that you want to cover – especially if you're feeling under pressure as it's easy to forget things.
- Help your boss to help you by giving them the information they need.
- Find out if there are any training courses that may help you cope better – like time management or problem solving. If you need training for an area of work that is causing you stress your boss may be able to organise this for you.
- Follow up – arrange a meeting to make sure that you and your boss are happy with how things are progressing and that your stress levels have gone down!

### Talk with your occupational health representative

If your company has a counselling or occupational health service then use it. They are there to help you and the service is confidential. Research shows that people who experience work-based stress benefit from these services.

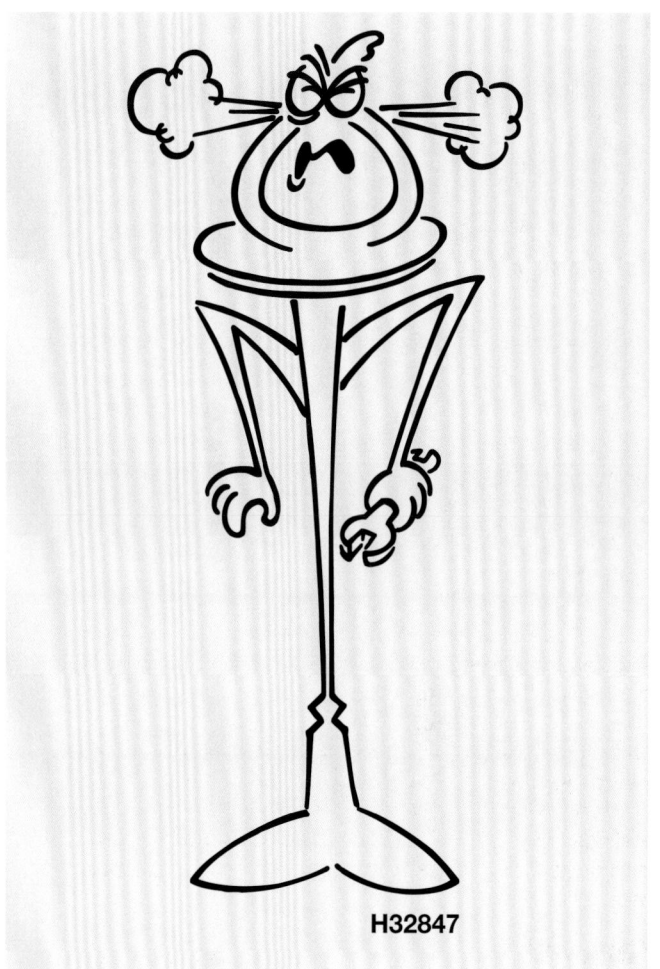

**H32847**

Occasionally we all drive at high revs. Too much of it and you'll blow a gasket

If you don't want to speak directly to your boss you could raise the issue with a staff or trade union representative who can speak to your employer on your behalf.

### Talk with a health professional

You can speak to a GP or practice nurse for advice and support, or contact NHS Direct (see *Contacts*). You can also ask your pharmacist for advice. Feeling run down, headaches, indigestion and sleeping problems can often be stress related and your pharmacist can give advice and over the counter treatment that may help, without the need for a prescription. They may also give you information and offer lifestyle advice on diet and getting active to help manage your stress levels in the long run.

## Feeling depressed or anxious?

Sometimes stress can feel overwhelming. This may trigger you to feel anxious or depressed. You can get help and support to deal with this. Speak to a GP, practice nurse or pharmacist. They can give you advice on how to cope and discuss treatments like exercise referral, other therapies or medication which may help.

PART 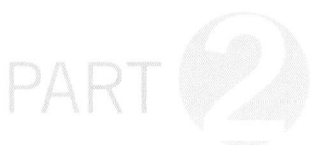 # Relaxation exercises

Reading a book on how to play the piano will not turn you into a concert pianist. Practice makes perfect, and this is the same with learning how to relax without resorting to alcohol or drugs.

- Make sure you will be alone, it will not help if you are constantly disturbed by requests for another drink of water or to answer a telephone.
- Either lie on a bed or sit in a chair with your head and arms supported and feet on a stool. Settle down and rid your mind of any thoughts which increase your anxiety.
- Concentrate on the positive words such as 'relax' or 'unwind'.
- Gentle music may help but is not essential.
- Breathe in deeply and hold your breath. Gradually release your breath and, as you do so, let your body sink into the chair or bed.
- Focusing your tension and release into specific parts of your body can be very effective.
- Concentrate on your right hand, make it into a fist, tightly clench it, then release it. Do it again. This time concentrate on the tension in your hand and as you release it notice the difference in the way it feels from when it is clenched and when it is relaxed.
- Do the same with your arms. Flex them and feel the tension build up as you bend your elbow. Imagine you are pulling a heavy weight. Hold the tension for a while and then relax.
- As you relax breathe out. At the same time reinforce the relaxation by thinking positive thoughts, 'I feel better', 'I am relaxing'.
- By concentrating on the difference between the relaxed and tensed state of your muscles and linking it to your mental state there will be a logical sequence of reinforcement.

Use a set pattern, for instance:
- Restore the normal state after each action. After tensing a muscle always return to a relaxed state.
- Do you feel the effect? Concentrate on the difference.
- Use a pattern for breathing. Always breathe in as you tense and breathe out as you relax your muscles.
- Even if you think you have completely relaxed a muscle try to release it that bit more.
- Take your time. It will become easier to achieve a state of relaxation more quickly as you become more adept.
- Use positive thoughts to augment your physical activity, 'relax', 'let go', etc.
- Repeat each individual exercise at least twice. You will be surprised at the level of relaxation you will achieve after each repeat.
- Use the same pathway for each part of your body, chest, neck, abdomen, legs and feet. You do not have to adhere rigidly to this system, you will soon find a pattern which suits you best.

Now is the time to reflect on the trivia which can cause such tension and how, with a little practice, they can be seen in their true light.

On the other hand you might still feel like pulling all your hair out by the roots, but at least you won't get out of breath.

PART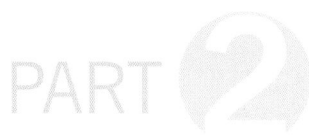

# Unexpected weight loss

Losing weight, or at least trying to lose weight, is very popular at the moment. This is perfectly reasonable if you are overweight, but there should be a good reason why you are seeing the pounds drop off. A significant loss of weight (over 4.5kg (10lbs) in 10 weeks) for no good reason is not normal. Increasing exercise will decrease your weight so long as you are not eating more than usual. Cutting down on alcohol if you have been drinking too much will also trim your waistline. But if you are losing weight but cannot pin down exactly why, you should be aware of some medical conditions which include weight loss in their list of signs and symptoms.

Do you have an increased thirst, pass water more often and feel generally tired? Some hormone deficiencies such as diabetes can cause weight loss with these symptoms. This condition tends to run in families, so if a close relative suffered from diabetes it will increase your risk. A simple test can be performed by your practice nurse.

Feeling restless, sweating profusely, feeling weak and having difficulty sleeping may be the signs of a hyperactive thyroid gland, which is producing too much thyroxine. This will cause weight loss by increasing your basic metabolic rate. Again, a simple blood test can check this for you.

Some rare infections like tuberculosis and even rarer disorders of the immune system such as AIDS can also cause weight loss. It is possible for your doctor to check for these conditions in a number of ways, including blood tests and X-rays.

Persistent diarrhoea with unusually pale stools may mean you are not absorbing your food properly. This may be due to an inflammation of the digestive system. Any marked changes in your bowel habit (how often you pass a motion) or any blood or tar-like substances in your stool, can be caused by inflammation or a tumour. This is not always accompanied by abdominal pain, although if pain is present, there is even more reason to get it checked sooner rather than later.

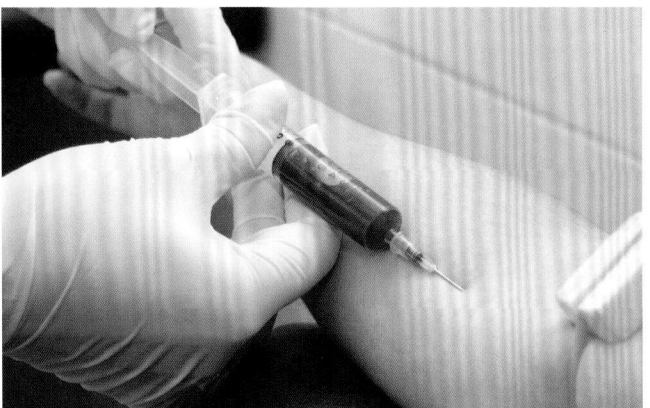

Photo: © iStockphoto.com

A simple blood test can identify a number of problems

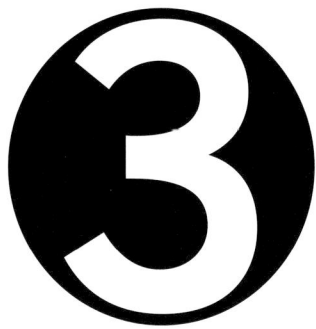

MAN MANUAL

# Heart and lungs

Photo: © iStockphoto.com, Chad McDermott

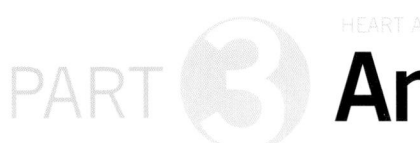

PART 3

# Angina (angina pectoris)

## Introduction

Angina is a pain or an uncomfortable, often vague feeling of pressure in the chest. It is a symptom that usually lasts only for a few minutes at the most and it will, in most cases, be relieved simply by resting. It is more common in men. In Britain, about 1 man in 10 will suffer angina at some time. Men with diabetes and men from the Indian subcontinent are more liable than others to suffer angina.

Angina is a symptom of the very common artery disease atherosclerosis which affects many arteries in the body, causing narrowing and partial obstruction to the blood flow. In this case, the arteries concerned are the coronary arteries of the heart. These arteries and their branches supply the heart muscle with the oxygen and fuel it needs to keep beating.

If these arteries can provide enough blood so that the heart gets the amount of fuel and oxygen it needs for its energy supply under conditions of exertion, the heart goes on beating painlessly. If the coronary arteries have been narrowed and can't get the blood to the heart muscle fast enough to meet the demand, abnormal levels of substances such as lactic acid collect in the muscle to the point of causing angina.

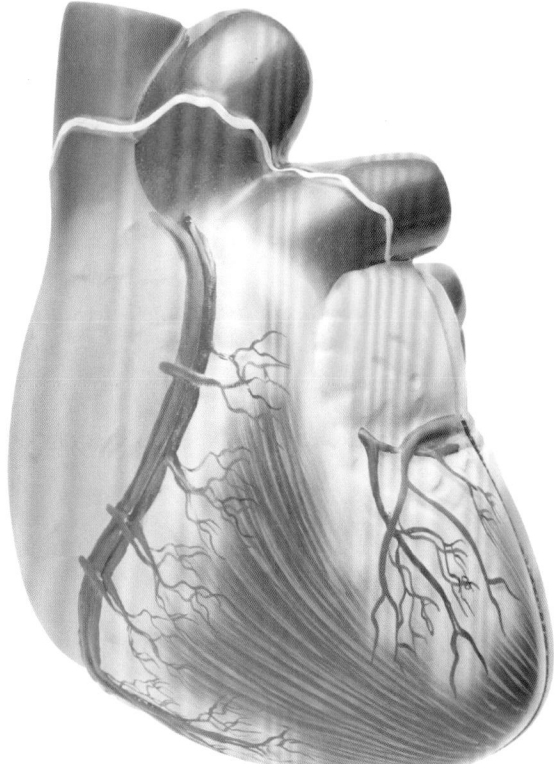

Heart, showing coronary arteries (red) and veins (blue)

Photo: © iStockphoto.com, Thomas Mounsey

## Symptoms

The pain usually comes on after a fixed amount of exertion for each man, such as walking a particular distance.

It may be of very variable severity, even in the same person, and may be affected by factors such as cold weather, a change of temperature as when going outside from a warm house, the strength of the wind, the state of your mind, and the length of time since your last meal.

The pain can vary enormously. It may be so mild as to be hardly a pain – more a feeling of uneasiness or pressure in the chest – or so severe as to stop you in your tracks.

It is often linked with breathlessness and belching but anti-indigestion treatments seldom help.

When the exertion ceases, the angina soon settles. It is quite common for angina to remain at a fairly constant level of severity for years.

Unstable angina is a severe and dangerous form of angina. Pain becomes more frequent and prolonged, and may occur at rest.

With unstable angina it becomes difficult to predict how much exercise will cause pain, and the risk of a heart attack is increased.

## Causes

Healthy coronary arteries can pass enough blood to allow the heart to reach its maximum output without pain. But narrowing of the coronary arteries will always mean that there is a limit to the rate blood can get to the heart muscle.

When a coronary artery, or a branch, is reduced in capacity by more than 50% any rise in demand often cannot be fully met.

A similar pain can be experienced elsewhere in the body under conditions of inadequate blood supply. If the main artery to the leg, for instance, is narrowed by atherosclerosis, pain occurs in the calf after walking a certain distance (claudication).

## Diagnosis

An ECG (electrocardiogram), taken during exercise, shows a characteristic pattern. Angina must be distinguished from the pain of a heart attack which often radiates up into the jaw, through to the back and down the left arm. It is associated with severe restlessness and distress and there will seldom be any doubt that something serious has happened.

The main difference between this pain and the pain of angina is the length of time it lasts. Generally speaking, angina ceases when you stop doing what brought it on. This can be the important difference between angina and a heart attack which usually lasts for hours and is not relieved by stopping any form of exercise.

Thankfully most cases of chest pain are due neither to angina nor to heart attack. Chest pain, however, should always be reported to your doctor. Unless the cause is obvious, it is not a symptom which can safely be ignored.

## Prevention

Once angina has been diagnosed it can be prevented by keeping within your exertional limits. But that's a bit like closing the stable door after the horse has bolted. Far better to prevent angina earlier in life by healthy living. This is going to be a mantra throughout this book, and no-one ever said it was easy,

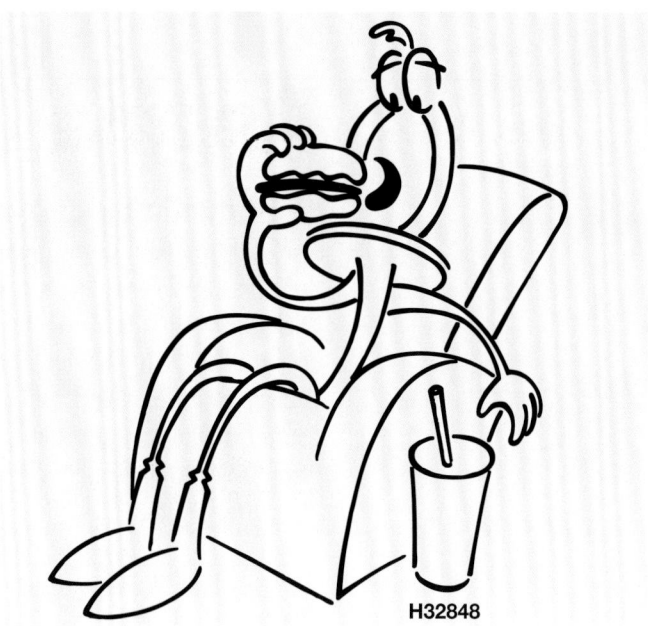

H32848

For optimum performance keep your fuel injectors clear of debris

but trying to avoid cigarette smoking, getting plenty of exercise and a good diet are the most important tips from our experts. In the case of angina, please don't try to 'walk through your pain barrier' as advised by less knowledgeable but well meaning people.

## Treatment

The drug glyceryl trinitrate (nitro-glycerine) is highly effective in controlling the pain of angina. The oral preparation may be taken in a tablet that is allowed to dissolve under the tongue and the pain is usually relieved in two to three minutes. The drug is also available in patches to be applied to the skin (transdermal patches) and sprays for under the tongue.

Glyceryl trinitrate should not be taken in combination with some other drugs. Ask your GP if you are unsure.

An effective treatment for angina is to have your narrowed coronary arteries widened by a procedure called coronary angioplasty.

A sausage-shaped balloon segment near one end of a very narrow tube is pushed into the narrowed part of the artery. The balloon is then inflated to widen the constriction before being removed.

The alternative to angioplasty, coronary artery bypass, now carries very little risk and the results are excellent. Segments of vein are used to provide a new channel by which the blood can be shunted past the blocked part of the artery.

Many surgeons prefer to connect a local artery from the chest wall, a mammary artery, to the narrowed coronary beyond the point of the block.

## Action

If you have chest pain on exertion, make an appointment to see your GP about it.

PART 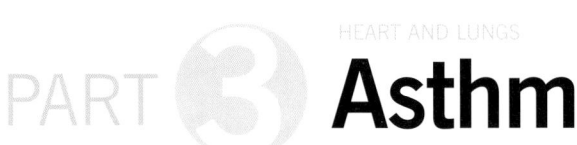 **3**

# Asthma

Asthma is often underestimated and can be a frightening condition where the airways of the lung constrict very quickly leaving the person coughing, wheezing and breathless. It is also common, starts at any age but most commonly in childhood. At least 1 in 10 children and 1 in 20 adults have asthma.

Asthma tends to run in families although many people with asthma have no other family members affected. Modern treatments are usually effective in controlling symptoms. With treatment, most people with asthma lead normal lives including school, work and sport.

In the past 20 years, asthma has become more common in all developed countries. In the UK, asthma cases and deaths as a result of asthma have doubled since the mid-1980s for reasons that are unclear. Thankfully, this is now on the decline. Each year in the UK, there are more than 85,000 admissions to hospital for the treatment of asthma, and about 100,000 people attend hospital for outpatient consultations for the disorder. Thankfully deaths are now on the decrease but are still at an unacceptable high of around 1500 per year.

## Symptoms

The common symptoms are cough and wheeze. Shortness of breath and a feeling of the chest being tight may also develop. The severity of symptoms can be quite variable between different people and at different times in the same person. Symptoms can range from mild to severe.

## Mild asthma

Some people just develop mild symptoms. For example, most of the time they have no symptoms. They may develop a mild wheeze and an irritating cough during a cough, cold, chest infection or in the hay fever season.

A child with mild asthma may have an irritating cough each night but is often fine during the day.

## 'Classical' asthma symptoms

Although symptoms do differ from person to person, the 'typical' person with asthma has bouts of wheezing and coughing that develop from time to time. Sometimes shortness of breath (breathlessness) also develops.

For many people there are spells, sometimes long spells, without symptoms. However, some people with asthma find that, without treatment, they are wheezy and breathless for some of the time on most days. Symptoms are often worse at night or first thing in the morning.

Children often don't have such classical symptoms. It may be difficult to tell the difference between asthma and viral infections in young children.

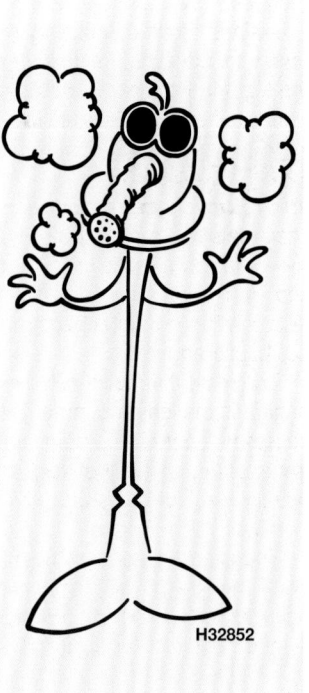

H32852

Getting enough air into your engine keeps you on the road. Don't ignore the signs of asthma, get your tubes checked

## Severe symptoms

A severe attack of asthma causes bad wheezing, a 'tight chest' and difficulty in breathing. Severe asthma attacks develop from time to time in some people who have classical symptoms of asthma. However, a severe attack may occur in people who normally have only mild asthma and occasionally in some people who have not had any symptoms for a long time.

One thing is certain, any asthma attack must be taken seriously, particularly if the person cannot speak, has blue lips, is breathing through pursed lips with almost silent breaths or is obviously exhausted from the effort of trying to breath.

## Causes

During an asthma attack, the muscle in the walls of the bronchi (airways) contracts, causing narrowing. The linings of the airways also become swollen and inflamed, producing lots of mucus that can block the smaller airways.

The symptoms of asthma may develop gradually and may not be noticed until a trigger provokes the first severe attack. Some people, for instance, find that they develop mild wheezing during a common cold or a chest infection, but usually this does not indicate asthma.

In some people, it can be an allergic response that triggers the asthma attack. Things that may trigger an attack of asthma symptoms include the following.

- Infections – particularly colds, coughs and chest infections.
- Pollens and moulds. The hay fever season is a common time for asthma to become worse.
- Exercise – some people only develop symptoms during sport, particularly when running in cold wind. However, sport and exercise are generally good for people with asthma and should be encouraged. Treatment can be taken before exercise to prevent symptoms developing.
- Certain medication. For example, about 1 in 50 people with asthma are allergic to aspirin which can trigger symptoms. Other medication that may cause asthma symptoms include anti-inflammatory painkillers and beta-blockers such as propranolol, atenolol or timolol. This includes beta-blocker eye-drops used to treat glaucoma.
- Emotion. Asthma is not due to 'nerves' but such things as stress, emotional upset or laughing may trigger symptoms.
- Certain fumes and chemicals such as cigarette smoke and pollution. The increase of air pollution may be a reason why asthma is becoming more common.
- House dust mite – a tiny creature that lives in mattresses and other fabrics around the home.
- Certain foods – this is uncommon and not thought to be of significance in most people.
- Allergies to pets.

Being affected by allergy conditions often runs in families and so may be inherited from fathers and mothers.

## Diagnosis

When you first go to the surgery, your doctor may arrange for you to have various tests to measure how efficiently your lungs are working. As part of these tests, your doctor may ask you to exercise for a few minutes in an attempt to induce a mild attack of asthma.

A device called a peak flow meter measures how fast you can

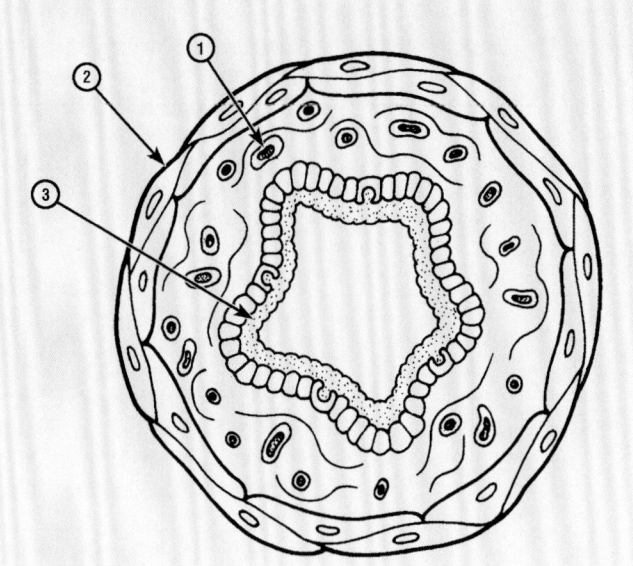

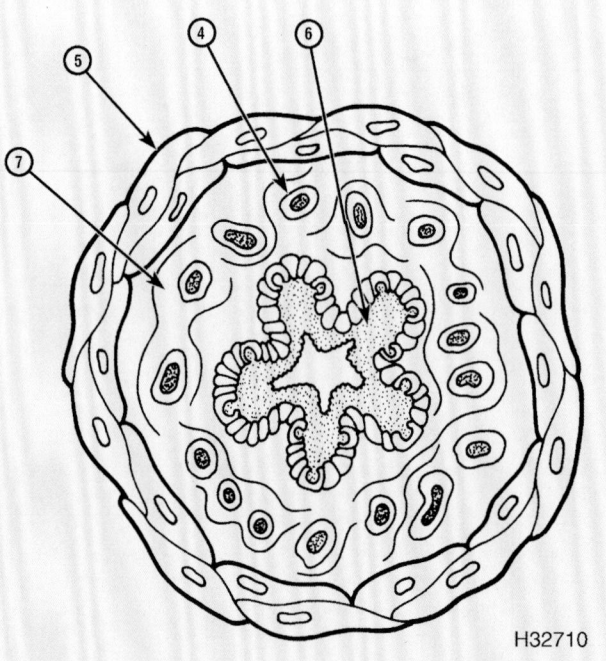

H32710

**Normal (top) and asthmatic airways**

1  *Normal blood vessels*
2  *Mucus*
3  *Uncontracted smooth muscle*
4  *Widened blood vessels*
5  *contracted smooth muscle*
6  *Excess mucus*
7  *Inflammation*

breath out which may be improved by inhaling a bronchodilator, which relaxes the airways. Your doctor may be able to diagnose asthma if your peak flow rate increases substantially after you have inhaled the bronchodilator drug.

Severe attacks may need you to go to hospital for treatment and further tests. If you are diagnosed with asthma, your doctor may suggest that you have further tests at a later date to check for allergies to substances that are known to trigger attacks.

If the timing and occurrence of your symptoms suggests that you have occupational asthma, your doctor will ask about substances used in your workplace to try to identify a specific trigger for your asthma.

## Prevention

There is no known way of preventing asthma but it is possible to reduce the number and severity of attacks.

Do not smoke. Smoking can make asthma worse. Children with asthma will benefit from a smoke-free home too as 'passive' smoking can also make asthma worse.

Treatment may vary from time to time. For example, increasing the dose of inhalers may be required for bad spells such as the

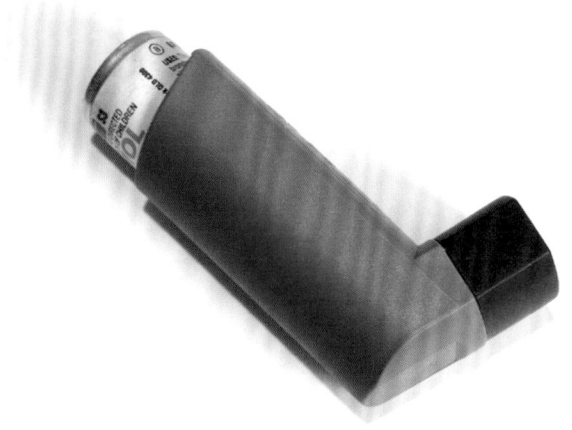

Photo: © iStockphoto.com, Nick Cowie

hay fever season, during chest infections, etc. Likewise, treatment may be reduced after being clear of symptoms for a long spell. As a general rule, if there have been no symptoms for 3 months or longer, some people may be able to reduce the dose of preventer inhaler. This is best done after discussion with a doctor or nurse.

Consult a doctor or nurse if symptoms are not fully controlled or if they are getting worse. For example: if a night time cough or wheeze is troublesome; if sport is being affected by symptoms; if peak flow readings are lower than normal; if a reliever inhaler is needed more often than usual. Adjustment in inhaler timings or doses may control these symptoms.

Make sure you know how to use the inhaler(s) properly. Do not be afraid to ask a doctor or nurse for advice if you think you are not using it to its best effect.

Seek medical attention promptly if a severe asthma attack develops that is not eased by a reliever inhaler. In particular, if you have difficulty talking due to breathlessness then urgent treatment is needed.

Influenza immunisation (the annual 'flu jab') and pneumococcal immunisation are commonly advised for people with asthma. These help to prevent some serious chest infections.

## Complications

A severe attack of asthma can be fatal and realizing that something is going wrong and calling for help is most important.

People with asthma can suffer from a collapsed lung – pneumothorax – which is potentially serious.

Asthma can lead to under-confidence and avoidance of sports, exercise and social gatherings, all of which can be helped by better use of medication.

## Treatment

Some people with asthma do not need treatment if they manage to avoid the triggers of their symptoms. However, there are so many triggers that it is very difficult to avoid them all, and for this reason treatment is often necessary.

Today, asthma attacks can usually be treated with short-acting drugs. In addition, long-term maintenance treatment can prevent asthma attacks developing. The current approach to asthma treatment is to give you the knowledge and confidence to be able to manage the condition yourself on a day-to-day basis, in partnership with your doctor.

The most important aspects of controlling your asthma effectively are the careful planning of drug treatment and regular monitoring of your condition.

The aim of all drug treatment is to eliminate symptoms and reduce the frequency and severity of asthma attacks so that visits to an accident and emergency department are no longer needed. Severe, potentially fatal attacks rarely develop without warning so recognising a serious change in your condition and taking prompt action by adjusting your treatment or contacting your doctor are essential to prevent an attack occurring.

### Types of drugs (medicines)

There are basically two types of asthma medicines.
● Relievers (quick-relief) drugs, which are used to relieve an attack of wheezing. Most relievers are bronchodilators. There are several different types of bronchodilator, all of which relax the muscles that narrow the airways and treat breathing problems as they occur. Relievers are usually effective within a few minutes if they are inhaled, but their effect lasts for only a few hours. They should be used as soon as symptoms develop or, if recommended by your doctor, before you start to exercise.
● Preventer drugs, which help to prevent attacks occurring. Most preventers of asthma are corticosteroid drugs, which slow the production of mucus, reduce inflammation in the airways, and make the airways less likely to narrow when they are exposed to a trigger substance. Nonsteroidal preventers, such as sodium cromoglicate and leukotriene antagonist drugs, are sometimes used to reduce the allergic response and to prevent narrowing of the airways. This type of treatment must be used on a daily basis and can take several days to become effective.

Both relievers and preventers are usually inhaled from a special device called a metered-dose inhaler, which delivers a fixed dose of the drug. Your doctor will show you how to use an inhaler. For acute asthma attacks, some people find drugs are most effective when inhaled using a spacer attached to

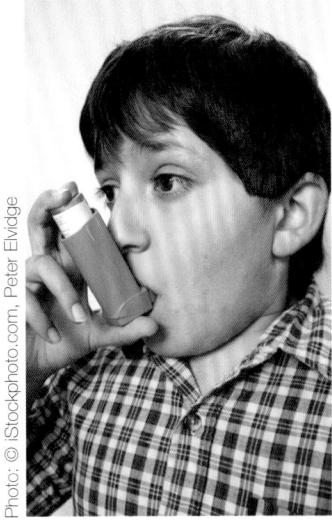

Photo: © iStockphoto.com, Peter Elvidge

the inhaler or through a device called a nebulizer. This device produces a fine mist of drugs to be inhaled through a mouthpiece or face mask.

Spacers are also useful if you find it difficult to synchronise your breathing in and releasing the drug. Children may need to use spacers.

People with long-term severe asthma may be given preventers in the form of low-dose oral corticosteroids rather than inhaled drugs. Oral corticosteroids may also be given to relieve severe attacks.

## Day-to-day care of asthma

You should take as much responsibility as possible for looking after your asthma, in partnership with your doctor, as it puts you in control of the condition instead of it ruling your life. Asthma may vary in severity from day to day or over longer periods. For this reason, you and your doctor will probably develop an asthma management plan which helps you to check on your progress make adjustments to your treatment accordingly. The key to controlling asthma is regularly checking your symptoms using a symptom diary and a peak flow meter, which determines the rate at which you are able to breath out.

If you are an adult newly diagnosed with asthma, treatment may start with a reliever drug only. Preventers may be added gradually if you find that you are using relievers more than a few times a week. Your doctor will closely monitor your progress over a period of time to decide on the best plan of treatment or whether it needs to be changed. If you use your peak flow meter to monitor your asthma every day, you will get an early warning sign of worsening of your condition and can adapt your treatment in accordance with the prescribed plan. Discuss your treatment plan with your doctor and ensure that you understand it. Your plan should include clear advice on what to do if you experience a severe attack of asthma.

There is no once and for all cure although recent advances in genetic engineering offer much promise. However, about half of the children who develop asthma 'grow out of it' by the time they are adults. For many adults, asthma is variable with some good spells and some not so good spells. The majority of adults with asthma are able to lead normal lives if they receive medical advice for their condition and then follow their treatment plans.

## Emergency treatment

If you have a sudden, severe attack of asthma, you should use your reliever inhaler as instructed by your doctor. If this treatment does not appear to be working, call for an ambulance immediately. If you have been given a reserve supply of corticosteroids as part of your treatment plan, take them as advised by your doctor. You should try to stay calm and sit in a comfortable position. Place your hands on your knees to help to support your back; do not lie down. Try to slow down the speed of your breathing to prevent yourself from becoming exhausted.

PART **3**

# Atrial fibrillation (irregular heartbeat)

## Introduction

The heart has its own natural pacemaker called the sinoatrial node. Its impulses are conveyed from there to another node at the junction between the upper and the lower chambers, called the atrioventricular node.

It is the atrioventricular node that determines the rate of contraction of the lower chambers, the ventricles, and thus the pulse rate.

Atrial fibrillation is a condition in which the upper chambers of the heart contracts at a very high rate and in an erratic manner. The result is an irregular beating of the ventricles, which is felt as a 'fluttering' in the chest.

The number of cases of atrial fibrillation in a population increases with age. People who already have heart disease are particularly vulnerable.

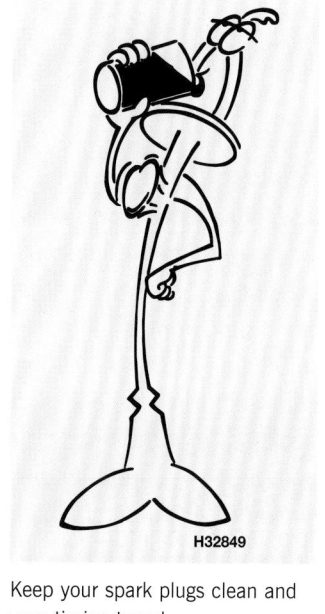

Keep your spark plugs clean and your timing tuned

## Symptoms

A 'fluttering' sensation in the chest is the commonest description. Atrial fibrillation is a completely irregular, but usually fast, heart beat rate. It is often in excess of 140 beats per minute, but the rate may be anywhere between 50-200 beats per minute. In the early stages, symptoms seem more prominent.

## Causes

Overactivity of the thyroid gland, excessive alcohol intake or inflammation of the heart muscle are all common causes

## Diagnosis

An electrocardiograph (ECG) is vital.

Blood tests can also be useful in the diagnosis. They may show anaemia, which may be complicating the situation, impaired kidney function, thyroid gland over activity (thyrotoxicosis).

## Prevention

Regular checks on blood pressure and treatment for raised pressure can reduce the chances of developing the heart problems that cause atrial fibrillation.

## Complications

The risk of stroke in people with atrial fibrillation is about twice that in the general population.

## Treatment

The first step is to be sure whether the cause of the atrial fibrillation is known and can be treated. If so, this may be all the treatment that is required.

Digoxin is a well established way of controlling atrial fibrillation, but beta blockers or the calcium channel blockers, or a combination of these drugs, can also help.

Cardioversion (electric shock to the heart under general anaesthetic) is most likely to be successful.

## Action

Make an appointment to see your GP.

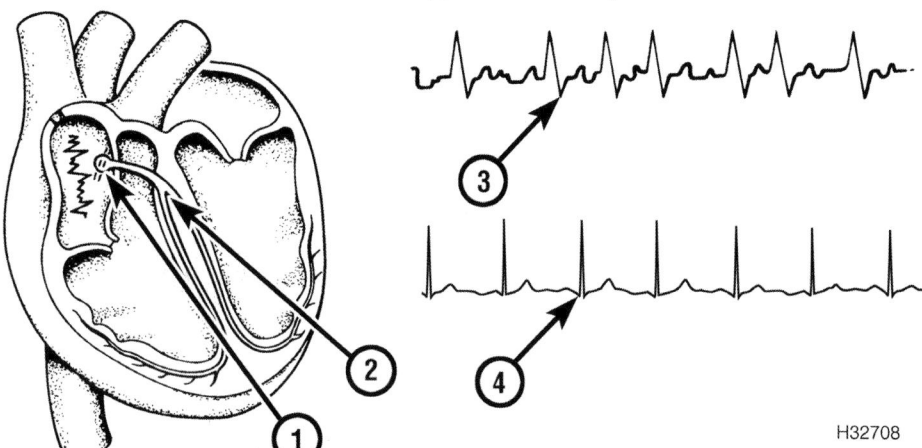

ECG trace showing atrial fibrillation

1   Sino-atrial node
2   AV node
3   Irregular heart beat
4   Normal heart beat

H32708

# PART  Breathlessness

## Introduction

Being breathless is a normal part of everyday life and for lots of different reasons. It is a natural response to the bodily system that detects that the oxygen in the blood has dropped. The carotid arteries in the neck have small clumps of cells called the carotid bodies. These are sensitive to the levels of oxygen in the blood passing upwards from the heart. If this blood is even slightly low in oxygen the carotid bodies will send messages, along nerves, to the vital breathing centres in the brain.

The result is an increase in the depth and rate of breathing. Breathlessness from unfitness from inadequate exercise is probably the commonest form of abnormal breathlessness.

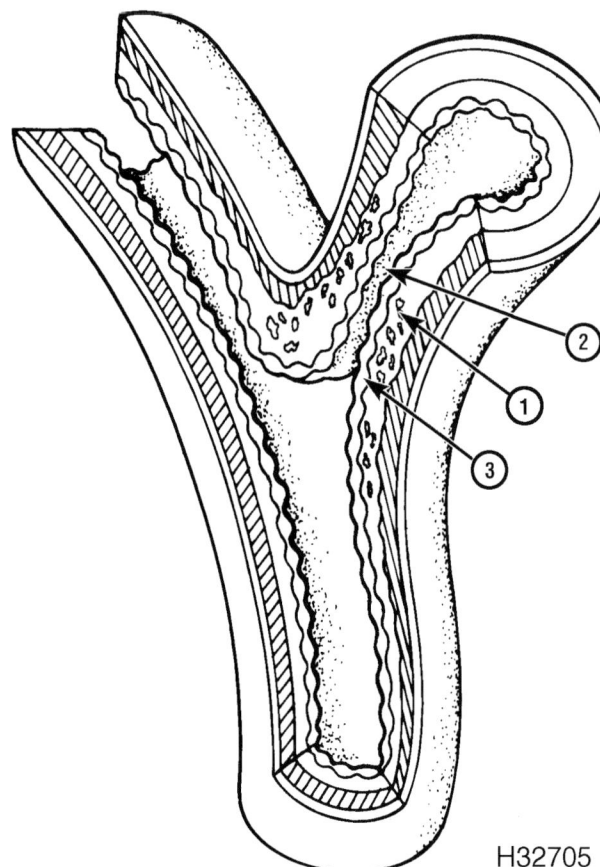

H32705

Section of artery showing signs of atherosclerosis

1   Fatty plaque
2   Narrowed channel
3   Fibrous cap

Atherosclerosis (disease of arteries) can lead to heart attacks, heart failure, strokes and other severe disorders. Almost any heart disorder can cause abnormal breathlessness, so atherosclerosis is, indirectly, a major cause of breathlessness.

People who are seriously unfit at a time in life when they ought to be fit are in some danger of developing diseases that will cause a much more serious form of breathlessness than ordinary puffing on the second flight of stairs.

## Symptoms

Breathlessness on only moderate exertion means either being unfit or unwell.

## Causes

Unfit breathlessness can always be corrected by sustained, graded exercise and by losing excess weight but breathlessness is sometimes an important sign of disease. Conditions that will always cause breathlessness for this reason include:

● Asthma.
● Lung collapse due to air leaking between the lung and the chest wall (pneumothorax).
● Acute bronchitis.
● Chronic bronchitis.
● A breakdown of the air sacs so that the area of tissue available for oxygen passage is much reduced (emphysema).

Smoking causes breathlessness in several ways. Cigarette smoke contains carbon monoxide, a poisonous gas that stops the blood from carrying oxygen effectively.

Breathlessness can sometimes be of psychological origin as part of a panic reaction.

## Diagnosis

Let's face it. We pretty much all know what being breathless is like. But if you find yourself suddenly becoming short of breath after light exercise then go and see your doctor. Your body is giving you a warning sign, don't ignore it.

## Prevention

Breathlessness from unfitness can always be reduced considerably if not totally prevented through exercise and losing weight.

If you've had no exercise in a while and you get breathless, pull on the trainers and give the man machine a good run. Start with some light exercise and work up. The British Heart Foundation can offer help and advice on getting and staying fitter.

## Treatment

The cause of the breathlessness needs to be diagnosed and treated.

## Action

Abnormal breathlessness should not be ignored. Make an appointment to see your GP.

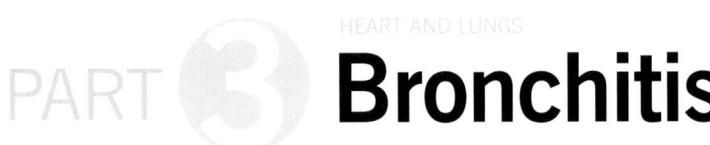

# PART **3** **Bronchitis**

## Introduction

**Cells which line the airways and help keep the lungs clean are damaged by cigarette smoke and industrial pollutants.**

Coughing is a natural reaction to irritation of the lung but in chronic bronchitis it is more or less the only way the lung can get rid of mucus.

People with chronic bronchitis cough up sputum on most days for at least three months of each year, usually the winter months. Most heavy smokers have chronic bronchitis, but refer to it simply as 'a smoker's cough'.

In the early stages, chronic bronchitis is a comparatively mild disease. But, with time and continued abuse, it is likely to progress to the condition called chronic obstructive airway disease (COAD), chronic obstructive pulmonary disease (COPD)

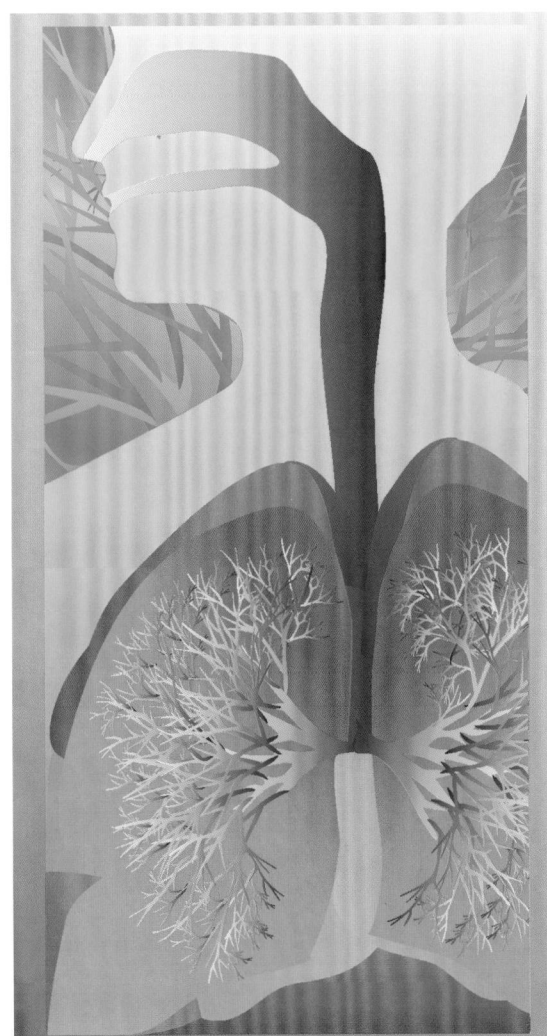

The lungs and bronchi

Photo: © iStockphoto.com, Julie Ridge

or emphysema. Large numbers of the tiny lung air sacs break down to form a smaller number of larger air spaces.

Smoking is especially dangerous in people with a persistent, productive cough. Chronic bronchitis and other forms of COAD / COPD affect 18% of male smokers.

## Symptoms

In acute bronchitis there is a cough, at first dry but later with sputum, maybe fever for a few days, breathlessness and wheezing. There may be some pain in the chest. Occasionally a little blood may be coughed up.

## Causes

Acute bronchitis in a previously healthy person is usually due to infection with a virus. In cigarette smokers this is often followed by additional infection by other germs that makes matters worse. Industrial atmospheric pollution may also be a cause.

Most experts are convinced that by far the most important factor in the causation of serious bronchitis is cigarette smoking.

## Diagnosis

Bronchitis causes characteristic sounds audible to a health professional on listening with a stethoscope.

In peak expiratory flow measurement in a normal person, asked to breathe out as forcibly as possible through the mouth, the rate of flow of the air rises rapidly to a peak and then declines steadily to zero. A normal person can breathe out at a peak rate of around 8 litres a second, but in certain lung diseases, such as bronchitis, because of narrowing or partial obstruction of the bronchial tubes, the figure is much lower.

## Prevention

You don't need an expert to work out the best way to prevent chronic bronchitis. Quit smoking, lay off the tabs, kick the wicked weed. See the section on stopping smoking in Part 2. However, you might need some expert advice on the best way to give up.

## Complications

The increased resistance to blood passing through the lungs imposes an additional load on the heart which responds by enlarging. Up to a point, the increased power of the enlarged ventricle enables the heart to compensate, but eventually the heart muscle fails and the blood returning to it from the rest of the body cannot be pumped fast enough.

## Treatment

Acute bronchitis is often treated with antibiotics and usually responds well, although it may be necessary to use oxygen in severe cases. There is no cure for chronic bronchitis, but not smoking can do much to improve it. Various other drugs can help.

## Action

Make an appointment to see your GP.

PART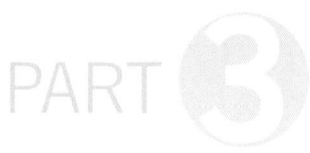

# Cholesterol and heart disease

*Prepared by Angie Jefferson, Consultant Dietician*

Cholesterol – we can't see it and we can't feel it, but we all have it and while we need some cholesterol for good health, most of us have too much which is where the problems start. The fact is that for most of us, our cholesterol levels are too high because of what we eat and how we live our lives. However the news is not all bad – we can take steps to lower our cholesterol levels and give ourselves a better chance of a long and healthy life with a lowered risk of developing heart disease.

## The facts

### Cholesterol

- Cholesterol levels are directly related to the risk of developing heart disease and strokes.
- People who are obese are not only likely to have high cholesterol, but are also likely to have poor glucose tolerance and raised blood clotting factors – greatly increasing the risk of heart disease and strokes.
- Half of all cases of heart disease are estimated to be due to having raised cholesterol levels.
- Two thirds of men and women have higher than ideal cholesterol levels.
- People with high cholesterol are more likely to get a build up of cholesterol in the arteries of the heart, brain, pelvic and abdominal arteries, causing heart attacks, strokes and contributing to impotence.
- 8 out of 10 people do not know they have raised cholesterol.
- Cholesterol levels can be lowered by dietary changes, in particular less saturated fat, using plant stanols or sterols, foods containing soya, oily fish, being more active and drug therapy.
- A proportion of people with elevated cholesterol levels will need medication.
- Losing weight reduces cholesterol, blood clotting and risk of heart disease. A 10kg weight loss is likely to result in:
  *A 10% fall in total cholesterol.*
  *A 15% fall in LDL (bad) cholesterol.*
  *A 30% fall in triglyceride levels.*
  *An 8% increase in HDL (good) cholesterol.*

### Heart disease

- Heart disease is the biggest single cause of death in the UK – the third highest rate in Western Europe behind Finland and Ireland.
- More than 65,500 men die of heart attacks each year (1 every 8 minutes).

- A British male of working age is twice as likely to die from heart disease as an Italian male.
- A Scottish man is 50% more likely to die prematurely from heart disease than a man in the south west of England.
- A manual worker is 58% more likely to die of heart disease than a non-manual worker.
- South Asian men living in the UK (Indian, Pakistani, Bangladeshi or Sri Lankan) have a rate of heart disease 46% higher than white men. And this difference is increasing!
- Despite more people surviving heart attacks, the number of people with heart disease is increasing in the UK – 1.5 million men in the UK have had a heart attack or live with angina.
- Death rates from heart disease have fallen but increasing rates of overweight and obesity could reverse this trend.

Get the picture? Looking after your heart and keeping cholesterol levels low is important for all men, of all ages. The facts are hard but there is nowhere to hide – cholesterol causes heart disease which kills men (and women) – and many of these deaths are unnecessary. You may believe that it will never happen to you – but the risk is real, it could happen to you, and sooner than you think, so the choice is yours whether to do something to look after yourself and reduce your risk or take your chances that everything will be alright.

## What is cholesterol?

Cholesterol is an off-white waxy substance – a type of fat, which is carried around in the bloodstream in particles called lipoproteins. There are two different types of cholesterol: Low Density Lipoprotein (LDL) cholesterol, often known as the 'bad' cholesterol, and High Density Lipoprotein (HDL) cholesterol, referred to as the 'good' cholesterol.

Around 80% of cholesterol is made by the body in the liver, using saturated fat from food as basic building blocks. LDL carries cholesterol from the liver to the tissues. HDL is able to recycle cholesterol from tissues that have too much cholesterol.

Cholesterol is also found in some foods, such as eggs, liver, kidneys, and prawns, but this tends to account for just 20% of the body's total. For most people, the amount of saturated

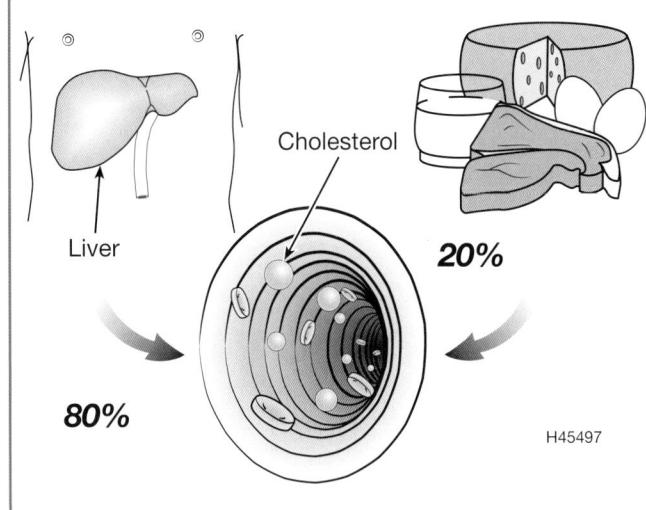

Cholesterol
Liver
20%
80%
H45497

Cholesterol is mainly produced by the liver and small amounts come from the foods that we eat

fat in food is therefore far more important than the amount of cholesterol.

- Low density lipoproteins (LDL or 'bad' cholesterol), carries cholesterol around the body and is the main source for cholesterol that builds up and blocks the arteries.
- High density lipoproteins (HDL or 'good' cholesterol), returns unused cholesterol to the liver for recycling, thus helping to keep cholesterol out of the arteries.
- Triglycerides, the fats that we recognise in our food and store under the skin. Like cholesterol, triglycerides from the gut (diet) or made in the liver are also carried on the lipoprotein particles in the blood.

The aim is to keep LDL levels lower and HDL levels higher. The ratio of LDL to HDL is important in assessing risk of heart disease.

## What does cholesterol do?

Cholesterol is a structural component of cells (think of the bricks and mortar in a wall) and so plays an essential role throughout the body. It is also used to manufacture vitamin D and hormones, such as testosterone and oestrogen, and to produce bile acids which help us to digest the fat that we eat. It only becomes a problem when there is too much in the wrong place – in the bloodstream.

## What is a normal cholesterol level?

When a blood test is taken it is normal to break the test down into several parts. The first is total cholesterol, which includes measures of both the LDL and HDL cholesterol fractions, and other minor lipoproteins. From a fasting blood sample (i.e. after not eating for 8 hours), the levels of total cholesterol, HDL and triglycerides are measured and then the level of LDL calculated from these. What is important are both the total values and the amount of the different fractions.

Current recommendations are for individual's levels to be:
- Total cholesterol (TC) less than 5.0mmol/l or 190mg/dl*
- LDL cholesterol (LDL-C) less than 3.0mmol/l or 115mg/dl
  Levels of HDL and triglycerides are not included in the current recommendations but a guide as to the correct levels is below:
- HDL cholesterol (HDL-C) greater than 1.0mmol/l or 40mg/dl
- Triglycerides less 2.3mmol/l

* **Note**: *In the UK lipids would usually be measured in millimoles (of cholesterol) per litre (of blood) (mmol/l), while milligrams per decilitre (mg/dl) is used in North America.*

These recommendations were made several years ago and are now under review. The new levels are likely to be for: total cholesterol to be less than 4.0mmol/l and LDL to be below 2.0mmol/l. If these figures are adopted then just 15% of men will have ideal cholesterol levels and just 2% a healthy LDL level.

## How does cholesterol link to heart disease?

If we are eating a healthy diet and living a healthy life the cholesterol produced by the liver is evenly balanced with the amount that the body can deal with, picture a see-saw – with the body on one side and the liver on the other, with the see-saw evenly balanced. But for most of us the amount of cholesterol produced by the liver is far bigger than the amount the body can handle and so the see-saw is out of balance.

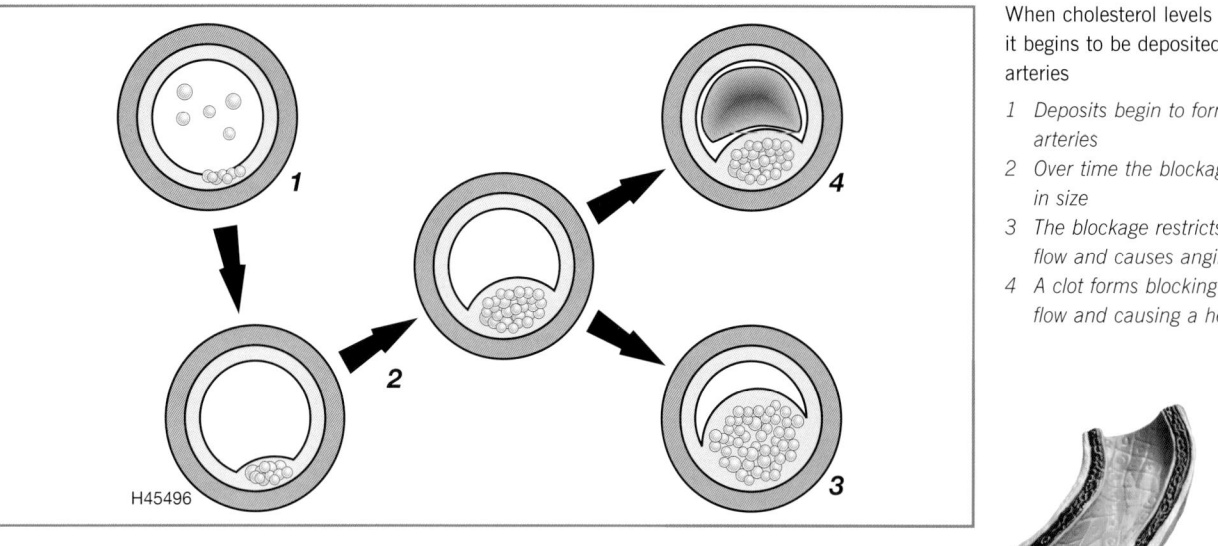

H45496

When cholesterol levels are high it begins to be deposited in the arteries

1 Deposits begin to form in the arteries
2 Over time the blockages build in size
3 The blockage restricts blood flow and causes angina
4 A clot forms blocking blood flow and causing a heart attack

Photo: © iStockphoto.com, Richard Scherzinger

When cholesterol levels are high it begins to be deposited inside the arteries – similar to the build up of lime-scale inside water pipes. This process is called atherosclerosis (or hardening of the arteries). Over time the blockage builds up and reduces the amount of blood flowing through the artery. Blockage in the arteries to the heart can cause angina – an uncomfortable feeling of pressure or pain across the chest, or even reaching out to arms, neck, stomach or jaw on emotional or physical exertion, due to insufficient blood reaching the heart muscle. The fatty blockage encourages blood to clot on its surface – like a scab on a cut. If the artery blocks completely, the heart muscle starved of blood dies (the heart attack) – or when the carotid arteries to the brain are blocked, the brain cells die resulting in a stroke. Arteries in the abdomen or pelvis are also affected, potentially affecting the kidneys, sexual function or leading to leg gangrene.

## What all men should know – it's not just about the heart!

Did you know that atherosclerosis can affect any of the arteries, not just those in the heart, but also those in the legs, brain, abdomen and pelvis? It is estimated that a quarter of all cases of erectile dysfunction (impotence) are caused by impaired blood flow to the penis.

So taking steps to lower cholesterol will not only look after your heart and circulation, but also increases the chances of you maintaining a healthy sex life into older age as well.

## Risk factors for heart disease

High blood cholesterol (also referred to as hypercholesterolemia) is one of the 'major risk factors' for coronary heart disease (CHD). But cholesterol isn't the only risk factor and it's important to consider the other risk factors as well. These include:

● Smoking – the best way to cut risk is to give up. Giving up alone is hard, but your GP or Practice Nurse is specially trained to help people quit and make the best use of aids such as nicotine patches or gum.
● High blood pressure (hypertension) makes hardening of the arteries worse and forces the heart and kidneys to work harder

than they should. High blood pressure can be lowered by weight loss, cutting back on alcohol, eating less salt and more fruit and vegetables.
● Overweight and obesity – dramatically increase the risk of developing heart disease. Losing weight is a priority to reduce cholesterol and other risk factors for heart disease.
● Physical inactivity – only one third of men are active enough for good health – i.e. undertake 30 minutes of moderate activity on at least 5 days each week. Be honest – at least 5 days a week? Most of us need to do a lot more, particularly if we need to lose weight.
● Diabetes – having diabetes greatly increases the risk of heart disease, especially if the diabetes is not well controlled.

Other lifestyle factors may also play a part in heart disease, including drinking too much alcohol, eating too much salt, and having raised levels of stress. And these factors don't simply add up – one factor will increase your risk, add in a second or a third and the risk multiplies. However, a raised level of cholesterol in the blood is the single greatest factor, contributing to almost half of all deaths from CHD.

## How do I get my cholesterol tested?

There are usually no symptoms of high cholesterol so the only way to know your cholesterol level is to have a blood test. In the recent National Diet and Nutrition Survey of UK adults, more than half of all UK men had high total cholesterol, more than 80% had raised LDL cholesterol and almost half had low HDL cholesterol levels.

Your options for a blood cholesterol test are:
● Ask your GP or practice nurse – where you know the test will

be reliable and your results can be interpreted along with any other risk factors you may have.

- Your workplace – may offer heart health checks through occupational health or private clinics.
- Some pharmacies will offer checks given by trained pharmacists.
- Home cholesterol kits can be purchased through pharmacies, but it is ideally recommended to obtain a test for a full lipid profile including both your total and LDL cholesterol. Home tests, which only measure total cholesterol levels, can be inaccurate unless used extremely carefully giving you a false reassurance that your cholesterol level is normal or worrying you if your result is very high. Many patient support organisations do not advise the use of home cholesterol test kits. If you do use a kit, it is worth checking your results with your pharmacist or GP to ensure you have an accurate result.

Ideally we should all get our cholesterol levels tested every 5 years or so, like our blood pressure, and more often if you've had a high test before. But you are especially recommended to ask your GP for a test if any of the below apply to you:

- There is a history of heart disease or raised cholesterol in your family.
- You have diabetes.
- You have high blood pressure.
- You already have coronary heart disease.
- You smoke.
- You are overweight/obese.
- You have peripheral arterial disease (hardening of abdominal or leg arteries).
- You have had a previous stroke.

Your GP or pharmacist should explain the results to you; let you know what the cholesterol levels mean, and if you have other risk factors.

## Why do men get more heart disease than women?

In general women tend to have higher levels of blood pressure, total and LDL cholesterol and a greater incidence of diabetes than men. However, before the age 65, four times as many men die from heart disease as women and 3-4 times as many men will have heart attacks.

This is due to several reasons. Before the menopause women are protected by the hormone oestrogen, which helps to keep HDL levels high – 3-4 times more men have low levels of 'good' HDL cholesterol compared to women. In addition women tend to smoke less and are more likely to store body fat around the hips (pear shape) rather than around the abdomen (apple shape). Abdominal fat is far more damaging to health than fat stored around the hips. Once women reach the menopause and oestrogen levels fall and LDL levels rise, rates of heart disease begin to increase.

## So what can I do to change my cholesterol levels?

Reducing cholesterol reduces risk of CHD. And the sooner you do this the better. The lower the cholesterol levels over your lifetime, the more your life long heart attack and stroke risk is reduced. Even a 10% cholesterol fall from a young age or a low level can reduce risk by more than a third.

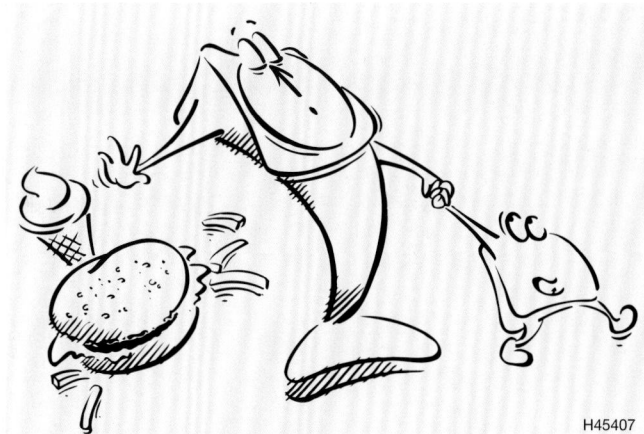

Your doctor may suggest lifestyle changes such as altering your diet to lower your fat, sugar and salt intake

A variety of things can affect cholesterol levels. These are things you can do something about:

- Changing diet – eating less saturated fats, increasing intake of fibre and wholegrain foods, using plant stanols or sterols, eating foods made from soya, and more fruit, vegetables and oily fish are all important.
- Losing weight – lowers LDL and triglycerides, and raises HDL cholesterol.
- Being active – regular activity lowers LDL and increases HDL cholesterol.
  There are other factors that can affect your cholesterol levels, but these are things you cannot do anything about:
- Age and gender – men have a higher risk for heart disease than women at virtually all ages. As both women and men get older, their cholesterol levels rise and risk increases. Men are more at risk of raised cholesterol than women. However women catch up – as many or more women will die of CHD.
- Heredity – your genes partly determine how much cholesterol your body makes. High blood cholesterol can run in families known as familial hypercholesterolemia (FH) or familial combined hypercholesterolemia (FCH).

Look after your heart and keep cholesterol levels low

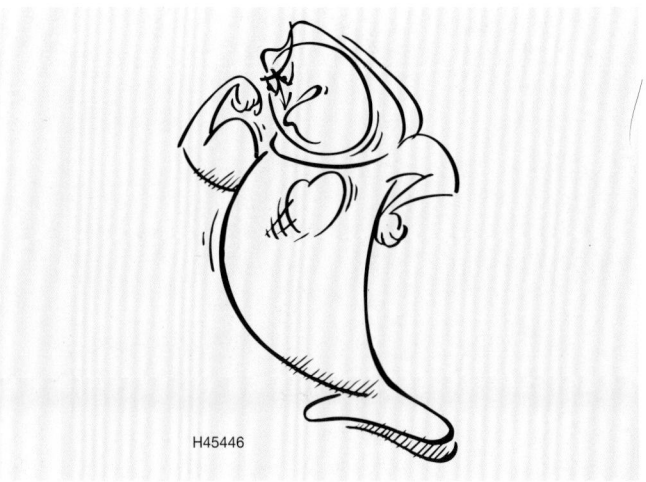

## Drug Treatments

Some people with very high cholesterol levels or who have several risk factors for heart disease may also need drug therapy prescribed by their GP. The decision to embark on prescribed treatment will be taken jointly by yourself and your doctor. The most commonly prescribed drugs are statins which reduce the amount of cholesterol manufactured by the liver, and as a result lower total and LDL cholesterol quickly and effectively. For best effects these need to be taken in conjunction with the lifestyle changes outlined here.

Since mid-2004, statins can now also be brought over-the-counter in pharmacist stores, or from web pharmacies. If buying in store the pharmacist is likely to ask you a few questions about your health to check that these are right for you. The dosage in the statins that you can buy from the pharmacist is lower than that which would be prescribed by your GP and so these should not be used to replace prescribed statins without prior approval by your GP.

For most people changing diet and lifestyle will allow them to reduce their cholesterol to an acceptable level. Even if prescribed drug therapy, it is still necessary to follow a healthy diet and lifestyle, if not the effectiveness of the drugs will be reduced.

## Eating for a healthy cholesterol

Changing your diet to lower your cholesterol need not be boring and tasteless, but may need a little more thought and planning than you are used to. Remember these are changes that you need to stick to so rather than getting all dramatic – make a number of small changes and then stick to them!

According to the 2002 World Health Report, published by the World Health Organisation, one third of deaths from heart disease are thought to be due to unhealthy diets, so getting it right could make a big difference.

## Demystifying fat

Dietary fat comes in different shapes and sizes, all of which have different effects on cholesterol levels. Fat is the most concentrated source of calories in the diet – providing 9kcals in every gram, which is more than alcohol (7kcal/g), protein (4kcal/g) or carbohydrates (4kcal/g). What this means is that if you eat a food that is very high in fat – e.g. butter or margarine, a small amount will add a lot of calories and fat to the diet. Every one of those tiny butter pats or tubs of margarine served in restaurants contains more than 8g of fat and over 75 calories – so just imagine what's in the large blob tucked into your jacket potato or in your plate of fish and chips. Much of the fat in our diet (70%), however, comes from invisible fats such as cakes, biscuits and fatty meat products.

A cholesterol lowering diet does not necessarily mean that you have to cut out all fats – it does however mean that you need to cut down on fat, especially saturated and trans fat, while using monounsaturated or polyunsaturated fats instead (see opposite). If you need to lose weight, keeping your intake of all fats low will make this easier.

You can learn a lot about the fat content of foods by checking the nutrition label on the side of the pack. This tells you the total amount of fat and, on many packs, also the amount of saturated fat in the food. Start to compare labels and choose brands with lower total and saturated fats.

As a general guide – if you are not overweight a maximum intake of fat is 95g per day and if you need to lose weight aim for less than this e.g. 70g fat per day. In terms of saturates a maximum of 30g saturated fat each day – although to lower cholesterol a maximum of 20g per day is a better target.

### News Flash
Decreasing dietary saturates (saturated fat) can help lower blood cholesterol.

## Saturated fats

Most people in the UK eat a diet that contains high levels of saturated fat, and this is a major reason why many of us have

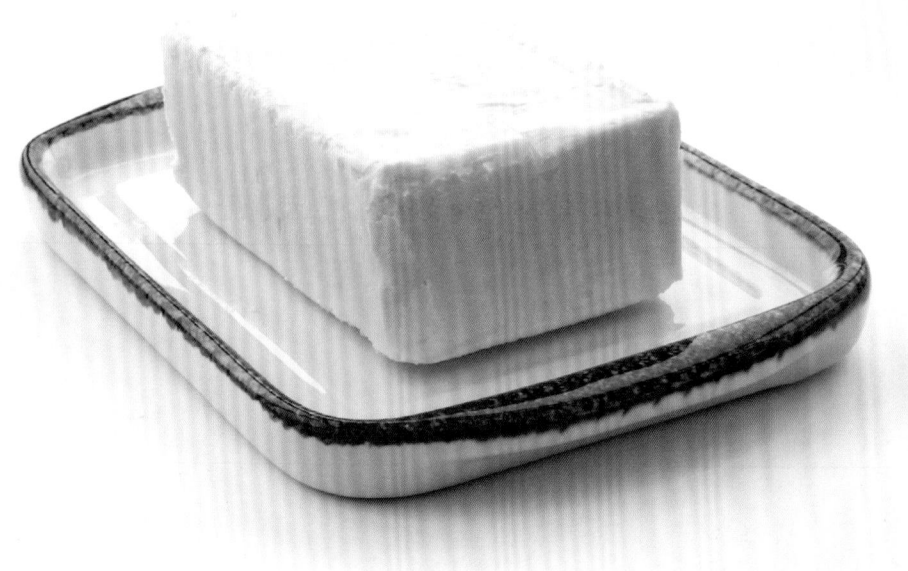

A small amount of butter adds a lot of calories and fat

Photo: © iStockphoto.com, Duncan Walker

high cholesterol levels. It's quite simple – the body uses saturated fats to manufacture cholesterol and so limit the saturated fat and the body makes less cholesterol. Foods high in saturated fat include: animal products such as fatty cuts of meat, sausages and meat products like pies and sausage rolls; full fat dairy products; butter, ghee, lard, cream; hard cheese; cakes, pastries and biscuits; chips and savoury snacks.

## Unsaturated fats – Monounsaturates and Polyunsaturates

Replacing saturated fats with either monounsaturates (MUFA) or polyunsaturates (PUFA) can reduce total and LDL cholesterol levels. MUFA offer some advantages over PUFA as they reduce total and LDL-cholesterol without adverse effects on HDL cholesterol or triglyceride levels.

## A guide to choosing fats and oils

| Saturated | Polyunsaturated | Monounsaturated |
|---|---|---|
| *Limit use* | *OK in moderation* | *OK in moderation* |
| Butter | Corn oil or spreads | Hazelnut or peanut oil |
| Ghee – butter or palm | Soya oil or spreads | Olive oil |
| Coconut oil | Sunflower oil or spreads | Rapeseed oil |
| Lard | Walnut or sesame oil | Mustard seed oil |
| Palm oil | Grapeseed oil | |
| Suet | Safflower oil | |
| | Plant stanol or sterol spreads | |

## Fat swaps

Reducing fat (saturated fat comes from spreads such as butter, milk, meat pies, cakes, biscuits, burgers and sausages) may make you may think you have to give up foods you eat and enjoy and there will be no pleasure left in eating. But it's worth looking at how a few food swaps can really make a difference in lowering the saturated fat.

| Instead of | Try this | Total fat saving | Saturated Fat Saving |
|---|---|---|---|
| Butter spread on 2 slices bread | Polyunsaturated margarine | 2 grams | 5 grams |
| 1 pork loin chop, grilled lean and fat | 1 pork loin chop, grilled lean only | 11 grams | 4 grams |
| 1 medium sausage roll (puff pastry) | Ham salad sandwich | 8.5 grams | 5 grams |
| 120g portion steak and kidney pie pastry top & bottom | 120g steak and kidney pie, pastry top only | 8 grams | 4 grams |
| BLT sandwich | Tuna mayonnaise sandwich – use low fat mayo | 7.5 grams | 3 grams |
| 1 tablespoon ordinary mayonnaise | 1 tablespoon lite mayonnaise | 11.9 grams | 1.8 grams |
| 30g packet crisps | 1 banana | 10 grams | 4 grams |
| 1/2 pint whole milk | 1/2 pint semi-skimmed milk | 5 grams | 4 grams |
| 1 jam doughnut | 1 slice of malt fruit loaf | 10 grams | 3 grams |
| Small (50g) bar dairy milk chocolate | 50g liquorice allsorts | 13 grams | 7.4 grams |
| Quarter pounder with cheese | Quorn™ burger | 21 grams | 9 grams |
| 1 takeaway large portion fries | 1 takeaway regular portion fries | 9 grams | 2 grams |
| 1 portion fried chips (265g) | 1 portion oven chips (265g) | 22 grams | 4 grams |
| Cheese and pickle sandwich | Egg mayonnaise sandwich – use low fat mayo | 10 grams | 10 grams |
| 40g portion cheddar | 20g portion cheddar | 7 grams | 4 grams |
| 40g portion cheddar | 40g portion half fat cheddar | 7 grams | 5 grams |
| 350g portion beef curry | 210g lentil curry dhal made with tomatoes and vegetable oil | 43.5 grams | 10 grams |

Fresh tuna is high in omega 3 fatty acids (the exercise catching them is good, too!)

Photo: © iStockphoto.com, Richard Gunion

## Fishy Business – omega 3 fatty acids and fish oils

The omega 3 fats found in oily types of fish are another type of polyunsaturated fat, but these ones are special. Omega 3 fats have a particular role in helping to keep the arteries supple and healthy, and make the blood less likely to clot inside blood vessels (clots cause heart attacks and strokes). Oily types of fish like herring, mackerel, sardines, salmon and fresh tuna are the best sources of omega 3s in the diet as the body is able to use these omega 3 fats directly. Try to eat these once or twice each week. If you have already had a heart attack or stroke, try to make this 2-3 times each week.

Non-fish sources of omega 3 fats include rapeseed oil, linseed, walnuts and seeds such as pumpkin seeds. Also some eggs – look on the box.

## Trans fats

Like saturated fats, trans fats can raise cholesterol levels. Trans fats are found in foods that contain processed (hydrogenated) fats, including some types of biscuits, cakes, fast food, pastry, margarine and spreads. So, as part of a healthy diet, try to cut down on foods containing hydrogenated or saturated fats and replace them with unsaturated fats. You will need to check the labels on these types of foods.

## Tips to cut fat

A quick reminder – the cholesterol in food only has a small impact on the cholesterol in the body – it is more important to concentrate on reducing total and saturated fats.

- Choosing how to cook foods well can make a big difference to your fat intake. Try to choose cooking methods such as microwaving, steaming, poaching, boiling or grilling, instead of roasting or frying and choosing lean cuts of meat and low-fat varieties of dairy products and spreads to help to reduce total fat.
- When using oils, always measure them out using a spoon rather than sloshing them into the pan – this way you will almost always use less.
- Buy a griddle pan to cook fish, chicken and lean steaks or burgers.
- Buy an oil in a spray can to use on salads.
- Cut back on cheese – enjoy a small amount of a strong cheese rather than a large serving of mild cheese.
- Have thicker bread and thinner spread.
- Always buy lean cuts of meat and cut visible fat off before cooking.

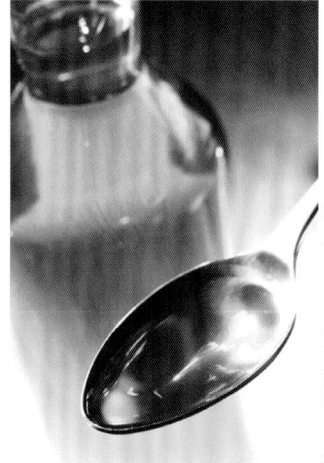

Photo: © iStockphoto.com, Ina Peters

## Carbohydrates

Although carbohydrate has no direct effect on blood cholesterol levels, increasing the amount of carbohydrate rich foods that you eat, while decreasing fat is usually encouraged; and after all is part of the message for general healthy eating. Choosing foods that are wholegrain – such as breads and breakfast cereals will help to keep your cholesterol low and help with weight control.

## News Flash

The inclusion of oats as part of a diet low in saturated fat and a healthy lifestyle can help reduce blood cholesterol.

Oats contain a particular type of fibre called soluble fibre which makes them special when it comes to cholesterol. Eating a diet rich in soluble fibre has been found to help reduce total and LDL cholesterol levels. And it's not just oats that contain soluble fibre, other good sources include pulses e.g. kidney beans, lentils and baked beans; oats, barley or rye; and fruits and vegetables.

## Fruit and Vegetables

Unless you have been hiding under a rock for the past few years you will know that eating plenty of fruit and vegetables every day is vital for great health. The average guide is to eat at least 5 servings each day which is equivalent to 400g, but estimates are that between one quarter and one half of deaths from heart disease in countries like the UK are due to eating less than 600g of fruit and vegetables every day – so for the best heart health at least 7 servings each day is required as recommended in some other European countries. Any fruit and vegetables provide lots of vitamins and minerals but different colours provide different amounts of 'antioxidants' which help to look after the heart. Including a variety of different colours and types will increase the range of nutrients you are giving your body.

## What is a serving?

An easy way to think of a serving is to think of the amount you can hold in your hand, but while this is easy with a bunch of grapes it is somewhat harder when it comes to frozen vegetables. Using the table will give you a start on different amounts of fruits and vegetables to choose. As often happens with guidelines there are a few exceptions and here are the ones to remember:

- Pure fruit juice can only be counted once a day, no matter how much you drink.
- Potatoes are counted as starchy carbohydrate so don't fit in the fruit and vegetable group.
- Pulses and beans can count too but can only be counted once a day.

## News Flash

The inclusion of at least 25g soya protein per day as part of a diet low in saturated fat can help reduce blood cholesterol.

| Fruits | Example of average portion |
|---|---|
| Medium sized fresh fruit | 1 apple, banana, pear, orange, nectarine |
| Small sized fresh fruit | 2 plums, 2 satsumas, 3 apricots, 2 kiwi fruit, 7 strawberries, 14 cherries, 6 lychees |
| Large fresh fruit | Half a grapefruit, 1 slice of papaya, 1 slice of melon (2 inch slice), 1 large slice of pineapple, 2 slices of mango (2 inch slice) |
| Dried fruit | 1 tablespoon of raisins, currants, sultanas, 1 tablespoon of mixed fruit, two figs, three prunes, one handful of banana chips |
| Tinned fruit (unsweetened) | Roughly the same quantity of fruit that you would eat as a fresh portion: 1 pear or peach half, 6 apricot half, 8 segments of tinned grapefruit |
| Juice | 1 medium glass (150ml) of 100% pure fruit juice, but juice only counts as once a day, no matter how much you drink |
| **Vegetables** | |
| Green vegetables | 2 broccoli spears, 8 cauliflower florets, 4 heaped tablespoons of kale, spring greens or green beans |
| Cooked vegetables | 3 heaped tablespoons of cooked vegetables such as carrots, peas or sweetcorn |
| Salad vegetables | 3 sticks of celery, 2 inch piece of cucumber, 1 medium tomato, 7 cherry tomatoes |
| Tinned and frozen vegetables | Roughly the same quantity as you would eat as a fresh portion: 3 heaped tablespoons of tinned or frozen carrots, peas or sweetcorn |
| Pulses and beans | 3 heaped tablespoons of lentils, kidney, cannelloni or butter beans or chick peas (Remember that beans or pulses only count as one of your 5 a day portions.) |

Soya and foods made from this humble bean can lower cholesterol. Gone are the days of soya being a food for health freaks sold in health food stores. Soya products are now widely available in supermarkets and include great tasting products such as milks (try the fresh varieties from the chiller cabinet – great for making smoothies and shakes), yoghurts, desserts, custards. Soya is also used to make tofu – sold in a block for stir fries or as burgers, sausages or ready meals. Soya protein is also added to some breads. In order to eat 25g of soya protein in a day you will need to include a soya product on several occasions e.g. a soya smoothie for breakfast, a tofu burger for evening meal and toasted soya bread for an evening snack.

## Plant Stanols and Sterols

Products containing plant stanols or sterols are designed specifically for people with raised cholesterol. Plant stanols and sterols are extracted from vegetable oils, concentrated and then added back into low fat spreads, yoghurts, bars and milk. One shot pots of yoghurt style drink containing a day's worth of plant stanols or sterols have recently arrived on the shelves, making using these everyday a little easier.

Clinical trials have clearly shown that daily consumption of stanols or sterols can reduce LDL cholesterol by approximately 10-15%, and this is in addition to any reductions achieved by other dietary modifications or the cholesterol-lowering medications known as statins. They have no effect on HDL cholesterol. It is important to check the label and only use the amounts recommended. Tests have shown that using more than this will not increase the cholesterol reduction that you achieve. However they only work while you take them, so daily use is recommended for the best results.

## Frequently Asked Questions

There are bound to be some myths or ideas about cholesterol that you pick up from the media, friends, advertising or just general reading. Check out the questions below and the evidence for or against their truth.

### Does garlic reduce cholesterol?

Minimally. Some studies have suggested that garlic may reduce cholesterol levels but there is not enough quality evidence to show that it has any effect.

### Does too much caffeine increase cholesterol levels?

Despite numerous studies there is little evidence to link caffeine and cholesterol levels. It is advisable to limit coffee consumption to 2 or 3 cups per day for other health reasons and enjoy a variety of drinks to keep fluid intake up, not just coffee.

### Fish oil supplements – do they work the same as oily fish?

If you have already had a heart attack or any form of cardiovascular disease, then you should include large portions of oily fish 2 to 3 times per week; or it can be taken in equivalent fish oil supplements (check they contain 0.5-1.0 grams omega

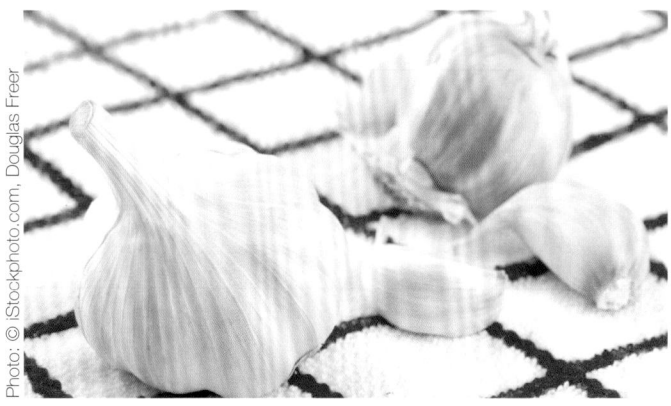

Photo: © iStockphoto.com, Douglas Freer

3 fatty acids per day) or rapeseed oil. Both eating oily fish and taking fish oil supplements appear to reduce heart disease.

### Do probiotics help prevent raised cholesterol?
Although probiotic bacteria can possibly help with gut function and immunity there is little evidence supporting a role for them in cholesterol lowering. One shot probiotic drinks look very similar to those containing plant stanols and sterols – so check carefully to avoid confusion.

### Does alcohol affect cholesterol levels?
Small amounts of alcohol (1-2 units a day) may slightly boost HDL levels. However, alcohol is high in calories so can contribute to overweight which will raise cholesterol negating effects on HDL. Alcohol has a direct effect on triglycerides so if yours are raised you need to cut right back on alcohol.

## Summary
Raised blood cholesterol is one of the most important risk factors in predicting coronary heart disease. But lowering it is quite achievable, you don't need to be a killjoy and give up all of your favourite foods. Think of it positively and take the opportunity to try all those foods you may not have tried before and that can help lower your cholesterol. See the 10 points below. However one pretty important fact to recognise is that this diet is for life, a week won't do or even a few months. To maintain healthy levels of cholesterol and help work on maintaining weight, you need to recognise this is a permanent change.

We all know that small changes can make a difference and following any of the points summarised here is a good start, but the more of them you are able to do, the bigger difference it will make.

- Only buy a margarine or spread that says high in monounsaturated fat (MUFA) or polyunsaturated fat (PUFA).
- Try to use olive oil for cooking and nut oils for salad.
- Get used to carrying fruit or vegetables with you or having them handy at home. Biscuits and cakes are usually more readily available and can make an easy tempting alternative.
- Ask your local food outlet where you go for meals or snacks to always have some fresh and tasty fruits and vegetables very visible.
- Do some food swapping – those pies and pastries are loaded with saturated fats and a bap, wrap, baguette or sandwich is usually a better choice if you watch the amounts of cheese and mayonnaise.
- Make up your own sandwich with thick slices of bread; choose a moist filling so you can leave out the spread or mayonnaise.
- A small change in cooking habits – measuring the unsaturated fat you use, grilling, steaming or microwaving can go quite a way to reducing saturated fat.
- What about giving some soya products a try – chilled fresh soya milk is an easy start; to drink, add to cereal or a quick smoothie. Add tofu to a stir fry or try food that uses a tofu base such as tofu sausages or burgers.
- When you think of food, think activity – try to fit in a quick walk at lunchtime, or in the evening whenever you can. Why not try an activity you haven't tried before.
- Always have breakfast – wholegrain cereal, porridge with fruit or wholegrain toast. If you don't like wholegrain try a 'half and half' variety.

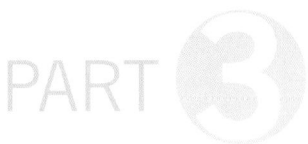

PART **3**

# Heart attack

## Introduction

An acute myocardial infarction (heart attack) is what happens when the blood supply to a part of the heart muscle has been cut off by blockage of one of the coronary arteries.

When blood is restricted or cut off the cells start to die.

Heart attack is the final result of a disease of the heart arteries (coronary artery disease) called atherosclerosis. About five people in every 1000, mostly men, suffer a heart attack in the UK each year.

## Symptoms

A heart attack can involve:

- Crushing central chest pain (often described as a 'vice around the chest').
- Breathlessness.
- Clammy skin, sweating and pale complexion.
- Dizziness, nausea and vomiting.
- Restlessness.

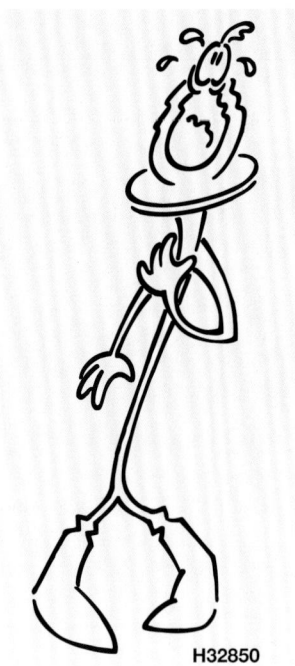

H32850

Much worse than a blockage on the M25

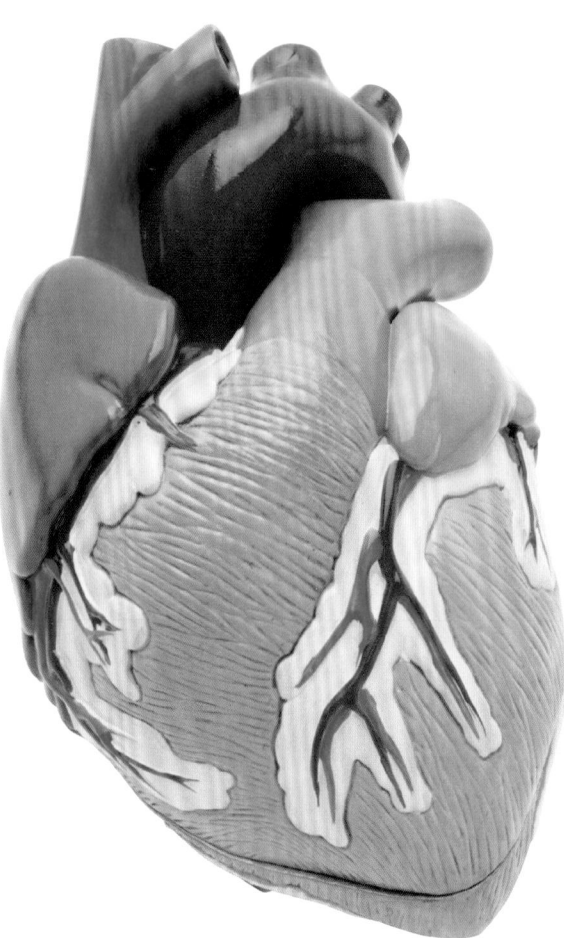

Photo: © iStockphoto.com, Kenneth C. Zirkel

Heart and blood vessels – arteries in red, veins in blue

The pain often travels to the neck, jaws, ears, arms and wrists. Less often, it travels to between the shoulder blades or to the stomach. The pain does not pass on resting as in angina (see *Angina*).

Severe pain is not always present. In less major cases pain may be absent and there is evidence that up to 20% of mild heart attacks are not recognised as such, or even as significant illness, by those affected.

## Causes

Blockage of the coronary arteries caused by a clot (thrombosis) from fatty material caught in the blood.

When total blockage occurs, part of the heart muscle loses its blood supply and dies. Depending on the size of the artery blocked, a larger or smaller portion of the heart will be affected.

Risk factors include:
- Smoking cigarettes.
- Being overweight.
- Abnormally high blood pressure.
- High blood cholesterol level.
- A diet high in saturated fats (animal fats).
- Diabetes.
- A family history of heart disease.
- Lack of regular exercise.

## Diagnosis

The ECG (electro cardiograph) draws a tracing of the electrical changes occurring in the heart with each beat. It also shows which part of the heart muscle has been damaged.

A blood test will look for certain heart muscle proteins that are only found in high levels immediately after a heart attack. These are also useful in confirming the diagnosis.

## Prevention

The best way to avoid a problem is to stop it happening. Regular body maintenance using the right fuels and getting regular run-outs will help. Here are some pointers:
- Your diet should include a high proportion of fruit and fresh vegetables.
- A small amount of alcohol – such as one glass of wine a day – may be helpful.
- Stop smoking, increase exercise if sedentary and avoid saturated fats.

## Complications

Immediate complications are:
- Dangerous irregular heart rhythms and very fast or very slow rates.
- Dangerous drops in blood pressure.
- Fluid build-up in and around the lungs.
- Clots forming in the deep veins of the legs or pelvis (deep vein thrombosis).
- Rupture of the heart wall.

Later complications are:
- Ballooning (aneurysm) of the damaged heart wall, which becomes thin and weak.
- Increased risk of another heart attack in the future.
- Angina.
- Poor heart action causing breathlessness and build-up of fluid in the ankles and legs (oedema).
- Depression, loss of confidence, loss of sex drive, and fear of having sex which is common and unfounded.

## Treatment

See *Cardio-Pulmonary Resuscitation (Kiss of Life)* in Part 1.

Clot-dissolving injections are now routinely used in hospital. These can break down the clot in the coronary artery and allow the damaged heart muscle to recover, sometimes completely. They must be given within 24 hours at the most. Because the heart rhythm may become temporarily abnormal as it recovers, this treatment is best given when the heart rhythm can be continuously monitored on an ECG. This can be done in an ambulance or in hospital.

In an uncomplicated recovery it is normal to be home within a week or less. Work can be restarted 4–12 weeks after the attack, depending on the level of physical exertion involved with the job. Driving can restart after one month, but DVLA and the motor insurance company must be informed of the heart attack.

Rather than avoiding any exercise it is now known that a return to normal levels of activity – this includes sex – helps prevent any further attacks.

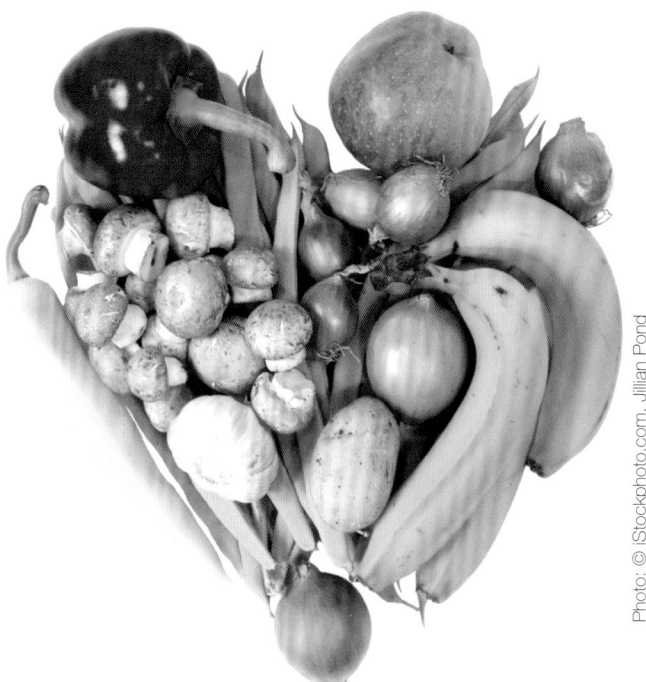

Photo: © iStockphoto.com, Jillian Pond

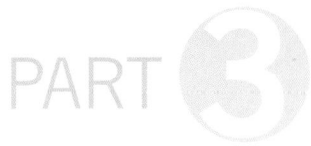

PART 3

# Heart failure

## Introduction

A frightening term but heart failure actually means that the heart is not pumping quite as efficiently as it could, not that the whole thing has collapsed.

Heart failure can be treated once it is recognised.

## Symptoms

Breathlessness, particularly when lying down flat is the most distressing symptom (many people find a couple of pillows helps). A wheezing or bubbling noise may sometimes be heard which clears on sitting up.

Breathlessness can also happen during mild activity such as climbing stairs.

Fluid may build up in the ankles causing swelling. This will be most noticeable in the evening after a day of walking or sitting.

## Causes

A number of things can cause the heart not to work efficiently. Leaking heart valves from an infection like rheumatic fever or a previous heart attack are among the most common causes. Sometimes this affects one side of the heart more than the other and the symptoms can be slightly different, but breathlessness is often the result.

## Prevention

There are lots of ways of reducing your risk from heart disease. If you haven't already, go back and read the expert tips on diet and exercise in Part 2. Your body will only function with the right fuel and then being thoroughly run in.

## Complications

Lack of treatment may cause the heart to become further weakened making the breathlessness even worse.

## Self care

There is no good reason for avoiding exercise and keeping active is important so long as it doesn't put too much strain on the heart.

Swollen ankles will benefit from putting your feet up while sitting down.

Cut down on your salt and/or use salt substitutes.

## Treatment

Modern medicines make an enormous difference not only to the quality of life but also life expectancy.

## Action

If you think you are suffering from heart failure from the symptoms described, call NHS Direct, your GP or dial 999 or 112 in an emergency.

A severe onset of breathlessness, particularly in a person with previously diagnosed heart failure, is a medical emergency – dial 999 or 112.

PART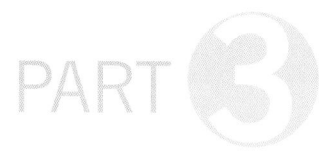

# Lung cancer

## Introduction

Most people think of the lungs as two plastic bags or balloons. Nothing could be further from the truth. Lungs are complex structures with more similarity to sponges than balloons. The main pipe (bronchus) connects both lungs to the airway in the throat. It splits lower in the chest, branching increasingly until tiny blind-ending pockets are reached. These are the alveoli where oxygen is exchanged for carbon dioxide across the thin membranes. Cancer can arise in the fine tubes but mainly in the larger tubes, the bronchi.

The correct medical term for lung cancer is bronchial carcinoma, a cancer of the large tubes of the lung. The lining cells of the air tubes in healthy lungs are tall (columnar) and the surfaces nearest the inside of the tube are covered with fine hairs (cilia) which move together. Imagine a wind blowing across a field of ripe corn. The movement of the cilia acts to carry dust, smoke particles and other foreign material upwards and away from the deeper parts of the lungs. This is essential to keep the lungs clear of debris and potentially harmful particles.

Smoking cigarettes damages the ability of the lining cells to do their jobs. First, the cilia disappear, then the number of cells increases, and finally the cells become flattened, so that the columnar lining is replaced by an abnormal scaly layer. Some years later this layer may develop into bronchial carcinoma.

Lung cancer is uncommon before the age of 40. Only about 1 case in 100 is diagnosed in people younger than 40. The great majority of cases (85 per cent) occur in people over 60.

The outlook in lung cancer is not good. After diagnosis of the disease only 20 per cent are alive a year later, and only 8 per cent, overall, survive for five years.

Smoking cigarettes damages the ability of the lining cells to do their jobs. Some years later this layer may develop into bronchial carcinoma

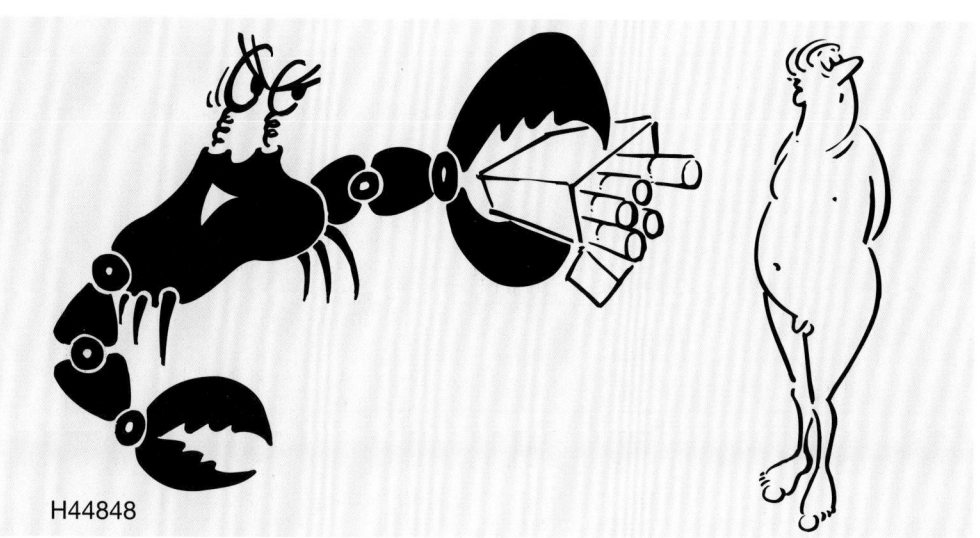

H44848

## Symptoms

Lung cancer usually shows itself with a productive cough, often with a little blood in the sputum. There may also be breathlessness. Pain in the chest is common, especially if the cancer has spread to the lung lining (pleura) or the chest wall.

Unfortunately the tumour may show no signs until late in its development. Watch out for:

- A persistent cough.
- Coughing up blood-stained phlegm (sputum).
- Shortness of breath.
- Chest discomfort.
- Repeated bouts of pneumonia or bronchitis.
- Loss of appetite.
- Loss of weight.

These don't necessarily mean you have cancer, but they need your doctor's attention in case you need further tests.

## Causes

It is almost entirely due to cigarette smoking, either directly or through passive smoking. The rate of lung cancer in non-smokers rises significantly if they are regularly exposed to other people's cigarette smoke.

## Diagnosis

Unfortunately diagnosis tends to be late in the day and can be fairly obvious from the symptoms you describe to your doctor. X-ray examination will often confirm the diagnosis, although sometimes it is also necessary to examine the inside of the bronchi with an instrument called a bronchoscope. If a tumour is seen, a sample (biopsy) is usually taken for examination to see what type it is. Cancer cells can sometimes be found in the sputum.

## Treatment

Treatment will depend on the type of cancer, how developed it is and your general state of health. Surgery, radiotherapy and chemotherapy may be used alone or together to treat cancer of the lung.

- Surgery: removal of part or all of the lung.
- Radiotherapy: the use of radiation treatment to destroy cancer cells.
- Chemotherapy: the use of drugs that kill cancer cells.

Nobody is trying to kid you that any of these treatments guarantee a cure, but early detection of the cancer can make all the difference.

Better still, reduce your risks of getting lung cancer in the first place by stopping smoking.

> First the good news: Lung cancer in men caused almost entirely by smoking is preventable and on the decrease. Now the bad news: Young men think they are immune.

> Around 80 000 people develop lung cancer in the UK each year and most of them are men. Yet of all the cancers it has to be one of the most preventable.

## The Smoking Gun

It's not difficult to work out what causes it. If you don't smoke, your chances of getting lung cancer are very small. Start early, die early and the amount of tobacco you smoke also shifts you that bit closer to the great scrap-yard in the sky.

Filters and low tar protect you? Aye, and sugar-coated cyanide won't kill you either. Wise up and stub it out.

So go for pipes and cigars? No way, they just give you a feeling of false security. Cut down then? No, that doesn't work either. You gradually creep back up. Stop completely.

All over the UK men are getting the message. That's why lung cancer in men is on the decrease. You can be one of them.

> You do not get permanently fat when you stop but you do enjoy your food more.

## How to quit the weed

- Nicotine patches and other ways of helping you to stop can be obtained through your GP. These can be very successful in easing the craving for nicotine.
- Get in touch with self-help groups or organisations which supply information.
- If you can't do it for yourself, do it for your partner or kids.

## Quit plan

- Set a day and date to stop. Tell all your friends and relatives, they will support you.
- Like deep sea diving, always take a buddy. Get someone to give up with you. You will reinforce each other's will power.
- Clear the house and your pockets of any packets, papers or matches.
- One day at a time is better than leaving it open-ended.
- Map out your progress on a chart or calendar. Keep the money saved in a separate container.
- Chew on a carrot. Not only will it help you do something with your mouth and hands, it provides a great chat up line for women. 'What's up Doc?'
- Ask your friends not to smoke around you. People accept this far more readily than they used to do.

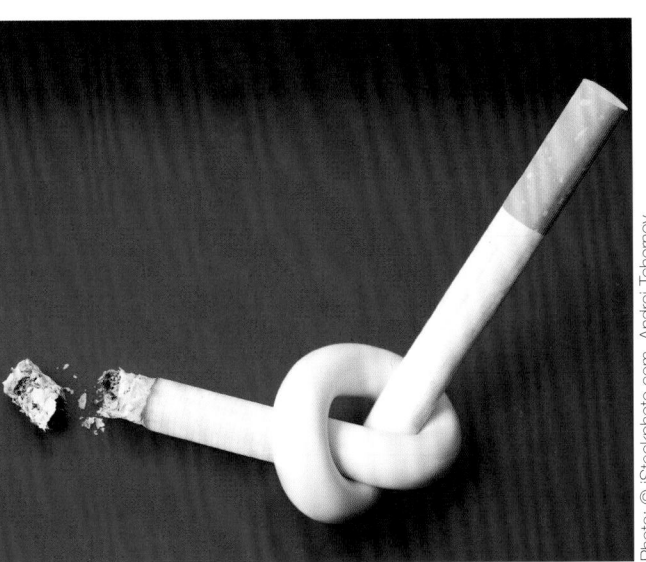

Photo: © iStockphoto.com, Andrei Tchernov

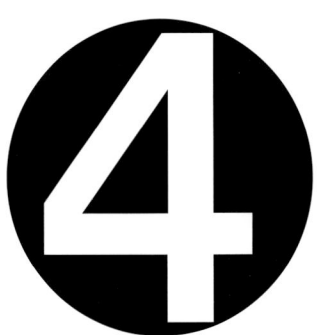

# Circulation

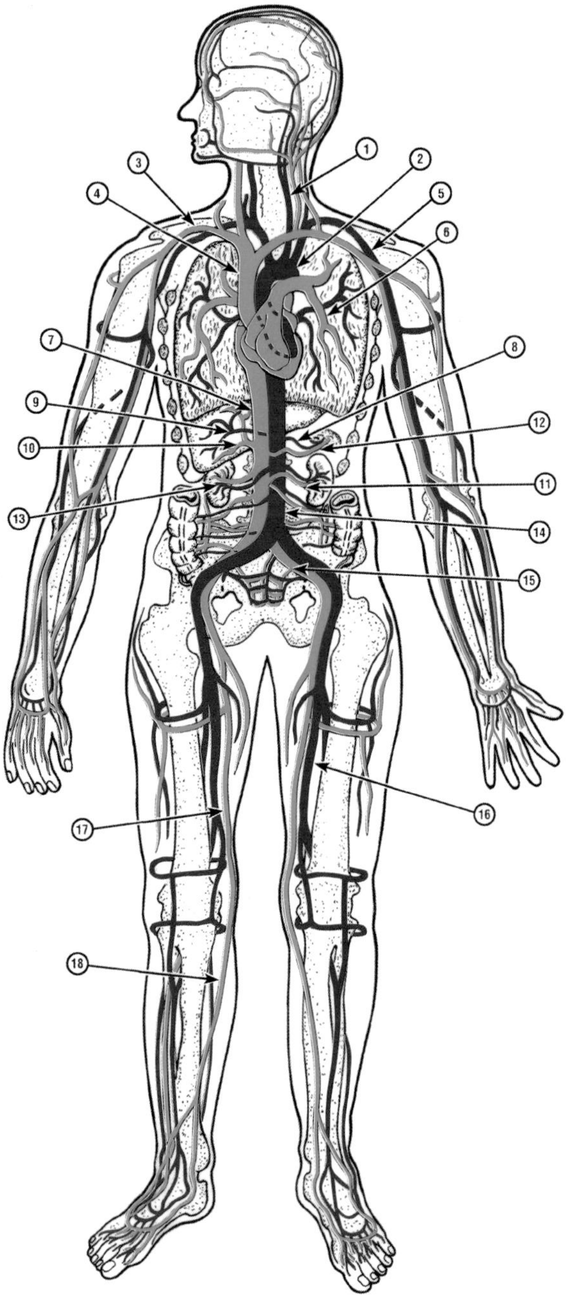

The major blood vessels

1 Carotid artery
2 Ascending aorta
3 Sublcavian vein
4 Superior vena cava
5 Subclavian artery
6 Pulmonary artery
7 Inferior vena cava
8 Splenic artery
9 Hepatic artery
10 Hepatic vein
11 Renal vein
12 Splenic vein
13 Renal artery
14 Abdominal aorta
15 Common iliac vein
16 Femoral artery
17 Femoral vein
18 Great saphenous vein

# Anaemia

## Introduction

Anaemia, which is due to a lack of iron, is a frequent cause of tiredness. Red blood cells which transport oxygen around the body need iron as part of this transport system.

Basically the body balances the amount of iron lost through turnover of the blood cells with the amount taken in with the diet. If there is too much lost and or not enough eaten you will become anaemic.

Young people can outstrip their iron supply particularly during the growth spurt around puberty.

Older people with poor diets can also suffer from anaemia and this may be overlooked and their tiredness and confusion put down simply to age. Fortunately, it can be recognised and treated quite easily.

## Symptoms

- Skin, lips, tongue, nail beds or the inside of eyelids can be pale in colour although this doesn't really happen until your iron stores are quite low.
- Tiredness and weakness.
- Dizziness or fainting spells.
- Breathlessness, particularly following exercise.
- Fast heartbeat felt in the neck or chest (palpitations).

## Causes

The usual cause of anaemia is lack of iron or vitamin B12 in the diet. It can also arise following blood loss (e.g. frequent nose bleeds). Conditions such as coeliac disease, some kidney problems and rheumatoid arthritis increase your risk of anaemia.

Bleeding into the bowel will cause anaemia so it should be checked out immediately. There may be changes in the appearance of your motions, usually a black tar like substance and you may lose weight for no apparent reason.

## Prevention

Being anaemic is not just about looking slightly pasty faced. Our tip for tip-top blood is to eat a balanced diet to supply all the minerals you need. Young boys going through their growth spurt need to make sure they are eating enough bread and other iron containing foods.

Meat is a major source of iron which is great news for carnivores, but if you are a vegetarian, you'll need extra iron containing foods – spinach and dark green veg is good – and may even benefit from iron supplements.

## Complications

Anaemia itself is not usually life threatening but it can cause accidents through tiredness and lower your defence against minor illness.

## Treatment

If you suspect you are anaemic and there is no obvious reason for being so do not start iron supplements until you have had blood tests performed and your doctor has advised you. Taking iron before the test makes it difficult to tell why you became anaemic in the first place.

If anaemia is confirmed by a blood test, your doctor may prescribe iron tablets or injections or, occasionally, vitamin B12 injections. You can also help yourself by eating plenty of iron-rich foods, such as red meat, wholemeal bread, dried fruit and leafy vegetables.

## Action

Make an appointment to see your GP.

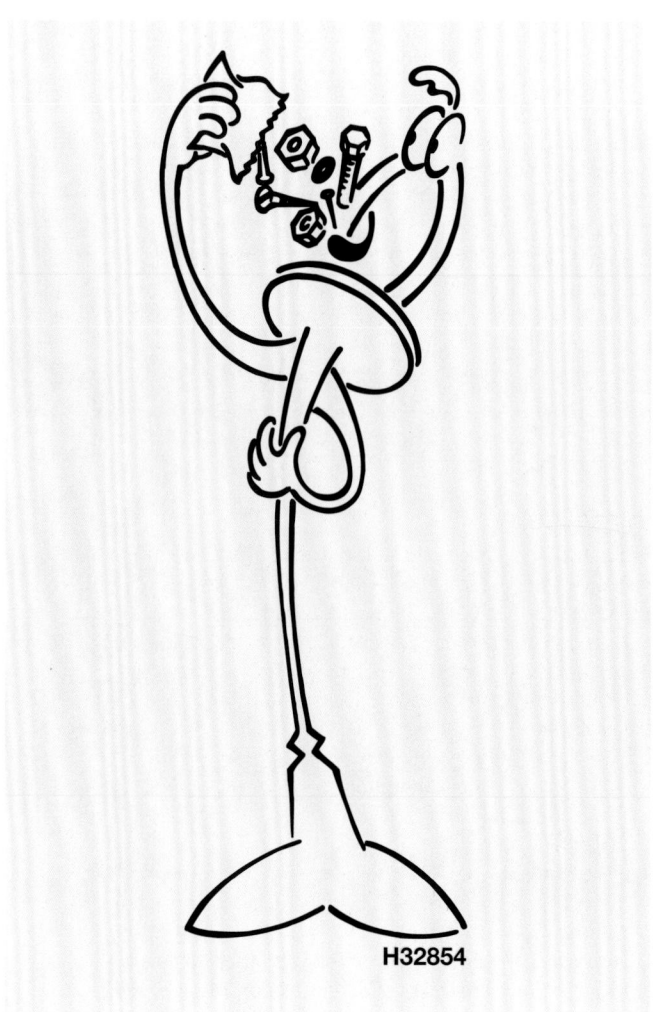

H32854

Fuel quality is essential in getting top performance in any model

# High blood pressure (hypertension)

## Introduction

Myths surround every aspect of blood pressure. It helps to know what is being measured in the first place. Blood pressure (BP) is always written as two numbers thus: 120/80. Neither of these numbers has anything to do with your age, height or weight. They are simple measurements of the heart's ability to overcome pressure from an inflated cuff placed around the arm or leg.

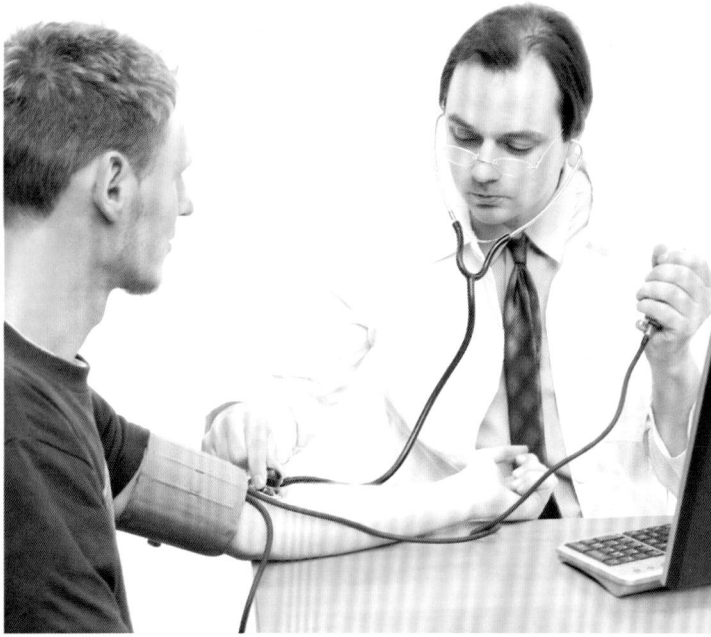

Photo: © iStockphoto.com, Kati Neudert

As the cuff is slowly deflated, the sound of the blood pushing its way past is suddenly heard in a stethoscope placed over the artery. This is the maximum pressure reached by the heart during its contraction. As the pressure is further released the sound gradually muffles and disappears. This is the lowest pressure in your blood system. Putting the two pressures over each other gives a ratio of the blood pressure while the heart is contracting (systolic) over the pressure while the heart is refilling with blood ready for the next contraction (diastolic). The lower pressure actually represents the pressure caused by the major arteries contracting, keeping the blood moving while the heart refills.

There is no 'normal' blood pressure as it constantly changes within the same person and depends on what they are doing at the time. A blood pressure above 140/90 for anyone at rest should be investigated.

## Symptoms

Hypertension is called the silent killer for good reason. Most people do not realise that they are suffering from high blood pressure until something serious happens.

As the pressure steadily rises, damage occurs to the arteries, kidney and heart. For this reason alone it is worth having your blood pressure checked every year or so when you are over the age of 45 years.

There may be some warning signs such as blood in your urine or loss of vision right at the edges (tunnel vision).

## Causes

Hypertension can be linked to genetic factors, and this risk is increased by high salt intake, fatty food, obesity, stress, alcohol abuse and lack of activity.

Hypertension can also be caused by other medical conditions, which have an effect on blood pressure. Kidney problems are a good example of this.

## Prevention

Just taking a look at the causes will mean that prevention explains itself. Cut down on the salt, reduce your body weight and fat intake, drink alcohol in moderation and stay active. Of all the prevention you can take, exercising three times a week until the point of breathlessness is perhaps the easiest and has the most dramatic effect for decreasing your risk from hypertension.

## Complications

Stroke and heart attacks are two of the most common complications from hypertension. It can also damage the kidneys and liver.

## Self care

Once diagnosed with hypertension apply all the advice as for prevention. Your doctor may well find that through losing weight, increasing activity and reducing alcohol intake you can do without the medication to bring down your blood pressure.

### Note

A single reading of blood pressure is unreliable. At least three readings over a few weeks are required. Simply having your blood pressure checked can make it rise in some people (called the white coat effect). Self testing using machines from the pharmacist is a good idea.

## Action

Make an appointment to see your GP.

PART 4

# Leukaemia

## Introduction

Despite the fear which surrounds  this particular cancer, leukaemia is now more treatable than most cancers affecting men, especially when caught early.

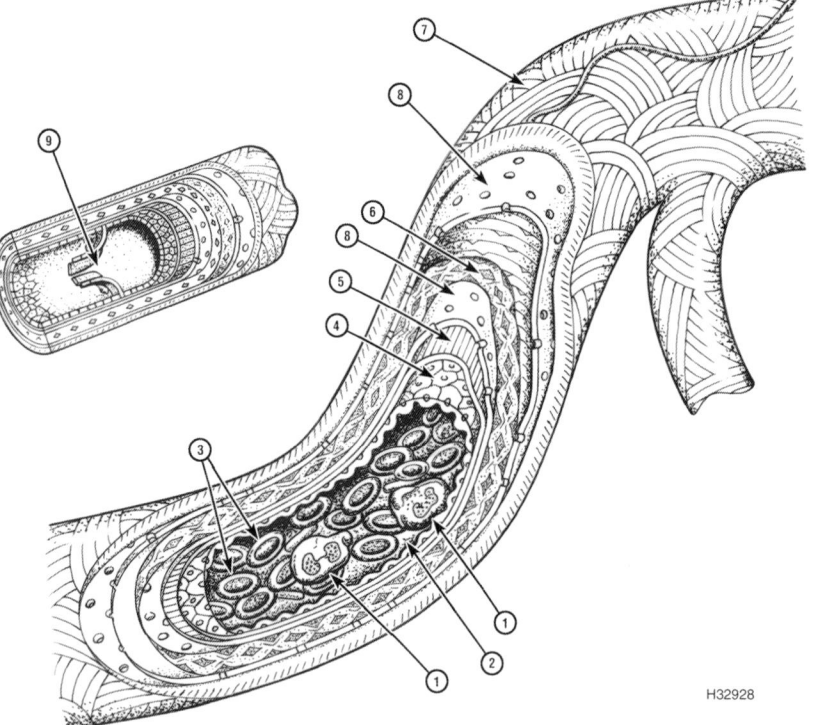

Blood vessels construction – artery (right) and vein

1   White blood cells
2   Platelets
3   Red blood cells
4   Tunica intima (inner layer)
5   Tunica intima (outer layer)
6   Tunica media
7   Tunica adventitia
8   Elastic layer
9   Non-return valve

H32928

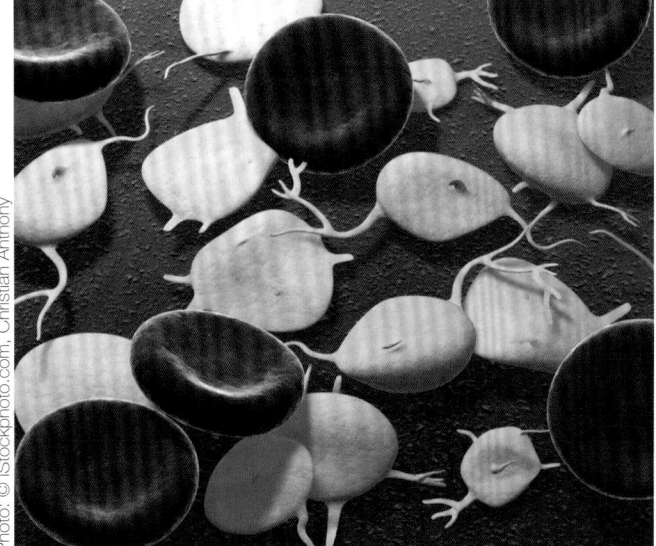

Photo: © iStockphoto.com, Christian Anthony

Blood cells

Blood is made up of basically two types of blood cells – red and white – although this is very simplistic as the white blood cells are actually a complex group of different types of blood cells. Blood is made up in the main by red blood cells, but cancer involves almost exclusively the white blood cells and the term leukaemia comes from two Greek words meaning 'white blood'.

The number of different white cell types is reflected by the types of leukaemia. Leukaemia is not one disease, but a group of different diseases. What they have in common is an abnormal production of white blood cells. Blood cells are produced in the marrow of many bones. Leukaemia is a disorder of the blood-forming cells in which certain groups of white blood cells reproduce in the bone marrow in a disorganised and uncontrolled way.

Perhaps the most serious effect of this uncontrolled growth is the progressive displacement, and interference with, the normal constituents of the blood. This can have serious implications for normal bone marrow constituents that are crowded out, such as those concerned with red blood cell production, blood clotting and producing the cells of the immune system that protect against infection.

What tends to emerge is a complex picture and leukaemia is not the same, therefore, in every person. They are all serious conditions – some more so than others – which, unless effectively treated, can cause anaemia from a shortage of red blood cells, severe bleeding from interference with blood clotting elements such as platelets, or infection from the loss of normal immune system cells. They also respond differently to treatment, with real cures possible in many cases.

There are two main groups:
- Acute leukaemias. Which are in general the more dangerous.
- Chronic leukaemias. In which the outlook is usually much better.

Leukaemias can also be split into two large categories depending on their origin:
- Acute lymphoblastic (lymphocytic) leukaemias. Predominantly affecting young children.
- Acute myelogenous (myeloid) leukaemias. Mainly affecting adults. These arise in the bone marrow itself.

# Symptoms
There are important differences in the way the two basic types of leukaemias – acute and chronic – make themselves felt.

### Acute leukaemias
As the name suggests, they start suddenly and the man will generally become ill in a matter of days. Symptoms vary but they include:
- Pallor.
- Fever.
- Various infections.
- Influenza-like symptoms, a feeling of great tiredness, sore throat.
- Bleeding from the gums and into the skin with unexplained bruising.
- Loss of appetite and weight.
- Lumps in the neck, armpits and groin caused by the lymph nodes becoming larger.

Blood checks may show a severe anaemia, with a significant lack of red blood cells and usually large numbers of white cells in early stages of development. Recognising these cells by microscopy is vital as it will help to decide the best course of treatment.

### Chronic leukaemias
A slow, insidious onset with gradually developing lassitude and fatigue set these leukaemias apart from the acute forms. Increasing size of the spleen can cause a dragging feeling with pain in the upper left side of the abdomen. There is slow loss of weight, aching in the bones and possibly nose bleeds or blood in the urine. Some men find warm rooms hard to bear and may sweat heavily, especially at night.

# Causes
Generally, no specific single cause is known. It seems likely that, in most cases, a number of different factors combine, or interact, to cause the disease. These factors include genetics, radiation, environmental chemicals, and cancer-causing viruses.

On the other hand, the cause of some leukaemias is understood. All leukaemic cells in people with chronic myeloid leukaemia, for instance, contain an abnormal chromosome called the Philadelphia Chromosome. This is derived from a broken-off piece of chromosome 9 attaching itself to a broken chromosome 22. The result is a gene which generates a protein that disrupts stem cell function in the bone marrow.

The association between leukaemia and radiation is well recognised. There is an increased incidence in people who have had a large single dose of radiation, not least those involved in war-time radiation, and in those who have had repeated smaller doses (as in medical treatment). The size of the risk is directly proportional to the total dose of radiation. Even so, even a large dose of radiation does not necessarily cause leukaemia – it only increases the risk. The name of the game is to avoid radiation or expose yourself to it as little as possible.

Chemicals such as benzene can damage bone marrow function. This damage is followed by leukaemia.

Sadly, treatment with some anti-cancer drugs can also increase the risk of developing leukaemia.

# Diagnosis
A great deal depends on your symptoms and your doctor's examination. A full examination of your blood sample, and often of a sample of bone marrow too, will be made. The microscopic appearance of the white cells, together with a chromosomal analysis of the abnormal blood cells, will help establish the diagnosis.

# Treatment
Chemotherapy is still the mainstay and saves thousands of lives. It is especially effective in chronic leukaemias and often maintains life for many years. Removal of the spleen is often advised in chronic leukaemias.

Good news for people with acute leukaemias as well. Around 50 to 60 per cent of patients enjoy a remission on chemotherapy. Tackling the anaemia, bleeding tendency and infections which can complicate the condition is essential, and this will usually involve blood transfusions and antibiotics. Other treatments include bone marrow transplants, radiotherapy and white cell transfusions.

Undoubtedly the biggest leap forward has come from bone marrow transplants, which are increasingly used to treat leukaemia. The graft provides the person with cancer a fresh supply of stem cells acting as the source of a continuing supply of healthy new red and white blood cells.

The donated marrow is obtained from a matched donor such as a sibling. First the abnormal bone is destroyed using total body radiation in combination with the drug cyclophosphamide. Then marrow is sucked out of the marrow cavity of the pelvis or breastbone of the donor and injected into one of the recipient's veins. The marrow cells are carried by the bloodstream to the recipient's bone marrow, where they settle and begin to produce new cell lines (clones) by normal reproduction.

In certain forms of leukaemia it is even possible to take marrow from a person in remission, store it, expose the person to heavy radiation and then replace the original sample to start up the marrow function again.

# Lymphoma

## Introduction

Lymphoid tissue has a number of roles in the body, not least to attack infections. Most of this takes place in the lymph nodes ('lymph glands') and the spleen. White blood cells, 'lymphocytes', are the most important part of the immune defence system.

Once it was thought that all white blood cells were the same, but now we know there are two broad classes of lymphocytes, T cells and B cells, which produce antibodies to attack bacteria and viruses. Lymphomas are cancerous lymphocytes, mainly B cells.

There are two kinds of lymphoma: Hodgkin's lymphoma (also called Hodgkin's disease) and non-Hodgkin's lymphoma, which used to be called lymphosarcoma. The lymphatic tissue in Hodgkin's lymphoma contains specific cells – Reed-Sternberg cells – that are not found in any other cancerous lymphomas or cancers. These cells distinguish Hodgkin's from non-Hodgkin's lymphomas. Non-Hodgkin's lymphoma usually consists of identical B lymphocytes which may have come from one single abnormal cell. It can affect any part of the body's lymphatic system, but varies in the speed at which it grows and spreads.

## Symptoms

One of the problems with Hodgkin's lymphoma is the lack of early signs or symptoms. Enlarged lymph nodes in various places around the body such as in the neck or armpits give some warning and should not be ignored. Weakness, tiredness and a reduced ability to fight off infection tend to come on later in the course of the condition. Younger men tend to develop the cancer most, but the good news is that it is very treatable, especially with early diagnosis.

Non-Hodgkin's lymphoma tends to have widespread, painless, firm enlargement of lymph nodes with lumps under the armpits, neck, abdomen or groin. There is also tiredness, loss of weight, and sometimes fever with night-time sweats. These enlarged nodes may put pressure on various structures of the body. This may cause various effects, which include:

- Pressure on the spinal cord with difficulty in moving or pain.
- Swallowing problems.
- Breathing difficulty.
- Vomiting from blockages in the bowel.
- Swelling of limbs from too much fluid.

## Cause

Lymphomas do not seem to have any direct cause. There appears to be a genetic factor, as it can be more common in some families.

## Diagnosis

Although the symptoms tend to be vague, the diagnosis is partly made on the clinical signs and symptoms. It may be confirmed by one or more of the following:

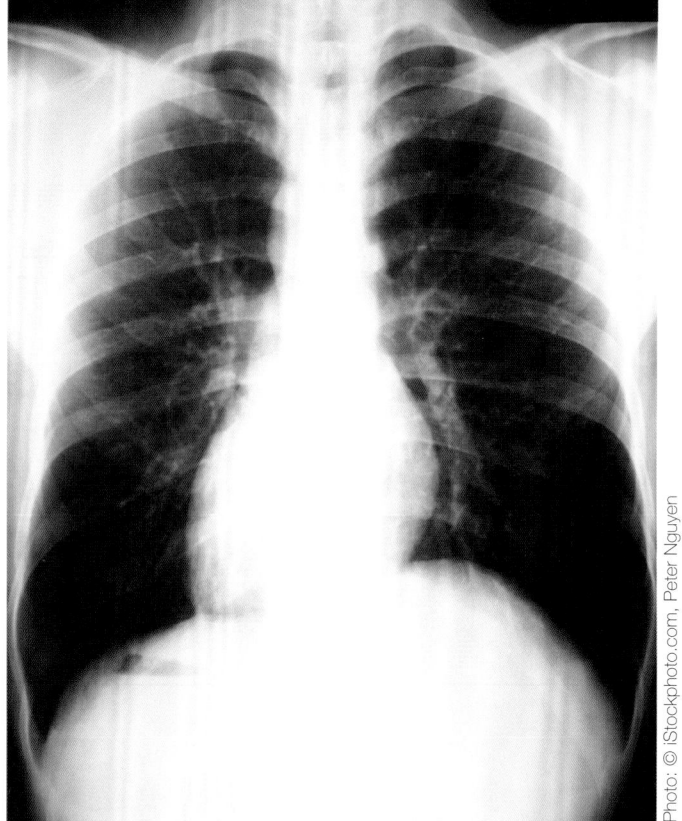

Photo: © iStockphoto.com, Peter Nguyen

- Blood tests, especially checking out the types of cells present.
- Chest X-ray.
- CT scan (computer assisted X-ray examination).
- MRI scan (magnetic resonance imaging which does not use X-rays and can better visualise more detail of the body).
- Microscopic appearance of tissue from a lymph node biopsy – a small sample of tissue taken either by using a fine needle or during surgery.

## Prevention

Unfortunately we don't know enough about lymphomas to give good advice on prevention, other than avoiding the obvious agents that can cause cancer. Much more important therefore is early diagnosis and seeing your doctor.

## Treatment

This will depend very much on how early the cancer is diagnosed. When treatment is required, radiotherapy is often best as in many cases this alone is enough.

In more severe cases other forms of treatment must be added. Chemotherapy with various combinations of drugs may be given every four weeks for six months. The results are often excellent, but the earlier the diagnosis is made, the better.

# Raynaud's phenomenon

## Introduction

Raynaud's phenomenon is a disorder affecting the small arteries supplying fingers and toes, in which exposure to cold causes them to go into spasm so that blood flow is restricted.

## Symptoms

Raynaud's disease usually affects both hands. The toes are less often affected. In cold conditions, there is tingling, burning and numbness in the affected parts and the fingers are very pale from lack of blood.

As slow blood flow is resumed and the oxygen is withdrawn from the blood, the characteristic purplish colour of deoxygenated blood (cyanosis) is seen. When the parts are warmed and the spasm of the blood vessels passes off, the vessels open widely, allowing a flush of fresh blood to pass. In this stage, the fingers or toes become red.

## Causes

Raynaud's phenomenon often occurs in men with underlying illnesses affecting the arteries, it sometimes affects those using vibrating power tools or pneumatic drills.

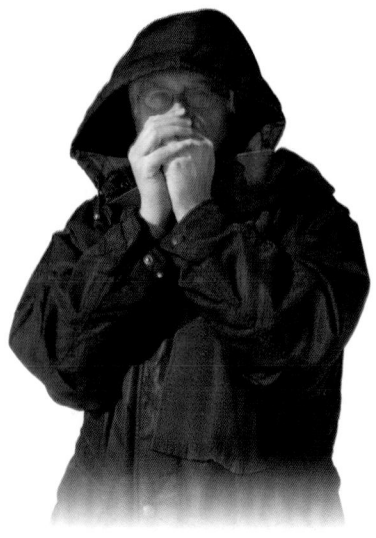

Photo: © iStockphoto.com, Ray Wrona

## Diagnosis

This is based on the characteristic physical signs (colour changes) that occur on exposure to cold.

## Prevention

People suffering from Raynaud's disease must avoid cold and keep the extremities well insulated. Cigarette smoking is especially dangerous as it increases the constriction of the small arteries.

## Complications

In the early months or years, no physical change occurs in the affected blood vessels, but in severe cases the vessel walls may eventually become thickened and the flow of blood permanently reduced.

## Treatment

Raynaud's phenomenon is treated by correcting the cause, if this is possible, but treatment of the symptoms may also be necessary. Various drugs to relax the smooth muscle in the walls of the arteries are useful in Raynaud's disease.

Cutting of the sympathetic nerves which supply the blood vessel wall muscles (sympathectomy) can be helpful, especially when the disease affects the lower limb.

## Action

Make an appointment to see your GP.

PART **4** # Sweat

## Introduction

Sweat is a mixture of water, salts and a little protein. It is produced by the skin's sweat glands which are found all over the body but tend to be more concentrated in areas like the hands. Although the skin is a major detoxifying organ the production of sweat is mainly part of temperature control. The evaporation of the water has a dramatic cooling effect, especially if there is free movement of air over the skin.

Clothes act as 'double glazing' trapping air heated by the body. Sweat evaporation is also prevented which is why totally impervious material like plastic produces dampness.

We can lose very large amounts of body water by sweating in high temperatures or during a fever which must be replaced as the body cannot withstand dehydration for more than a day or so.

## Symptoms

Profuse sweating can be embarrassing but rarely dangerous unless there is also significant dehydration. Lack of sweating can cause overheating.

## Causes

The main cause is a high environmental temperature but it can also occur with a fever. It is important to reduce the amount of clothes to allow this sweat to evaporate and cool the body as the brain in particular cannot tolerate high temperatures. A fan can help cool someone that much quicker.

Inappropriate sweating can occur from alcohol abuse and anxiety.

The smell of under-arm sweat comes from bacteria which like warm damp environments, not from the sweat itself which has little or no smell.

## Prevention

Right, no sweat. That really is a tall order for our tradesmen. It might be embarrassing, always happening at the worst times, but sweating is vital. Fresh sweat should have no smell, so the most important tip is to wash regularly to prevent stale sweat. Sparing use of antiperspirants will help, but many so-called deodorants simply mask the smell and do not stop sweating. Dress appropriately for the weather and lose excess weight, it'll stop your body working so hard and having to get rid of excess heat. Rinsing sweaty hands in a dilute solution of aluminium chloride (from your pharmacist) will stop sweating for many hours, useful if you are a politician 'pressing the flesh'.

It is possible to have a surgical block on the nerves which stimulate the sweat glands. This is a last resort.

## Complications

Dehydration causes confusion, exhaustion and heart failure. Chronic dehydration can also damage the kidneys.

## Self care

A day's hard work in a hot environment can need up to a gallon of water to replace sweat alone. Water lost as sweat must be replaced by unadulterated water, not alcoholic drinks which simply make the dehydration worse by stimulating the kidneys to get rid of even more water.

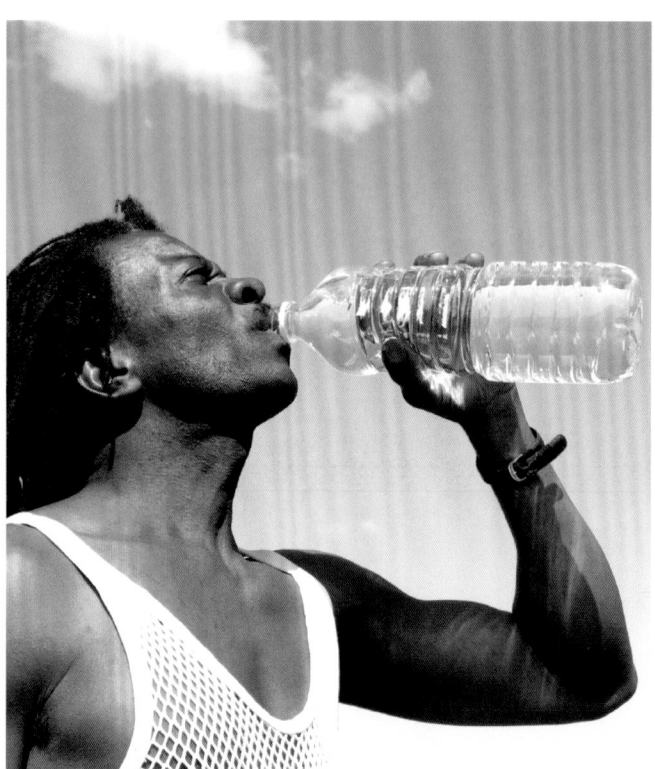

Keep your water intake up

Photo: © iStockphoto.com, Lise Gagne

# 5 Brain



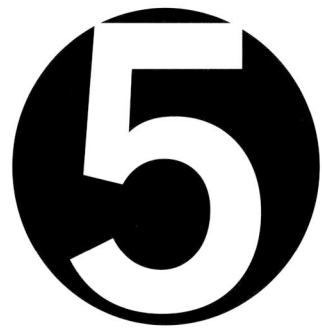

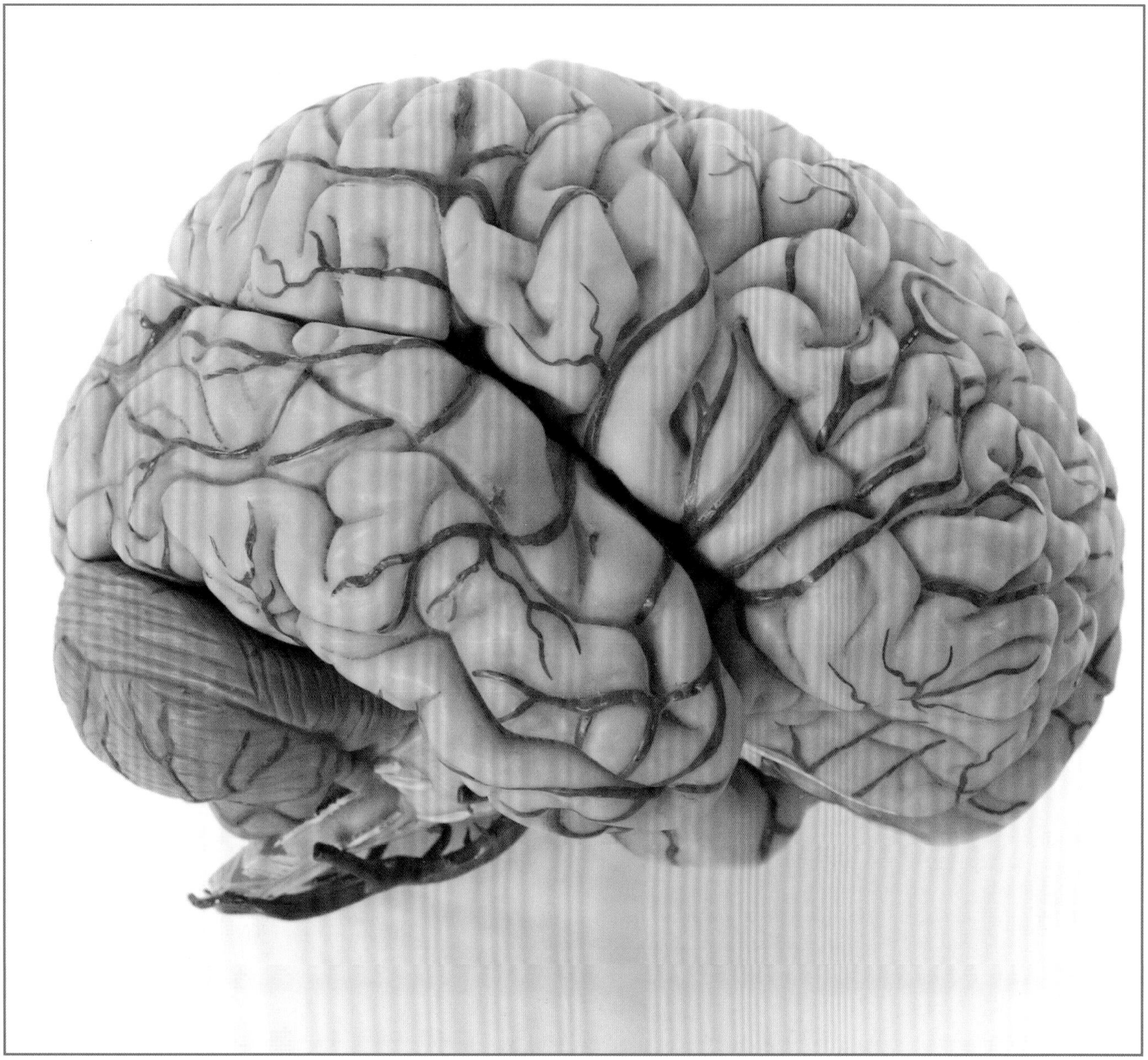

Photo: © iStockphoto.com, Mark Evans

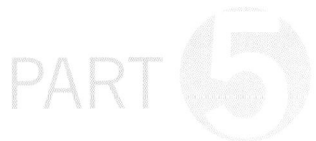

# Dementia

The term 'dementia' is used to describe the symptoms that occur when the brain is affected by specific diseases and conditions. These include Alzheimer's disease and stroke.

Dementia is progressive, which means the symptoms will gradually get worse. How fast dementia progresses depends on the individual. Each person is unique and will experience dementia in their own way.

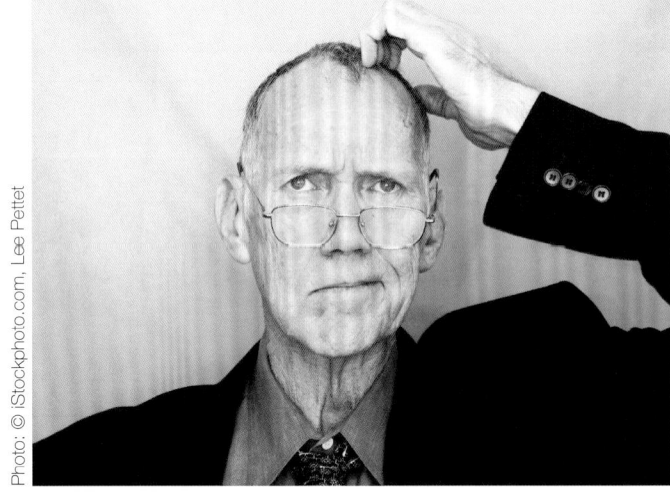

Photo: © iStockphoto.com, Lee Pettet

## Symptoms of dementia include
● Mood changes – particularly as parts of the brain that control emotion are affected by disease. People with dementia may also feel sad, frightened or angry about what is happening to them.
● Communication problems – a decline in the ability to talk, read and write.
● Loss of memory – for example, forgetting the way home from the shops, or being unable to remember names and places. What dementia is not is simple forgetfulness. We all forget things and this usually increases as we get older; dementia is not a normal part of ageing.

In the later stages of dementia, the person affected will have problems carrying out everyday tasks and will become increasingly dependent on other people.

## What are the odds?
The older you get the more common dementia is. The well-established prevalence rates for dementia in the UK are:

| Age (years) | Prevalence |
| --- | --- |
| 40-65 | 1 in 1000 |
| 65-70 | 1 in 50 |
| 70-80 | 1 in 20 |
| 80+ | 1 in 5 |

## Types of dementia

Alzheimer's disease is the most common form of dementia. Although there is some disagreement over the precise numbers, the proportions of those with different forms of dementia can be broken down:

| Disease | Proportion of people with dementia affected | About the disease |
| --- | --- | --- |
| Alzheimer's disease | 55% | This is the most common cause of dementia. During the course of the disease, the chemistry and structure of the brain changes, leading to the death of brain cells. |
| Vascular disease | 20% | If the oxygen supply to the brain fails, brain cells may die. The symptoms of vascular dementia can occur either suddenly, following a stroke, or over time, through a series of small strokes. |
| Dementia with Lewy bodies | 15% | This form of dementia gets its name from tiny spherical structures that develop inside nerve cells. Their presence in the brain leads to the degeneration of brain tissue. Memory, concentration and language skills are affected. |
| Fronto-temporal dementia (including Pick's disease) | 5% | In fronto-temporal dementia, damage is usually focused in the front part of the brain. Personality and behaviour are initially more affected than memory. |
| Rarer causes | 5% | There are many other rarer causes of dementia, including progressive supranuclear palsy, Korsakoff's syndrome, Binswanger's disease, HIV and Creutzfeldt-Jakob disease (CJD). People with multiple sclerosis, motor neurone disease, Parkinson's disease and Huntington's disease can also be at an increased risk of developing dementia. |

## What happens in Alzheimer's?

In 1906, the German neuropathologist Alois Alzheimer was the first to observe plaques and tangles during the post-mortem study of a woman, aged 51, who had had dementia. He noted deposits, 'plaques', of what he called 'a peculiar substance' scattered all over the brain and 'dense bundles' or 'tangles' of fibrils within brain cells, many of which had died.

These 'plaques' consist of aggregates of a protein called beta-amyloid, a protein that is formed throughout our lives by many cells in our body. The amyloid plaques are toxic to nerve cells, and dead and dying nerve cells can usually be seen surrounding the plaque.

The 'tangles' seen in Alzheimer's disease consists of thousands of entangled paired helical filaments of a protein called tau.

In a normal brain cell, tau forms an essential part of the cell's skeleton. The tau in tangles, however, is in an abnormal state where it no longer stabilises the skeleton but instead forms tangles of fibrils that eventually accumulate in such amounts that they burst the nerve cell, causing it to die.

## What happens in other dementias

With vascular dementia the blood supply to the brain is restricted and nerve cells become hyperactive. In this state the nerve cells start to release excess amounts of neurotransmitters, the chemicals that usually send messages between neurons, which in these excessive amounts begin to damage surrounding cells.

Lewy bodies (named after the doctor who first identified them in 1912) are tiny, spherical protein deposits found in nerve cells. Their presence in the brain disrupts the brain's normal functioning, interrupting the action of important chemical messengers, including acetylcholine and dopamine.

Lewy bodies are also found in the brains of people with Parkinson's disease (PD), a progressive neurological disease that affects movement. Some people who are initially diagnosed with PD later go on to develop a dementia that closely resembles DLB. Researchers have yet to understand fully why Lewy bodies occur in the brain.

Dementia with Lewy bodies (DLB) is sometimes referred to by other names, including Lewy body dementia, Lewy body variant of Alzheimer's disease, diffuse Lewy body disease, cortical Lewy body disease and senile dementia of Lewy body type. All these terms refer to the same disorder.

The term 'fronto-temporal dementia' covers a range of conditions, including Pick's disease, frontal lobe degeneration and dementia associated with motor neurone disease.

All are caused by damage to the frontal lobe and/or the temporal parts of the brain. These areas are responsible for our behaviour, emotional responses and language skills.

## Treatment and cure?

There is no known cure for Alzheimer's disease and other types of dementia.

There are drugs available that may alleviate some of the symptoms. Some complementary therapies may also help to improve quality of life.

No drug treatments can provide a cure for Alzheimer's disease. However, drug treatments have been developed that can temporarily slow down the progression of symptoms in some people. Most work in a similar way and are known as acetylcholinesterase inhibitors. There is also a newer drug which works in a different way to the others.

Public interest in complementary therapies is growing at a significant rate, easily outpacing the research conducted into their safety and effectiveness. People are often attracted to the 'natural' and safe image of these therapies, particularly in treating chronic medical conditions, for which conventional treatments are often less than completely effective. There is little high-quality research into the treatment of dementia with complementary and alternative medicine. However, a number of therapies are providing some interesting preliminary results.

All types of dementia are progressive. This means that the structure and chemistry of the brain become increasingly damaged over time. The person's ability to remember, understand, communicate and reason gradually declines. How quickly dementia progresses depends on the individual. Each person is unique and experiences dementia in their own way.

### Staggering statistics

- It is estimated that there are 775,000 people with dementia in the UK.
- It is forecast that there will be 870,000 people with dementia in the UK by 2010 and 1.8 million by 2050.
- Currently there are an estimated 24 million people worldwide with dementia. Two thirds of these live in developing countries. This figure is set to increase to more than 80 million people by 2040. Much of this increase will be in rapidly developing and heavily populated regions such as China, India and Latin America.

### Common myth

Dementia just happens to old people. Dementia can strike much younger people. It's much rarer but over 18,000 people with dementia in the UK are aged under 65 years.

## Preventative maintenance

### Health warning

- Despite many claims to the contrary, we know of no fail-safe ways of avoiding dementia.
- There is no known cure for Alzheimer's disease and other types of dementia.

### Risk factors for dementia that we can't change

Research tells us that the most significant risk factors are those we cannot change.

- **Age** is the most significant known risk factor for dementia. Dementia affects one in 20 people over the age of 65 and one

in five over the age of 80. But dementia is not restricted to older people – there are over 18,000 people under the age of 65 with dementia in the UK. Dementia is not a normal part of ageing.

- **Genetic inheritance** influences our risk of developing many diseases. The role of genetics in the development of dementia is not fully understood. However, in the vast majority of cases, the effect of inheritance seems to be small. A person's chances of developing Alzheimer's disease if their parent or other relative has Alzheimer's disease are only a little higher than if there are no cases of Alzheimer's in their immediate family.
- **Women** are more likely to develop Alzheimer's disease than men, even if we discount their longer life expectancy. Men are more likely to develop vascular dementia at an earlier age than women.
- A high proportion of people with **Down's syndrome** go on to develop Alzheimer's disease at an early age. This means that people with Down's syndrome are at particular risk of developing dementia.
- **Other medical conditions** may put people at a higher risk of developing dementia. These include multiple sclerosis, Huntington's disease, and HIV infection.

### Changes to our lifestyle that might affect our risk of dementia

There are lifestyle changes that we can make that may reduce our risk of developing dementia.

Research evidence increasingly suggests that there are strong links between a healthy heart and a healthy brain.

However, anyone can develop dementia, including those who follow a low risk lifestyle. It is not possible to guarantee that you won't develop dementia if you change your lifestyle and reduce your risk.

But keeping your mind and body active and healthy is the best way of protecting your brain. Other factors, such as education and early nutrition, need to be considered at a more general level.

### Top tips for changing your lifestyle . . .

- Don't smoke.
- Reduce your intake of salt and saturated fat.
- Take regular exercise.
- Drink alcohol in moderation.
- Eat plenty of fruit and vegetables.
- Eat oily fish once a week.
- Have a GP check your blood pressure and cholesterol levels.
- Avoid head injuries (wear a helmet for cycling or motorcycling; don't box).
- Enjoy an active social life, interests and hobbies.

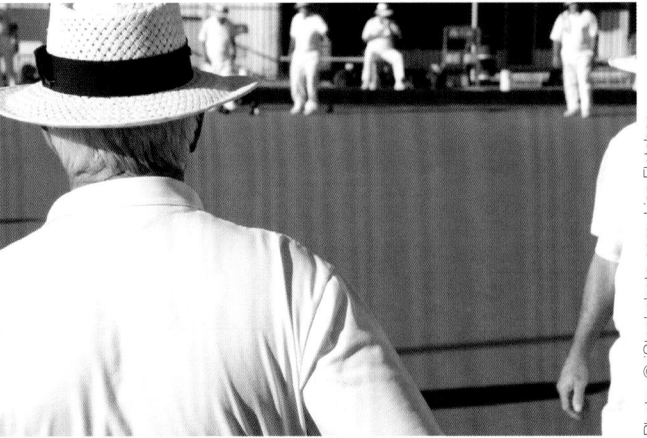

Photo: © iStockphoto.com, Lisa Fletcher

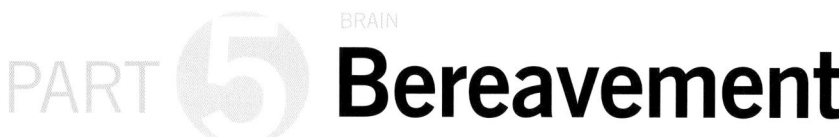

PART **5** BRAIN

# Bereavement

## Introduction

Death is inevitably upsetting and may occur at any age, even in childhood. As we grow older, our contact with personal loss increases, but it may never get any easier to deal with.

## Death in old age

The loss of an elderly relative or friend is supposed to be less painful. People will attempt to console you with well-intended comments such as, 'Well, she had a good innings'. Heads will nod, but a long innings often gives more reason to hope that death will never come.

## Scale of misery

Psychologists often refer to a scale that rates life events in terms of the stress they can cause. The death of a spouse or child comes at the very top.

## Predictable response

The scale is useful because it helps to demonstrate how you may feel when you have lost a loved one. The stages of the 'grieving reaction' are listed below. While the order of these stages remains the same for almost everyone, the severity and duration of each will vary from person to person.

- **Denial**: 'It can't be true. There's been some mistake.'
- **Anger**: 'It must be the doctor's fault. Why did they leave me?'
- **Guilt**: The next emotion, self-guilt, can be the most destructive. 'How could I be so idiotic? It's all my fault.' People will find the most unlikely things with which to whip themselves unmercifully. This stage can last a long time even when people rationalise the cause of their misery.
- **Acceptance**: After a variable amount of time there comes a period of acceptance. There is no fixed time for this period, which can even depend upon the community. People generally will profess to have come to terms with their loss before they have actually done so.
- **Coming to Terms**: Well-meaning folk will tell you that you'll get over it. The truth is that you never 'get over' a major life event. What happens is that you come to terms with it; the pain diminishes gradually with time. It is not a smooth progression, however, and anniversaries, returning to places, or even casual mention of the person or some object or event will release waves of heartache.

## Just to help me sleep

People close to the recently bereaved can be so shocked by the effect on their loved one that they may ask for, or even demand, sedatives from the doctor. Your doctor is highly unlikely to give in

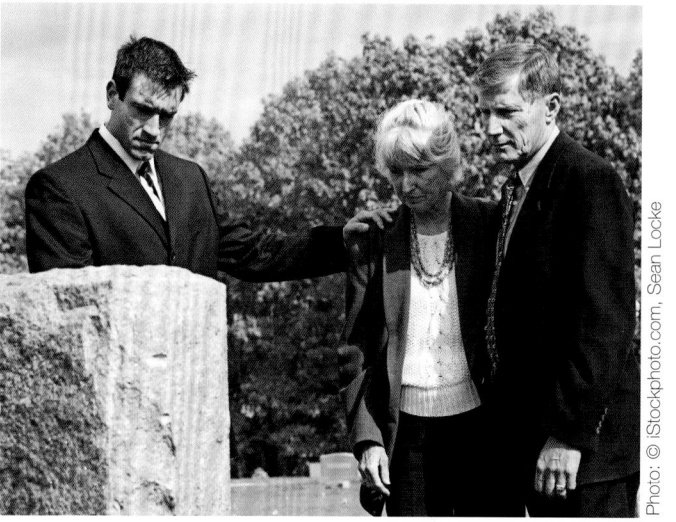

Photo: © iStockphoto.com, Sean Locke

to these demands. There can be no doubt that drugs will numb the pain of grief. Unfortunately, grief will not be denied; and if it is not allowed to take its course with the support of friends and relatives, it will resurface after the drugs and the support have gone.

People in grief then find themselves alone but with the heartache they should have had when help was at hand. People often talk of such an experience as 'floating above the events' only to come down with a thump later on.

## Effects underestimated

Most people underestimate the effects of bereavement on a person, until it happens to themselves. Some effects can be so bad that the bereaved person often will not realise that loss of interest in job or family, constant pacing of the floor, spontaneous weeping or complete loss of appetite are all normal and common manifestations of grieving.

People close to the bereaved person may also become impatient as time wears on, again underestimating the extent of the effects of grief and the length of time they can be felt.

It is at this point that true friends are worth their weight in gold. To know when to leave the person alone and when to sit and listen, often to the same story over and over again without interruption, is a gift that few people have nowadays.

Bereavement can even affect the memory, and people will say they experienced a 'complete blank' for a period following the death. Almost every facet of life can be and is affected – only the scale and duration varies between people.

Thankfully, there are professional agencies that specialise in bereavement counselling and can be contacted through your GP. Nobody pretends that strangers are as good as friends or relatives, but they can often help people who have difficulty coming to terms with their loss.

# Brain cancer

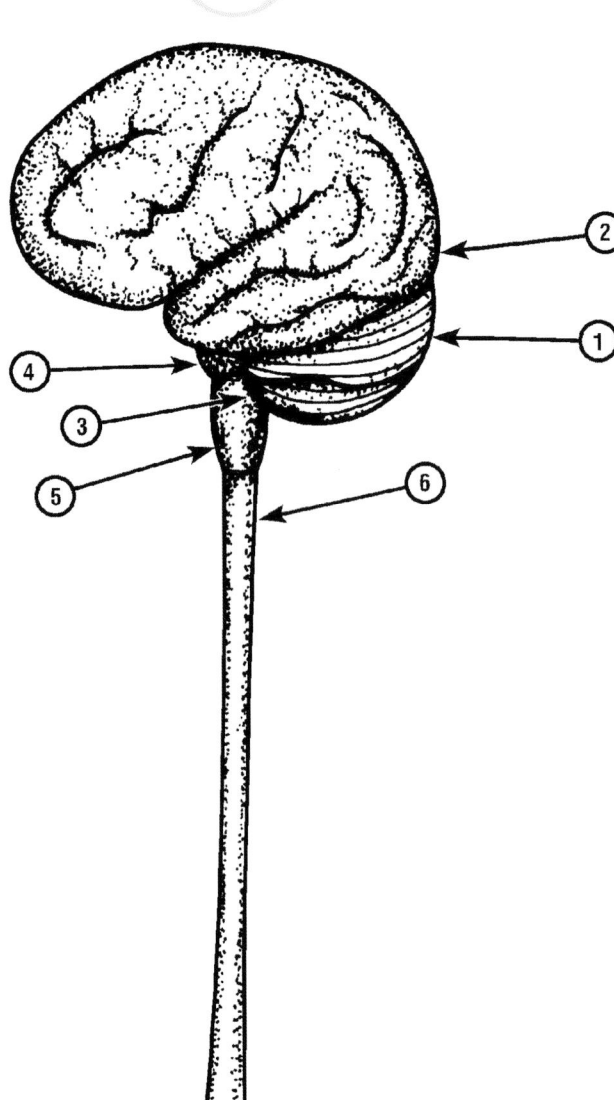

The brain is more than just a huge number of nerve cells. It has a complex support structure of blood vessels and coverings, not to mention bone, which forms an intricate scaffolding within the skull.

For reasons not entirely known, nerve cells of the brain do not form cancers. Cancers arise in the structures supporting the brain such as:

● Brain coverings, the meninges (meningioma).
● Neurological supportive tissue, the glial cells (glioma).
● Blood vessels (haemangioma).
● Bone of the skull (osteoma).
● Pituitary gland (pituitary adenoma).

By far the most common kind of brain cancers are those spreading to the brain from another malignant tumour in some other part of the body such as the lung, breast or prostate gland.

More rare forms of brain cancers are of congenital origin (craniopharyngioma, teratoma) and are due to abnormal development while in the womb.

## Symptoms

Unlike some other kinds of tumours, the signs and symptoms of a growing tumour within the skull are often indirect and not always obvious until a fairly late stage. A progressive rise in the internal pressure within the skull, either from the growing mass or from interference with the normal circulation of the cerebrospinal fluid, can put pressure on parts of the brain or its blood supply. This can produce symptoms such as:

● Severe, persistent headaches resistant to even powerful pain killers.
● Persistent dizziness.

For reasons not entirely known, nerve cells of the brain do not form cancers

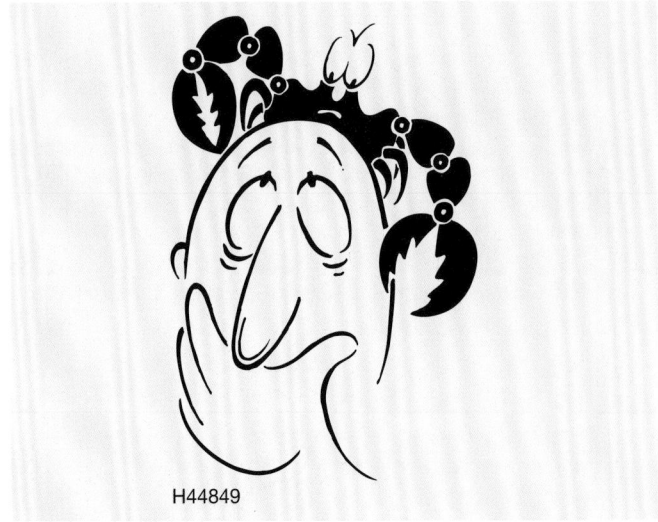

H44849

H32715

The brain and spinal cord

1 *Cerebellum*
2 *Cerebrum*
3 *Hindbrain*
4 *Pons*
5 *Midbrain*
6 *Spinal cord*

- Vomiting which is sometimes sudden, unexpected and often without any feeling of 'sickness' (nausea).
- Seizures (fits), either major seizures or local twitching. Any seizure in a person previously free from them must be checked out by a doctor.
- Loss of part of the field of vision. This can mean poor vision to the side, central loss where you need to look slightly to one side to see properly or loss of vision in one eye.
- Hallucinations, particularly of strange tastes or noises.
- Drowsiness, especially with no good reason and with difficulty to rouse. This can happen in the middle of the day.
- Personality changes or abnormal and uncharacteristic behaviour such as sudden irrational anger or weeping. Emotional 'flatness' where there is a lack of response to other people can also be a symptom.

Even so, if every person who had a headache was suffering from a brain tumour there would be standing room only in the hospital neurology units. Headache may be a symptom but only a tiny proportion of even severe headaches are due to brain tumour. A new, persistent and severe headache without any obvious cause can be a different kettle of fish, and in that case you should seek medical attention.

## Causes

Like many cancers brain tumours can often be very preventable. Cancer from the lung can spread to the brain at an unfortunately early stage in the condition. Lung cancer, and therefore secondary cancer to the brain, is preventable by simply stopping smoking.

Cancers arising within the brain itself are thankfully less common but the causes are unknown. Although radiation from mobile phones has attracted much attention, any link with primary brain tumours is not yet confirmed. Banning their use while driving may make more sense than simply preventing accidents, as reducing your exposure to any intense radiation from whatever source must be a good idea.

## Diagnosis

Most of the diagnosis comes from the symptoms and signs. As the skull is pretty tough and inflexible, any growth inside tends to raise the pressure inside the skull and can cause high blood pressure as the heart tries to force blood into the skull against this back pressure. Checking the retina at the back of the eyes using an ophthalmoscope (a flat telescope) is vital as it is in direct connection with the brain and the only visible way of checking from outside. In one quarter of cases of brain tumour and in most of those with raised pressure within the head, the parts of the optic nerves visible within the retina are obviously swollen (papilloedema).

Most people will also be checked by special X-ray or other non-invasive tests such as CT or MRI scanning.

## Treatment

Once considered virtually impossible, many tumours can now be successfully treated, especially the non malignant variety. The outcome depends on the location, type and degree of malignancy of the tumour. Many brain tumours are not malignant. Treatment is by surgical removal, often supplemented by radiotherapy.

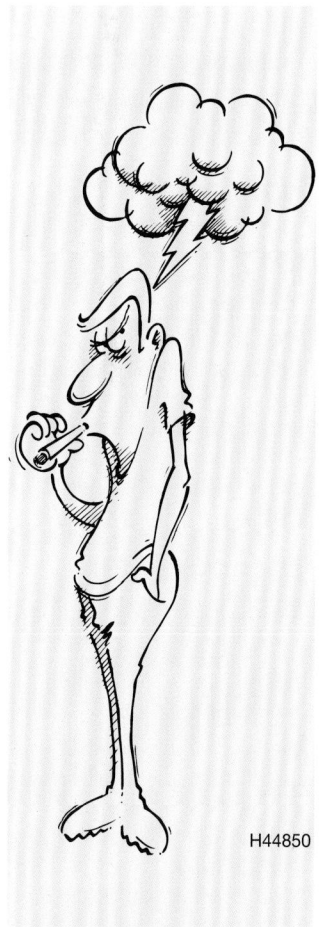

H44850

Lung cancer, and secondary cancer to the brain, is preventable by simply stopping smoking

# Hangovers

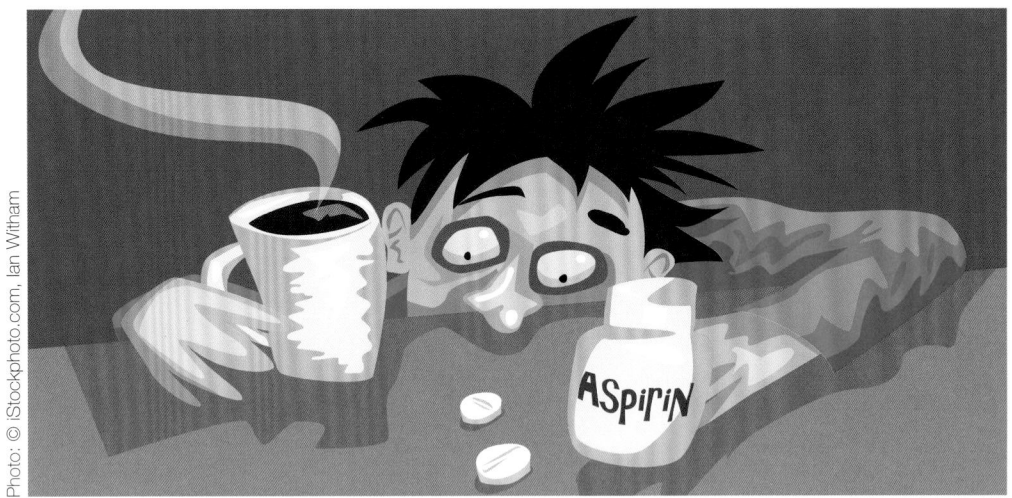

Photo: © iStockphoto.com, Ian Witham

## Introduction

A hangover can be so bad you actually think there is something seriously wrong with you, especially if it is the first time it has ever happened.

## Symptoms

Headache, nausea, tiredness and thirst are the commonest symptoms.

## Causes

Dehydration is the main cause. Alcohol acts as a diuretic stimulating the kidneys to lose water. Some alcoholic drinks contain toxins which act as mild poisons. Red wine in excess tends to cause headaches for this reason. Sleep while intoxicated is always poor as the alcohol interferes with the normal sleep pattern. This causes a feeling of not having slept the next morning.

## Diagnosis

Finding that more alcohol stops your hands shaking or cures a hangover headache, not to mention the need for more sleep later in the day, are all warning signs of possible addiction.

## Prevention

Every man who's ever had grape or grain pass his lips is an expert on hangovers. Unfortunately most of their advice is best ignored. Clearly the best way to avoid a hangover is not to drink to excess. Drinking a few glasses of water before going to bed will also help.

While drinking try alternating alcoholic and non-alcoholic drinks throughout an evening, or switch to less or non-alcoholic drinks towards the end of the night.

If you do find yourself with a hangover, drink plenty of water, take a painkiller and if possible have a nap later on to make up for the poor quality of sleep.

## Complications

Hangovers are rarely dangerous but routinely taking the hair of the dog to ease the symptoms can lead to alcohol abuse.

People underestimate just how long alcohol stays in the blodstream after a night's drinking and may well be still over the legal limit for driving the next day. Alcohol abuse is commonly linked to violence, suicide, self harm and visits to casualty

## What service to use

See your pharmacist but consider seeing your GP if you feel that alcohol is running your life rather than the other way round.

## Action

If you are suffering hangovers regularly it is highly likely that you are abusing alcohol and may be becoming dependent on it. If people are commenting on your drinking, you are becoming defensive over it, your work or home relationships are suffering or you are drinking early in the day you should contact support groups such as Alcoholics Anonymous, or contact your GP or pharmacist for advice.

On board computers and high tech electrical systems don't work well after a soaking

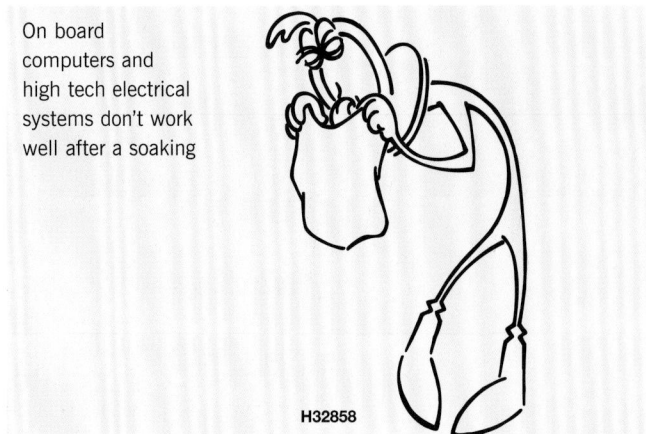

H32858

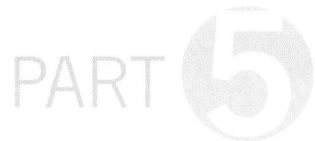

# Memory

## Types of memory

Memory is central to how we function. It doesn't take a great deal of reflection to realise that there are different types of memory that we use in different ways.

Psychologists have found it useful to define five main categories of memory:

- **Short-term**: this is our memory for things we don't need to remember for very long, such as telephone numbers, the beginnings of sentences, or mental arithmetic.
- **Procedural**: memory for skills such as swimming, driving a car or riding a bike.
- **Episodic**: memory for personal experience, such as your first day in a new job, your wedding day, a holiday, what you were doing when you heard Diana, Princess of Wales, had died in a car crash.
- **Semantic**: the body of information, facts and figures about the world that you have acquired through education and experience. Here you remember Diana's death in a different way, as historical fact rather than personal experience.
- **Prospective**: memory for things that have to be done in the future, such as keeping a doctor's appointment or switching off the oven.

## Memory and the brain

The brain co-ordinates and controls all the activities of the body and the mind, from breathing and moving to thought, emotion and memory.

It does this by receiving information from the body, and the world outside, processing it and then producing the appropriate response, based on a lifetime's experience.

For example, if the phone rings, your ears relay the sound to the brain in the form of electrical signals that pass from one nerve cell (neuron) to another. The sound is recognised (which, of course, involves memory), and the brain then sends a message back to your muscles, telling them to pick it up. Because we are human there is another dimension to this action – we can choose whether or not to take the call – which involves more brain activity.

Working out just how the brain manages to carry out all these tasks is probably the biggest challenge in science today.

Where memory is concerned, there is no one part of the brain that stores memories. It looks as if memory arises from the interplay of many different brain regions.

No one really knows what a memory is. The most accepted theory is that of a 'trace' but what does a trace consist of?

A trace is not a specific substance like a protein or even a group of neurons. What seems most likely is that long-term memories are stored in a dynamic pattern of connections like a network of neurons throughout many regions of the brain. When some stimulus triggers a memory, what it does is 'light up' the network corresponding to that memory in the brain.

It's claimed that memory loss appears with age.
A theory that fills me with rage.
At fifty-two my memory's great,
Which brings me on to my pet hate:
It's claimed that memory loss appears with age.
A theory that fills me with rage.
At fifty-two my memory's great,
Which brings me to my pet hate:

### Why do we forget?

There are two theories of forgetting (or failure of retrieval). Our memory traces may just fade away with time, like ink in bright sunlight. Or they may be 'overwritten' by more recent information. The evidence suggests that both occur.

Strangely, perhaps, it is hard to forget procedural skills (you always remember how to swim or ride a bike). It may be that such memories are stored in a different way or place in the brain to make them easily accessible.

## Making the most of your memory

You can improve your memory – whatever your age.

What we do know about memory suggests that there are four key elements to developing its powers. All memory techniques rely on them to a greater or lesser extent:

### Attention

So many memory lapses occur because people just don't pay attention when the material to be memorised is first presented. For example, when being presented to someone new, they are thinking about what to say, or wondering what impression they are making, instead of trying to take in the person's name. And when you put something important away, really think about what you are doing and don't get distracted.

### Interest

The mind dismisses boring material as irrelevant. But boredom is relative – if you must memorise something, find a way of making it interesting to you. Make it into a story, or imagine asking critical questions of the person presenting it.

### Organisation

Memory works best if new material is linked to something already known – maybe the man you've just been introduced to has the same name as your brother or an old school-friend? Use this as a hook to recall the name in future.

### Practise

There is nothing like 'hands on' experience to improve the memory – the mind gets the subconscious message that this material is important if you keep forcing it to recall. So if you learn a new word – foreign or otherwise (someone's name, say) use it straight away in a written or spoken sentence and repeat often.

## Top ten memory tips

### Make the most of external memory props

These are things such as diaries, wall planners, electronic organisers, Post-it notes, 'to-do' lists – even knots in your hanky or notes written on your hand.

### Leave a message

If you are at work when you remember something you must do when you get home, call home and leave a message about it on your answering machine, or e-mail yourself at home.

### Learn some poetry off by heart

The late poet laureate Ted Hughes said that the secret of learning poetry is a combination of visual imagery and careful listening to the underlying sound pattern. He suggested splitting the poem up into phrases and extracting a key word from each phrase, for which you make a vivid visual image, linking it firmly to the one which went before. Try it with the first four lines of William Blake's *Auguries of Innocence*:

> *To see a World in a Grain of Sand*
> *And a Heaven on a Wild Flower*
> *Hold Infinity in the Palm of your Hand*
> *And Eternity in an Hour*

The key words could be 'world', 'grain of sand' and so on. You could perhaps imagine a tiny globe suspended in a sand grain to start off with. Notice how the rhythm within the lines helps, as do the rhymes in lines one and three, and two and four. Literary verse, with its strong rhythms is easier to memorise than modern blank verse. But if you like the latter, your interest should help you learn it – relying mainly on visual imagery. And, of course, you should speak the verse aloud. Not only will this add to your pleasure, but it will help fix the poem in your mind.

### Get organised

Don't dismiss the old saying 'A place for everything, and everything in its place' as a memory aid. Put things in logical places – pills you take at bedtime next to your toothbrush, items for the following day in your bag, letters to post in a tray by the door. Be consistent about keeping things in their place so your memory creates strong associations between the item and its location.

### Little and often

If you have a lot of material to absorb – for a presentation, an

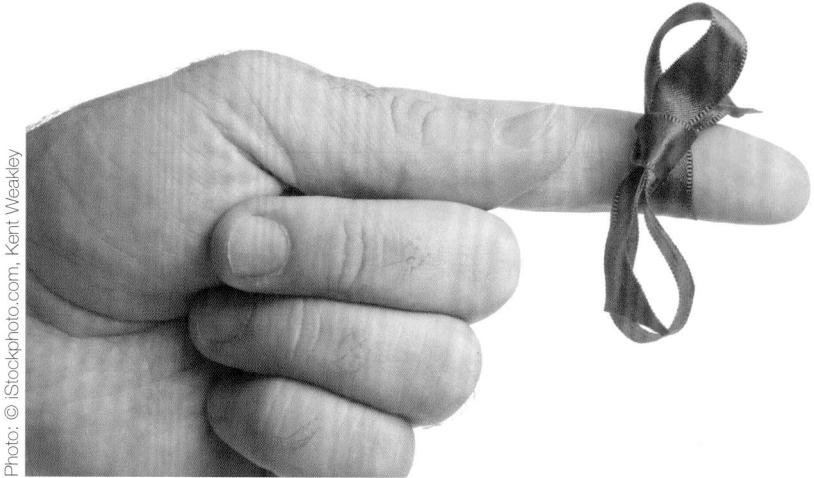

Photo: © iStockphoto.com, Kent Weakley

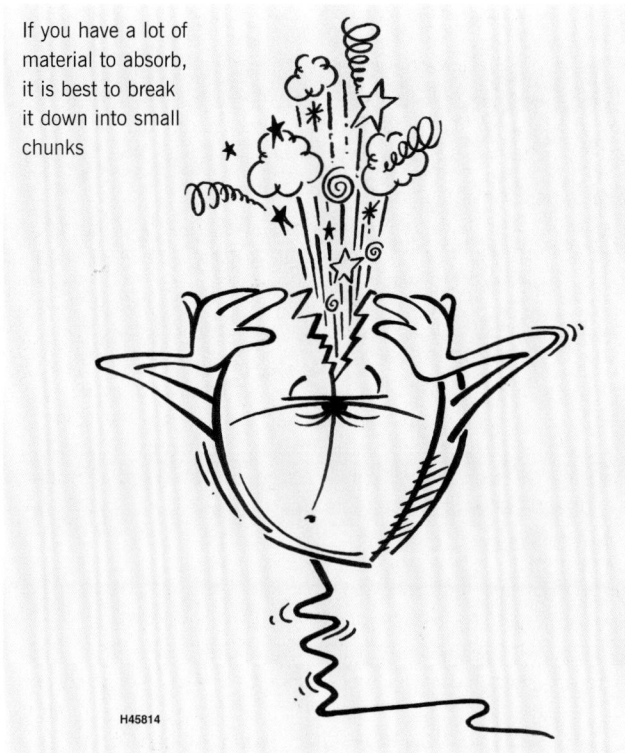

If you have a lot of material to absorb, it is best to break it down into small chunks

H45814

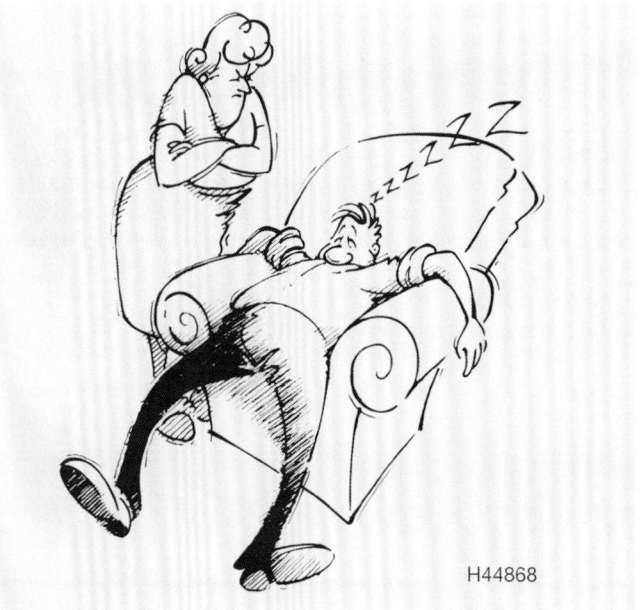

H44868

People differ in when they are most mentally alert

exam or a special project – it is best to break it down into small chunks and tackle it in several short, but frequent, sessions. Research shows that people remember more if they split seven hours of study over a week (an hour a day) than into longer, but less frequent, learning sessions of two or three hours.

### Lock away your diary
If you feel you are too dependent on external props such as Filofaxes and organisers, try creating a mental diary. Imagine the day (week, month or year) as a journey dotted with interesting locations – a river, a clump of trees, a castle and so on. Each feature corresponds to an hour of the day, so 2 o'clock is the entrance to a park, for example. Now make an image for each thing you have too remember – the dentist might be waiting for you, smiling with a flower in his buttonhole, by the herbaceous border near the park entrance – in other words, you are due to see the dentist at 2 o'clock. Try it for a day or a week and see if it gives you an enhanced feeling of control over your life.

### Get enough sleep
If you are studying, or generally being bombarded with information, don't lose out on sleep. While – amazingly – no one knows why we need to sleep, there is some evidence that it may play a role in learning. When students were deprived of sleep in an experiment they found it harder to recall complex material (although their ability to memorise simple lists was not impaired).

### Look for landmarks
It's frustrating and time wasting to forget where you parked your car or how to find your way out of an unfamiliar building. Try memorising landmarks – for instance, your car may face a tree or a sign. In a building, mentally trail a length of string behind you with features tied into it at specific places – a notice on the wall before you turn right, or a pot plant by that set of swing doors.

### Go with your biorhythms
People differ in when they are most mentally alert. Try learning a list of words and see when the peak time is for you.

### Keep a journal
Most of us take photos on holiday to preserve our memories – but why not try capturing the experience in writing too? The verbal dimension will strengthen the memory trace – which will add to your pleasure when you look back. A journal can have immense practical value for checking facts and details and may be a good place to work out problems and reflect on experience. It may even make you famous – for inspiration, look at the diaries of Samuel Pepys, Virginia Woolf, Alan Clark, Sir Roy Strong and Kenneth Williams.

## Little known facts
The brain itself has no pain nerve endings; the pain of a headache comes from the scalp.

## Staggering statistics
- The brain contains about 100 billion neurons (about the same as the number of stars in our galaxy, the Milky Way). All this in about 1.5kg (3lb) of greyish, porridge-like tissue.
- The rate at which neurons communicate varies between one signal every few minutes to about a thousand per second.
- Each neuron has between 1,000 and 10,000 synapses. The brain therefore has up to one million billion synapses.
- Dominic O'Brien, five times world memory champion, can memorise a single pack of shuffled cards in 38.29 seconds. Unfortunately for Dominic, who obviously enjoys a game of blackjack, he has been banned from all the casinos in the UK.

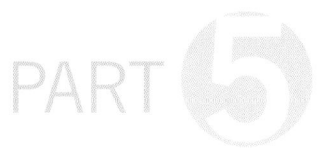

# Mental problems

## Introduction

Just as our physical health is linked to our genes and our lifestyle, so too is our mental health. For instance, through their genes, some people may be more susceptible to anxiety or depression. Others may develop a mental health problem as a result of child abuse, substance misuse or experiencing a traumatic event. All of us are vulnerable when it comes to major life changes – a death in the family, divorce or losing our job. Even positive changes, such as having a new baby or moving house, can be stressful and have a negative impact on our mental well-being.

Experiencing a mental health problem should not be a cause of shame any more than having pneumonia or breaking a leg. In fact, mental health problems are extremely common. Indeed, 1 in 4 of us will experience one at some point in our lives.

Although mental health problems affect both men and women, men are much less likely to seek help from their doctor. Men traditionally expect themselves to be competitive and successful, tough and self-reliant. They can find it very difficult to admit that they are feeling fragile and vulnerable. If they do see their doctor, they are more likely to talk about their physical symptoms than the emotional and psychological ones. As a result, many men do not get the help they need and make their problems worse by abusing alcohol and drugs.

Mental health problems include a wide range of conditions.

People don't like to talk about upsetting events

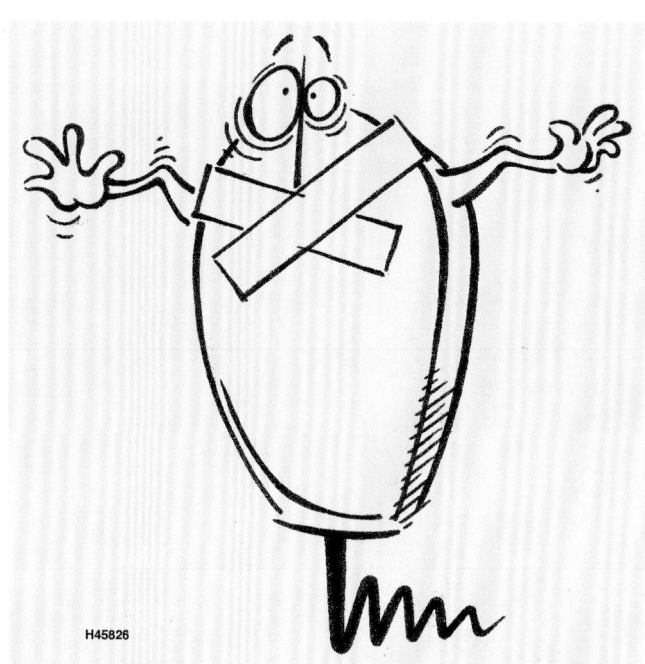

H45826

Some affect our sense of well-being, such as anxiety and mild depression. Other mental health problems can be more severe, such as schizophrenia, where a person can at times lose contact with reality.

Many mental health problems respond very well to treatment, so it is important to seek professional help. If you are feeling wretched, don't hold back – talk to your GP, a family member or friend.

# Anxiety

We all feel anxious when faced with situations we find threatening or difficult. In fact, fear and anxiety can be useful, as they help us to avoid dangerous situations, and give us the motivation to deal with problems and make necessary changes to our lives.

Sometimes it is obvious what is causing the anxiety, for instance worries about work or family. Anxiety can also be caused by using street drugs or even by the caffeine in coffee. Usually, when the source of stress disappears, so does the anxiety. However, if the feelings of fear and anxiety become too strong, or go on too long, they can stop us doing the things we want to do, and make our lives miserable.

A phobia is an extreme fear of particular situations – a social phobia is a fear of being in social situations – or particular things like spiders, which most people do not find troublesome. Sudden unexpected surges of anxiety are called panic and usually lead to the person having to escape as quickly as possible.

## Physical symptoms
- Palpitations.
- Sweating.
- Muscle tension and pain.
- Breathing heavily.
- Faintness and dizziness.
- Indigestion and diarrhoea.

## Mental symptoms
- Constant worry.
- Tiredness.
- Difficulty concentrating.
- Feeling irritable.
- Problems sleeping.
- Easily startled by unexpected sounds.

## Treatment
Although 1 in 10 people suffers from anxiety and phobias at some point in their lives, most do not seek treatment. Effective treatments include psychotherapy, group therapy, medications such as tranquillisers and anti-depressants, and learning relaxation techniques (see *Treatments and how they work*).

The important thing to remember is that having anxiety, and seeking help, is not a sign of weakness.

# Post Traumatic Stress Disorder (PTSD)

Any one of us can have an experience that is overwhelming, frightening and beyond our control. We could find ourselves in a car crash, witness a terror attack, or be a victim of violence. Most people, with time, get over the experience without needing help. In some, however, the traumatic experience sets off a reaction that can last for many months or years.

## Symptoms
In addition to the common symptoms of anxiety, people with PTSD may also:
- Have vivid memories, flashbacks and nightmares.
- Feel emotionally numb.
- Be constantly 'on guard'.
- Avoid places and people that remind them of the trauma.
- Have to keep busy to cope.
- Feel depressed.

These symptoms are a normal reaction to narrowly escaping death, and nearly everyone will have them for the first month or so. They actually help the person to come to terms with the traumatic experience.

For 1 in 3 people the symptoms do not go away, and they have problems coping with what has happened. This is more likely if the event was:
- Sudden and unexpected.
- Went on for a long time.
- Was man-made.
- Caused many deaths.
- Caused mutilation and loss of limbs.
- Involved children.
- The person was trapped and could not get away.

Because people do not want to be thought of as weak or unstable, PTSD is often unrecognised and untreated. Men are more likely to go to their doctor about the physical symptoms which accompany PTSD – palpitations, headaches and diarrhoea – than to seek help for the psychological symptoms such as depression and being 'on edge'. If a person has these symptoms for more than 6 weeks, it is important to see their doctor.

## Treatment
Anti-depressants can reduce the strength of PTSD symptoms and relieve any depression. Other effective treatments include Cognitive Behavioural Therapy (CBT), group therapy and complementary therapies (see *Treatments and how they work*). A newer technique, Eye Movement Desensitisation and Reprocessing (EMDR) uses eye movements to help the brain to process flashbacks and make sense of the traumatic experience.

# Depression

Depression is a common illness which causes a huge amount of mental pain. At some point in their life, 1 in 10 men will suffer from depression. Men who live alone, have no friends around, are stressed, have other worries or are physically run-down are more at risk. Depression is responsible for high rates of sick-leave and can be a potentially fatal disorder – most people who kill themselves have been depressed.

Everybody, at times, feels down and unhappy. Usually there is a good reason, often more than one reason. At other times, unhappiness can come 'out of the blue'. Generally these feelings don't last longer than a week or two, and don't interfere too much with our lives. However, if they don't go away, become severe or start to interfere with life, you may have a 'depressive illness'. You may not realise how depressed you are because it has come on gradually. You may be determined to struggle on and cope with feelings of depression by keeping yourself very busy.

Depression has nothing to do with being weak or unmanly. Even powerful people can become depressed. Winston Churchill called his depression his 'black dog'. Depression can also run in

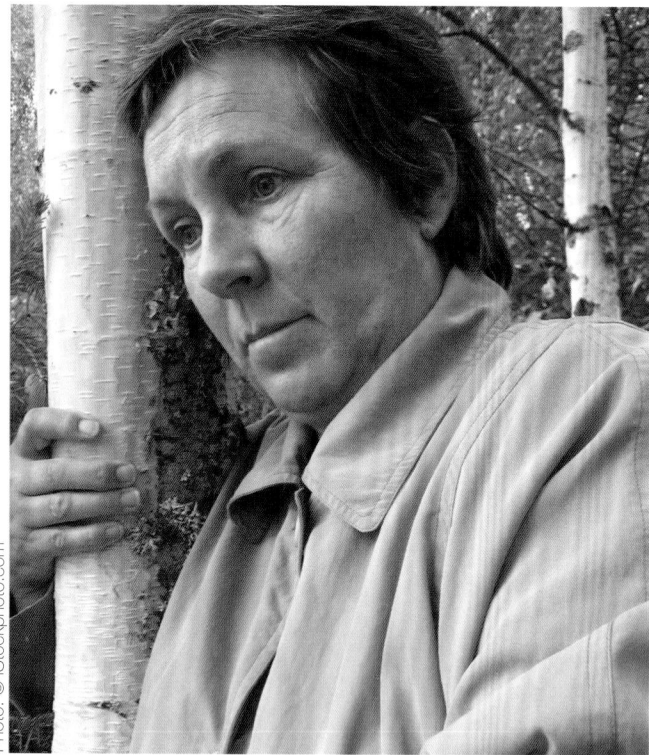

Photo: © iStockphoto.com

families. If one of your parents was severely depressed, you are 8 times more likely to become depressed yourself.

Gay teenagers and young adults may be more vulnerable to depression because of the stress of 'coming-out', victimisation and bullying.

### Psychological symptoms
You may:
- Feel unhappy most of the time (particularly in the morning but you may feel a little better in the evening).
- Lose interest in life and can't enjoy anything.
- Find it hard to make decisions.
- Find it hard to concentrate.
- Feel restless and agitated.
- Feel tense and anxious.
- Feel irritable.
- Feel worthless and hopeless.
- Feel guilty.
- Feel utterly tired.
- Lack motivation.
- Cry for no apparent reason.

### Physical symptoms
You may:
- Have difficulty getting to sleep, and/or wake early or during the night.
- Lose your appetite and therefore weight.
- Experience physical pains and constant headaches.
- Lose interest in sex.

### Treatment
Treatment can include, psychotherapy, counselling and anti-depressants.

The organisation Relate offers relationship counselling, and

Cruse offers bereavement counselling. A small number of people may need more specialist help and will be referred by their GP to a psychiatrist or member of the community mental health team.

### How to help yourself
There are also many ways you can help yourself:
- Don't bottle things up – talk to someone about how you are feeling. This is the mind's natural way of healing.
- Keep active and exercise.
- Eat properly.
- Avoid drugs and alcohol – they actually make depression worse.
- Learn relaxation techniques.
- Make lifestyle changes.
- Try to do something you enjoy.
- Keep hopeful – depression can be a useful experience. You may come out stronger, see situations and relationships more clearly, and be able to make important decisions and changes in your life which you had been avoiding.

# Eating disorders
Everyone has different eating habits and there are a large number of 'eating styles' which can allow us to stay healthy. However, some eating habits can actually damage our health. These are called 'eating disorders', and the most common are Anorexia Nervosa and Bulimia Nervosa.

Although girls and women are 10 times more likely to suffer from anorexia and bulimia, boys and men seem to be getting eating disorders more often. Anorexia is a serious illness which can damage your heart, lungs and bones. It has the highest death rate of any psychological disorder.

Anorexia usually starts in the teenage years and affects around one 15 year-old boy in every 1,000. Bulimia often starts in the mid-teens, but people don't usually seek help for it until their early to mid-twenties because, unlike anorexia, they are able to hide it.

### Symptoms (for men in particular)
- Eating less and less.
- Worrying more and more about your weight.
- Using harmful ways to get rid of calories, such as vomiting and using laxatives.
- Exercising more and more to burn off calories.
- Using slimming pills, or smoking more to keep your weight down.

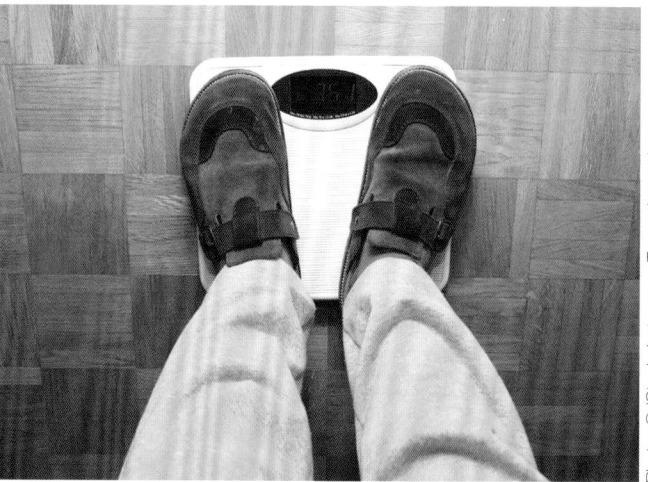

Photo: © iStockphoto.com, Tomaz Levstek

- Losing interest in sex.
- Erections and wet dreams stop, your testicles shrink.
- Binge eating.

The symptoms of anorexia and bulimia are often mixed. The pattern of symptoms can change over time – someone may start with anorexic symptoms, but later develop those of bulimia.

Another eating disorder has recently been recognised – binge eating disorder. It involves dieting and binge eating, but not vomiting. It is much less harmful than bulimia and sufferers are more likely to become overweight.

### Possible causes
- Social pressure – occupations which demand a low body weight (or low body fat) – body building, wrestling, ballet, swimming and athletics – seem to make eating disorders more common.
- Control – your weight may be the only part of your life that you feel you can control.
- Puberty – anorexia can reverse some of the physical changes of becoming an adult – pubic and facial hair for example. This may help you put off the demands of getting older, particularly sexual ones.
- Family – saying 'no' to food may be the only way you can express your feelings or have a say in family affairs.
- Depression – people with bulimia are often depressed. Bingeing may start as a way of coping with feelings of unhappiness.
- Self-esteem – people with anorexia and bulimia often don't think much of themselves and compare themselves unfavourably with other people.
- Emotional distress – anorexia and bulimia can develop as a result of sexual abuse, physical illness, and important life events.

### Treatment
Most people with a serious eating disorder will end up having some sort of treatment, as the condition does not appear to get better on its own. Bulimia can sometimes be tackled using a self-help manual and some guidance from a therapist. However, anorexia usually needs more organised help from a clinic or therapist. Although half of people with anorexia make a recovery, on average they will be ill for five to six years. A full recovery can happen even after 20 years. About 1 in 5 of the most seriously ill may die.

Although Cognitive Behaviour Therapy and Interpersonal Therapy have been found to be beneficial for bulimia, many patients have responded to other therapy approaches, particularly forms of family therapy. In the case of anorexia, no particular therapy has advantages over others.

# Bipolar disorder (manic depression)
About 1 in 100 adults has bipolar disorder (manic depression). This means that they have periods of bad depression alternating with periods of feeling 'manic'. The manic episodes can be just as harmful as the periods of depression. The pattern of mood swings varies considerably from person to person, with some people experiencing high and low swings, others only manic episodes, and some mainly depressive episodes.

Bipolar disorder most commonly starts in the late teens or early twenties and affects nearly as many men as women. Research has shown that it does run in families. There is a

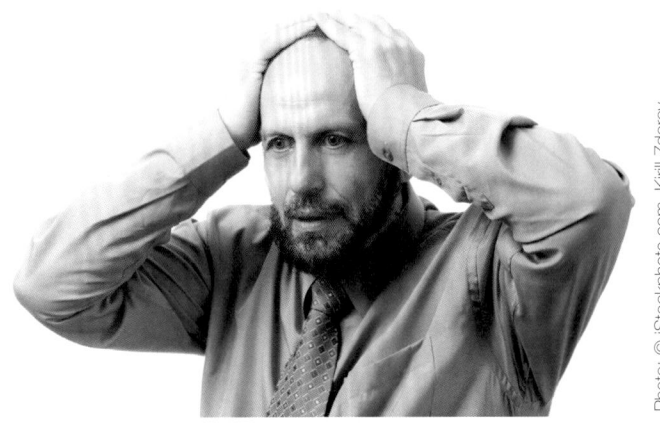

Photo: © iStockphoto.com, Kirill Zdorov

problem with the part of the brain that controls the general level of how we feel emotionally. This is why medication can control the symptoms.

### Symptoms of manic mood episodes
You may feel:
- Very happy and excited.
- Full of new exciting ideas.
- Irritated with other people (who don't share your optimistic outlook).
- Full of energy.
- Sure that there is no problem.
- That you don't need to sleep.
- That you want to talk to people much more.
- That you are very important.
- Less commonly, you may hear voices that other people don't.

When you are having a manic episode, you may not realise any thing is wrong. Others may notice that you:
- Behave in a bizarre way.
- Speak very quickly.
- Make odd decisions on the spur of the moment.
- Spend money recklessly.
- Are less inhibited about your sexual behaviour.
- Make plans which are grandiose and unrealistic to other people.

When someone recovers from a manic mood episode, they often regret the things that they did and said whilst 'high'. Without the right help, the condition can destroy your family, your relationships or your work. Therefore, it is important to recognise the signs that a manic episode is about to start. You can then get help before you are feeling so good that you don't see that there is a problem.

### Treatment
One of the main treatments for bipolar disorder is lithium, a natural substance found in the earth. Mood stabilising medications such as carbamazepine & sodium valproate can also help control manic and depressive mood swings. Psychotherapy and anti-depressants can be used to treat the depression. Psychotherapy and counselling can be helpful in the periods between mood swings.

# Schizophrenia
Schizophrenia is a serious and complicated mental health disorder that affects around 1 in 100. It affects men and women equally and seems to be more common in city areas and in some

minority ethnic groups. It is rare before the age of 15, but can start at any time after this, most often between the ages of 15 and 35.

1 in 10 people has a parent with the illness. Research suggests that genes account for about half of the risk of developing the disorder. The use of some street drugs, including cannabis, ecstasy, LSD, amphetamines and crack seems to increase the risk of developing schizophrenia in some vulnerable people. Suicide is also more common in people with this illness.

It is important to understand that:
- Schizophrenia is not a 'split personality'.
- People with schizophrenia are not necessarily dangerous.
- 1 in 5 people will recover completely.

**Symptoms are often described as 'positive' and 'negative'**

Positive symptoms:
- Hallucinations – you hear, smell, feel or see something that others cannot.
- Delusional ideas that make you feel persecuted or harassed.
- Muddled thinking and difficulty concentrating.
- Feeling that you are being controlled.
Negative symptoms. You:
- Lose interest in life.
- Lose interest in your personal appearance.
- Feel uncomfortable with other people.
- Lose insight.
- Feel depressed.

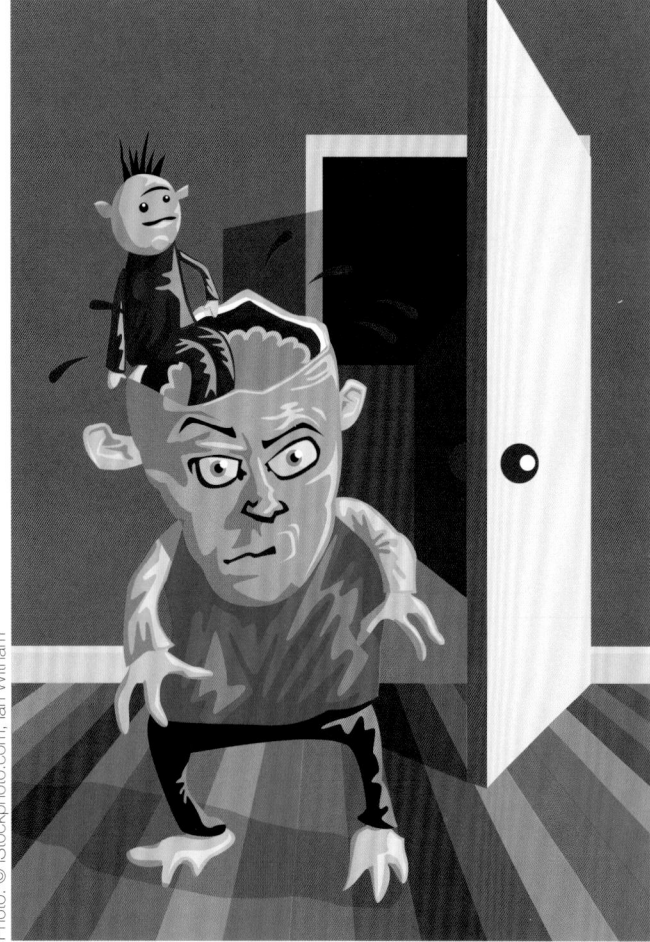

Photo: © iStockphoto.com, Ian Witham

### Treatment

The longer schizophrenia is left untreated, the greater its impact on your life. Antipsychotic medication should be started as soon as possible. This can help the most disturbing symptoms and make it possible for other kinds of help to work. Talking therapies include Cognitive Behaviour Therapy (CBT), counselling and supportive psychotherapy. You may not need to go to hospital, but will need to see a psychiatrist and a community mental health team.

## Possible causes of malfunction

### Genes

There is evidence that some people, through their genes, are more susceptible to certain mental health problems, including schizophrenia, bipolar disorder and depression.

### Relationships

We all need to feel loved and appreciated. It has been shown that, for men, relationship difficulties are the most common cause of mental health problems. Men are less able to cope with disagreements than women, and arguments can make men feel physically uncomfortable. By withdrawing, they avoid difficult discussions and confrontations. This can lead to his partner feeling more upset and ignored, and the problem escalates. The vicious circle can easily destroy a relationship.

Separation and divorce can be particularly hard for men and a relationship break-up often brings on mental health problems. Men who are divorced are most likely to kill themselves. Divorce is a form of bereavement that can mean the loss of a man's main relationship, as well as contact with his children. He may also have to move out of the family home, and may find himself with financial problems. It is therefore not surprising that separation and divorce often result in depression and other mental health problems.

### Bereavement

Grief takes place after any sort of loss, but most powerfully after the death of someone we love. After the initial shock and numbness, you may experience a sense of agitation and yearning for the lost person. Other common feelings are anger and guilt. After about two weeks the agitation can be replaced by sadness or depression which often peaks at about six weeks. If the depression continues to deepen, you may need anti-depressants, or to see a bereavement counsellor or psychotherapist.

### Pregnancy and children

More than 1 in 10 fathers suffer psychological problems after the birth of their child. Having a baby changes your life more than many other events. You may feel you are taking second place

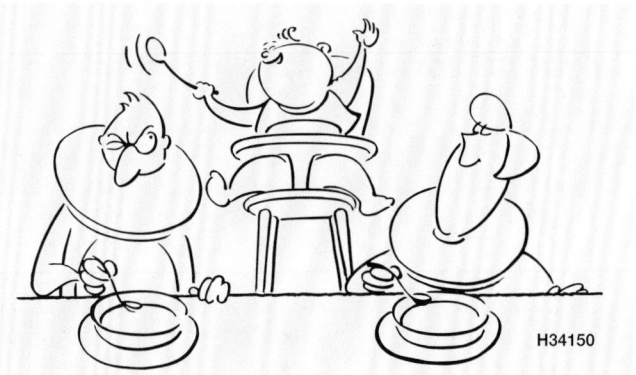

H34150

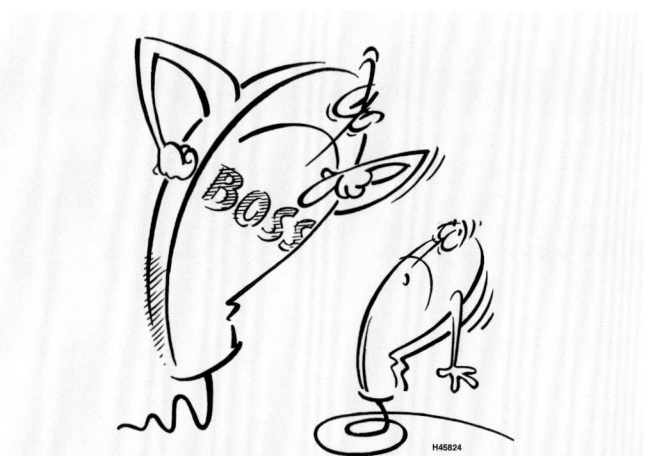

Difficult bosses who bully and criticise can result in feelings of tension and worry

in your partner's affections. You are likely to spend more time looking after your partner, and possibly other children, and you may be more tired than usual. On an intimate level, new mothers tend to be less interested in sex, which may make you feel rejected and unloved.

### Work

Work is generally good for our mental health. It provides a shape and meaning to our day and gives us the opportunity to make friends. Work can make us feel better about ourselves and is a reminder that other people value us. However, too much pressure and stress at work can combine with other problems, such as difficulties at home, and contribute to the development of depression and/or other mental health problems.

Jobs in which employees cannot use their skills, or which are repetitive, seem particularly likely to make people fed up with their work. Uncertainty about how well you are performing, or the future of employment contracts, can result in feelings of tension and worry, as can difficult bosses who bully and criticise.

### Unemployment and retirement

After relationship difficulties, unemployment is the most common cause of severe depression in men, with 1 in 7 becoming depressed six months after losing their job. This is not surprising, as work is often the main source of a man's sense of self-worth. The loss of a job can mean the loss of the symbols of success. From being in a position of control, a man may now face an uncertain future. Retirement can also be difficult for men who lose the structure of their day, and contact with colleagues.

### Mid-life

Some men appear to experience a crisis of confidence at mid-life (most commonly in the 40s to 50s), which may be accompanied by depression and other mental health problems.

### Alcohol and drugs

People use and misuse many different substances. These can be legal, such as alcohol, tobacco and solvents, or illegal such as cannabis, heroin and cocaine. Addiction occurs when a person develops a physical and/or psychological dependence, and has withdrawal symptoms if they do not use the substance.

Substance misuse and addiction are increasing in the UK, especially amongst young people. According to the Department of Health, around 1 in 8 men is physically addicted to alcohol.

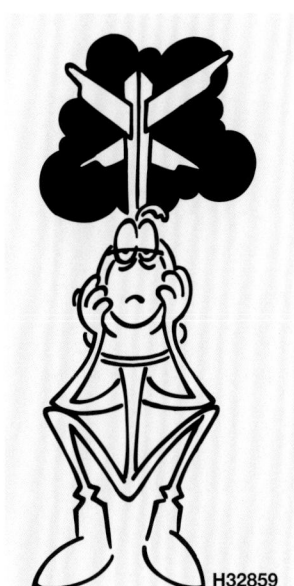

It is not suprising that separation and divorce often result in depression and other mental health problems

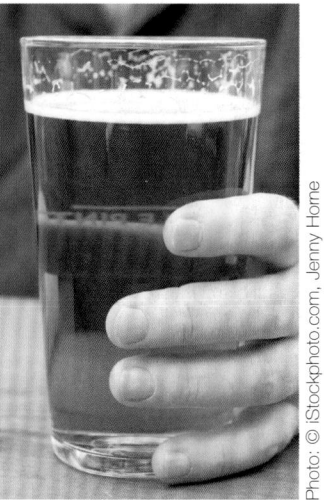

Photo: © iStockphoto.com, Jenny Horne

*When you're drunk it's hard to say 'preliminary' and 'stowaway',*

*And it'll come as no suprise that even worse is 'synthesize'*

*But what is even harder still?*

*'No thank you, I've had my fill'*

Alcohol acts on the brain like many other drugs. If you drink regularly, you will find that you need to drink more and more to get the effect you want. This is called 'tolerance' and is a powerful part of becoming addicted to alcohol.

Alcohol and drug misuse can lead to serious and permanent mental health problems:

- Dementia – memory loss like Alzheimer's disease.
- Psychosis – you may start to hear voices.
- Dependence – if you stop using the substance you get withdrawal symptoms such as shaking, nervousness and sometimes seeing things that aren't there.
- Schizophrenia – there is evidence that the use of cannabis is linked to the development of this serious mental illness in some vulnerable people.

- Suicide – 40% of men who try to kill themselves have had a long-term alcohol problem.
  Some facts about drinking too much alcohol:
- Alcohol increases the risk of depression.
- Regular drinking causes social problems – family arguments, domestic violence and poor work.
- Anxiety and depression will become worse if you drink alcohol.
- Binge drinking seems to be connected with an increased risk of death in middle-aged men.

The table gives a rough guide to the units of alcohol found in standard measures of different drinks.

So how much are you drinking?

| Beer, cider and Alcopops | Strength ABV | Half pint | Pint | Bottle/can (330ml) |
|---|---|---|---|---|
| Ordinary strength beer, lager or cider | 3-4% | 1 | 2 | 1.5 |
| 'Export' strength beer, lager or cider | 5% | 1.25 | 2.5 | 2 |
| Extra strong beer, lager or cider | 8-9% | 2.5 | 4.5 | 3 |
| Alcopops | 5% | – | – | 1.7 |

| Wines & Spirits | Strength ABV | Small glass/ pub measure | Wine glass | Bottle (750 ml) |
|---|---|---|---|---|
| Table wine | 10-12% | – | 1.5 | 9 |
| Fortified wine (sherry, martini, port) | 15-20% | 0.8 | 2-3 | 14 |
| Spirits (whisky, vodka, gin) | 40% | 1 | – | 30 |

### Street drugs

Using street drugs like cannabis (hash), speed (amphetamines), ecstasy (E), cocaine and heroin can seriously damage your health, and in some cases be fatal. Some facts:

- Mixing ecstasy and alcohol can lead to dehydration, coma and death.
- Cannabis can make you feel panicky, confused, tired and hungry. Smoking cannabis causes lung disease.
- Young adolescent men who smoke cannabis on a weekly basis are more likely to become dependent later on in life.
- 'Skunk', a particular strong form of cannabis, is particularly dangerous.
- Cannabis can trigger schizophrenia in vulnerable people.
- Amphetamines affect the heart and can cause death.
- Amphetamines can make you feel scared and anxious.
- LSD can cause terrifying experiences.
- Cocaine and crack cocaine can cause chest pain, difficulty breathing and are highly addictive.
- Heroin is highly addictive and can be fatal.
- Steroids can cause breast development in men, depression and hormonal problems.
- Serious infections, such as HIV and hepatitis, can be spread by sharing needles or 'equipment'.

The most common sign that you have a drug problem is that you find you need more and more of the substance to get the same effect and you cannot cope without it. If you think you have a problem speak to your doctor.

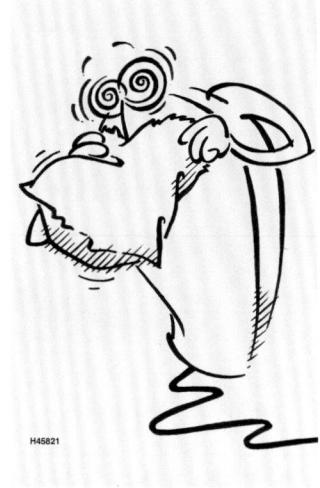

H45821

Using street drugs can seriously damage your health

### Physical illness

A serious physical illness can affect every area of your life – relationships, work, spiritual beliefs and how you socialise with other people. Being ill can make you feel sad, frightened, worried or angry. You will be particularly vulnerable to depression if the illness returns, for example, a recurrence of cancer or a second heart attack.

The emotional impact of a serious physical illness can be overwhelming.

You may feel out of control of your body and your situation generally. You may be uncertain about what exactly is wrong, anxious about the pain of surgery, the effectiveness of the treatment and the side-effects of medication. You may feel lonely and isolated from family and friends, because you may find it difficult to talk about the illness with those close to you. You may fear death.

Some drug treatments, such as steroids, and some physical illnesses, such as an under-active thyroid, affect the way the brain works and can cause anxiety and depression directly. Symptoms of depression can be similar to those caused by the physical illness.

Health professionals can help identify whether it is the illness, or the depression, which is causing the symptoms and what treatment is needed. They can explain your illness and its treatment, and help you to talk about your feelings.

## Self-harm

Self-harm is linked to emotional distress in people who have been struggling with difficulties for a period of time. Often there are problems with relationships, particularly in young people who feel that they are not heard, are powerless, and are bullied.

About 10% of young people harm themselves. Although self-harm is more common in females, men may be more likely to disguise it as accidents. Once someone has started to harm themselves, they tend to do it again quite quickly and 30% will repeat it during the following year. Self-harm is not an attempt at suicide. People who use violent methods to harm themselves, who are socially isolated, or have a psychiatric disorder, should be seen by a healthcare professional.

Self-harming can include:
- Overdosing.
- Cutting yourself.
- Burning your body.
- Banging your head.
- Throwing your body against something.
- Punching yourself.
- Sticking things in your body.
- Swallowing objects.

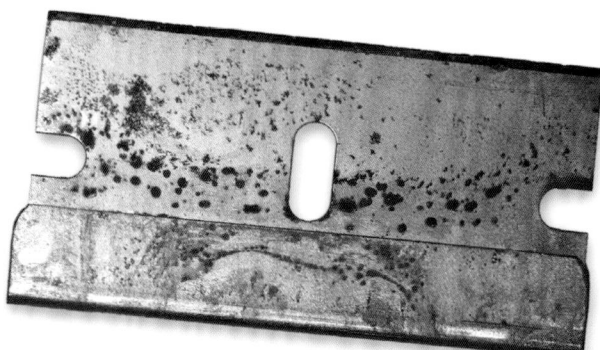

Photo: © iStockphoto.com, Christian Misje

## Suicide

Many people who kill themselves have been depressed. Men are 3 times more likely to kill themselves than women. Suicide is commonest amongst men who are separated, widowed or divorced and is more likely in someone who is a heavy drinker. 40% of men who try to kill themselves have had a long-standing alcohol problem. Men between the ages of 16 and 24, and 39 and 54, are particularly vulnerable.

We know that:
- 2 out of 3 people who kill themselves have seen their GP in the previous 4 weeks.
- Nearly 1 in every 2 people who kill themselves will have seen their GP the week before they take their lives.
- 2 out of 3 people who kill themselves have talked about it to friends or family.

As most men have to pluck up the courage to tell someone about the way they are feeling, it is very important to take anyone who talks about suicide seriously. If you are feeling so bad that you have thoughts of suicide, it is essential to talk to someone.

Most studies suggest that treatment is difficult. Talking about the problem can help clarify the problem areas. There are also a number of internet sites and telephone organisations for people who prefer to talk anonymously.

## Treatments and how they work

### Anti-depressants

These are drugs which relieve the symptoms of depression and other mental health problems, and have been used since the 1950s. The main types of anti-depressants available today are:
- Tricyclics.
- SSRIs (Selective Serotonin Re-uptake Inhibitors).
- MAOIs (Monoamine Oxidase Inhibitors).
- SNRIs (Serotonin and Noradrenaline Re-uptake Inhibitors).

Anti-depressants can take between 2 to 6 weeks to work. They are not addictive, although one third of people who stop taking SSRIs and SNRIs have some withdrawal symptoms (upset stomach, flu-like symptoms, and anxiety). They can have side-effects, particularly at the start of treatment, and you may be advised to avoid certain foods. Anti-depressants are not licensed for use in people under the age of 18.

Anti-depressants are used to treat:
- Moderate and severe depression.
- Severe anxiety and panic attacks.
- Obsessive compulsive disorders.
- Chronic pain.
- Eating disorders.
- Post Traumatic Stress Disorder (PTSD).

### Tranquillisers

These are drugs used to reduced anxiety and they can also help you to sleep. Common tranquillisers are diazepam, lorazepam and temazepam. Tranquillisers should not be used for longer than a couple of weeks, as they can become addictive.

### Antipsychotics

These are drugs used to treat the symptoms of the most severe mental illnesses such as schizophrenia and psychotic depression. Psychotic symptoms may include hallucinations and delusions. Newer antipsychotic drugs have fewer side-effects.

### Psychotherapy

Many men are reluctant to consider psychotherapy or counselling. But, these are powerful ways of relieving depression and anxiety and work well for many men.

There are many different types of psychotherapy. Some focus on feelings you have about other people and involve discussing past experiences. Others focus on changing problematic patterns of behaviour directly. Family and relationship therapy will try to include all the people involved in a relationship problem.

### Cognitive Behaviour Therapy (CBT)

Research shows that CBT is as effective as anti-depressants for many forms of depression, and is also one of the most effective treatments for anxiety. It can help you to make sense of overwhelming problems by breaking them down into smaller parts. CBT helps you change how you think and what you do, to make you feel better. It focuses on the 'here and now' problems and difficulties, and looks for ways to improve your state of mind now. It has been found to be helpful in:
- Anxiety, panic, phobias.
- Post Traumatic Stress Disorder.
- Depression.
- Bulimia.
- Schizophrenia.

CBT can be done individually, within a group and also from a self-help book or computer programme. Individual therapy may involve meeting a therapist for between 5 and 20 weekly, or fortnightly, sessions, each lasting between 30 and 60 minutes.

### Complementary therapies

Physiotherapy, osteopathy, massage, reflexology, acupuncture, yoga, meditation and Tai Chi can help relieve symptoms of anxiety and depression. St John's Wort is a herbal remedy, available from chemists, which has been shown to be effective in mild to moderate depression. If you are taking other medication, consult your doctor before taking St John's Wort.

## Here are some tips to help you maintain mental well-being

**Don't**
- Bottle up your feelings.
- Resort to using alcohol and drugs.
- Feel ashamed if you have a mental health problem.

**Do**
- Eat healthily.
- Exercise.
- Spend time with family and friends.
- Learn how to relax.
- Do things you enjoy.
- Take a break.
- Keep a check on your lifestyle.
- Have a purpose – work, volunteer, practise a hobby.
- Be patient with yourself if you have suffered a major loss.

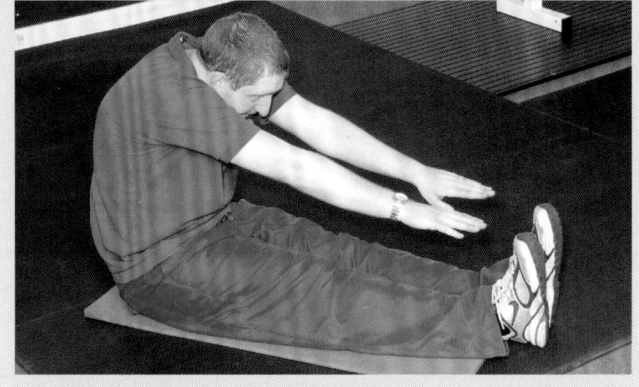

Doing any physical activity regularly, however gentle, can help

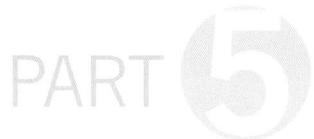

# Migraine

## Introduction

Migraine is common and runs in the family. As any sufferer will tell you, the migraine headache differs both in character and severity from an 'ordinary' headache.

## Symptoms

Visual patterns such as chequerboard or spots are often a warning of an impending attack. The headaches themselves can be quite debilitating, making the person sick and unable to concentrate.

## Causes

The exact cause is still not known, although there is some connection with the blood vessels of the head. Certain foods appear to trigger migraine. Red wine, blue cheeses and chocolate are all culprits. Stress, the weather and even hormonal changes have been known to increase the suffering.

## Prevention

Migraine is a tough nut to crack. Avoiding triggers such as red wine or blue cheese seems obvious but different things trigger different people. Try to keep a migraine diary, of both triggers and attacks, and take it with you when you go to the doctor. There are loads of treatments so the chances of something working are very high.

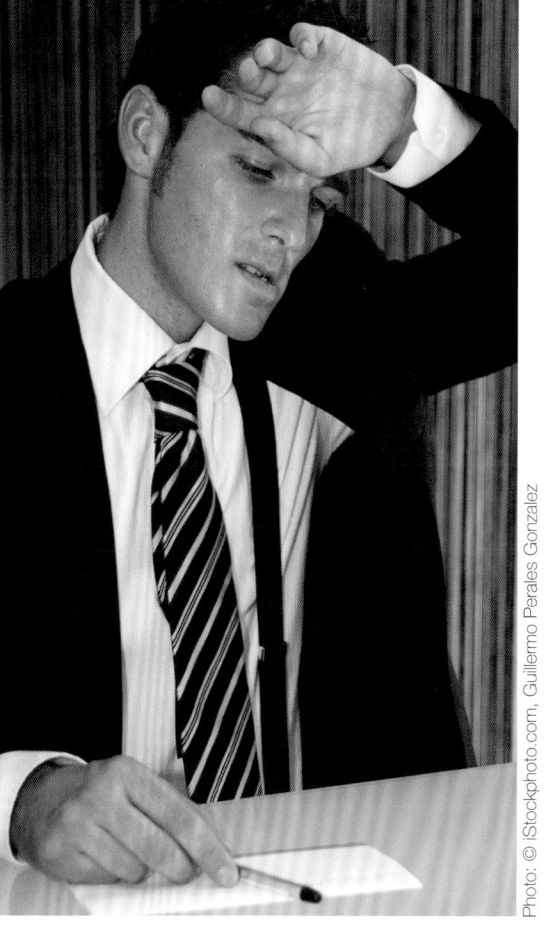

Photo: © iStockphoto.com, Guillermo Perales Gonzalez

## Complications

The greatest danger from headaches is missing the rare occasion when something more serious is the problem.

Your irritability increases and you find you have a greater risk of an accident, as well as abusing painkillers.

## Self care

Light can hurt the eyes and lying in a darkened room helps for some people, although modern thought is to avoid such isolation and instead get on with 'normal' life.

The attack can last from minutes to days. Painkillers work for many men, and there are treatments available from your doctor which may reduce or even prevent a full blown migraine attack.

BRAIN

# Stroke

*Words by Paula de Souza and Natika Halil*
*The Stroke Association*

A stroke happens when there is an interruption to the blood supply to the brain. Most strokes happen when a blood clot blocks the flow of blood. Less commonly a stroke can happen because of bleeding in or around the brain.

A Transient Ischaemic Attack (TIA) is similar to a stroke and is sometimes called a mini stroke. The symptoms are the same as stroke but they do not last as long, and the person recovers completely within 24 hours.

The common symptoms of a stroke or TIA are:

● Sudden numbness, weakness or paralysis on one side of the body.
● Sudden problem with speaking or understanding speech.
● Sudden blurring or loss of vision, particularly in one eye.
● Sudden dizziness or unsteadiness.
● Sudden memory loss or confusion.

There are no signs that a stroke is going to happen. When someone has the symptoms it is because the stroke or TIA is happening at that time.

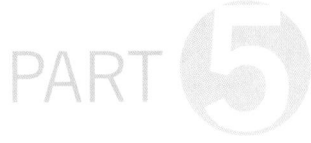

If you suspect someone may be having a stroke call 999 or 112 and get a medical help as soon as possible.

## Men and stroke

Stroke is a serious health issue for men. Each year in England and Wales, over 130,000 people have a stroke, and 57% of strokes in those aged under 75 occur in men. Although stroke is more common as we get older, it can happen to anyone. Almost 25,000 people aged under 65 have a stroke each year, accounting for 18% of all strokes.

## Psychological effects of stroke

Many people are aware of the physical effects of stroke such as one-sided weakness and loss of speech, but stroke can cause a range of psychological effects too. These effects can be because the stroke has directly affected the part of the brain controlling emotion or behaviour. Also, stroke happens very suddenly, and it can be hard coping with the emotional and physical after-effects.

### Depression

Depression is one of the most common problems after stroke, up to half of people who survive a stroke will experience some depression in the first year. Depression can affect anyone and it can develop immediately after the stroke happens, or weeks or months later. Being assessed and receiving the right help is crucial as managing depression can really make a difference.

Sometimes the stroke causes direct damage or chemical changes in the brain that can lead to depression. There can also be underlying physical causes for depression after stroke such as chronic pain. Depression often sets in once the initial period of recovery is over, and the person has become aware of how their lasting disability may affect their everyday life. With this, they may have to come to terms with the loss of some hopes and plans for the future, as well as having to adapt to a changed role in the family, and possibly the loss of a career. All this can affect confidence and self-esteem.

The symptoms of depression after stroke are the same as for depression generally and include:
- Feeling sad, blue or down in the dumps.
- A loss of interest in everyday activities.
- Feelings of worthlessness, hopelessness or despair.
- Anxiety or worry.
- Changes in sleeping pattern or appetite.
- Suicidal feelings.
- Low self-esteem.

The most effective treatment for depression is psychological intervention or counselling combined, if appropriate, with anti-depressant medication. Psychological and counselling services aim to encourage people to talk about their thoughts and feelings and help them to come to terms with what has happened.

Anti-depressant medication works by acting on the chemicals in the brain. Many anti-depressants are very effective and about two thirds of people who take them benefit. Anti-depressants take at least two weeks to work properly, and there are many alternatives to try if there is no improvement after this time.

### Personality changes

Where parts of the brain controlling personality and behaviour have been affected by the stroke, this can result in personality changes. Some people become impatient and irritable or withdrawn and introspective. Sometimes previous character traits can be reversed, with a mild mannered person becoming aggressive, a difficult person becoming more passive or a once sociable and lively person may become less sociable and withdrawn. More commonly, however, existing traits are exaggerated.

These psychological changes can be very difficult for family and friends to cope with, especially if the behaviour is aimed at one person only. Some stroke people are unaware that their behaviour has changed or that it is upsetting for their families. Sometimes explaining this to the stroke person is helpful. It is also important for family members to have support for themselves.

### Apathy

Apathy is a lack of motivation or enthusiasm. Someone with apathy may appear indifferent to everyday occurrences and unmoved by emotional events that would arouse strong feelings in other people, or in themselves previously. Often there is a loss of interest in things going on around, such as socialising or previous hobbies. Apathy can be a symptom of depression after stroke, or can be a symptom on its own, a result of the changes in the brain due to the stroke.

Many survivors with post-stroke apathy are happy to join in activities and are able to manage responsibilities, provided that they are assisted in getting started and setting goals. People with apathy depend upon kind encouragement from carers, friends and family to help them to make plans and overcome inactivity. As with many of the after effects of stroke feelings of apathy often begin to disappear through the recovery process, or if it is as a result of depression, as the depression begins to lift. If however after a period of time apathy linked to depression shows no sign of lifting, then anti-depressant medications and counselling may help.

### Emotional lability

Emotional lability is the term used when someone is more emotional and/or has difficulty controlling their emotions. Some people describe feeling as though all their emotions are 'much nearer the surface' or more exaggerated after their stroke. For example they may become upset more easily, or cry at things they would not have cried at before their stroke. Their emotional response is in line with their feelings, but is much stronger than before the stroke. For other people the symptoms can be more exaggerated, and some stroke people find that they cry for little or no reason. Less commonly, people laugh rather than cry, but again the emotion is out of place and does not match how they are feeling at the time.

These emotions usually come and go very quickly, which is unlike when someone feels upset and is crying. Some people may even swing from crying to laughing. Although the stroke person realises that their crying or laughter doesn't fit the situation, they cannot control it and this in itself can be very upsetting.

Emotional lability is generally worse soon after the stroke happens, but usually lessons or goes away with time as the person recovers from the stroke. If this doesn't happen, the GP may be able to help. Some medications that are also used to treat depression can help with the control of emotions even if the person is not depressed.

### Recovery and rehabilitation

As with all effects of stroke, these psychological effects can improve over time. As the brain heals and the stroke person comes to terms with what has happened and how life may have changed, effects such as depression can improve. Although most recovery from stroke happens in the first few months, there is no end to the recovery period and changes and improvements can still happen many months and even years later.

Unfortunately there is no way to predict how much recovery someone will make after stroke or how long that may take. For some people the damage done to the brain cannot be healed and they are left living with the effects of their stroke. Part of the rehabilitation process involves learning to adapt to how things have changed because of the stroke and there is help and support available.

## Available help

If you are concerned about any psychological changes after stroke, discuss these with the GP in the first instance.

The GP can advise on any medication that may be helpful, and make referrals to a clinical psychologist or counsellor if appropriate.

Relationship counselling, for example through an organisation such as Relate, can be helpful for the stroke person and their partner.

Support groups are a useful way of meeting people who have been through similar experiences. Contact The Stroke Association for details of groups near you.

## Helping yourself

There are many things that can be done to ease the psychological effects of stroke. Not all of the suggestions will suit everyone, but most people find at least one or two helpful.

### Startling Stats
- Stroke is a serious health issue. Each year in over 130,000 people have a stroke – that's one person every five minutes.
- Stroke doesn't just affect older people, it can happen to anyone. Almost 25,000 people aged under 65 have a stroke each year, accounting for 18% of all strokes.
- 57% of strokes in those aged under 75 occur in men.
- Stroke is the third largest cause of death in the UK, causing 9% of all deaths in men.

## Mental men myths

**Stroke only causes physical effects**

While stroke does cause numerous physical effects, many people experience psychological effects too, such as depression, apathy and personality changes.

**Stroke cannot be prevented**

There are many lifestyle changes you can make to reduce your risk of stroke. These include:

- Eating a healthy diet: cutting down on salt, sugar and fat, and eating plenty of fruit and vegetables.
- Taking regular exercise
- Giving up smoking
- Seeing your doctor regularly for check ups such as blood pressure, cholesterol and diabetes.

### Keep informed

Having information about stroke can be reassuring and if there is something you are not sure about, or you do not understand, don't be afraid to ask your doctor or carer to explain. The Stroke Association can also help with information about stroke and its effects.

### Social contact

Meeting people regularly, everyday if possible, is important, especially against effects such as depression. Talking to others can also be a big help.

### Hobbies and interests

Returning to hobbies and interests is an important part of the rehabilitation process after stroke. Many activities can be adapted to enable you to carry on enjoying them, and you could even look at trying new things.

### Exercise

Recent research shows that exercise is very beneficial in treating and preventing depression. Doing any physical activity regularly, however gentle, can help.

### Healthy diet

A poor diet can make you feel tired and run down. Try to eat regular meals with fresh fruit and vegetables every day.

## Further information

The Stroke Association is the only national charity solely concerned with combating stroke in people of all ages. Their vision is to have a world where there are fewer strokes and all those touched by stroke get the help they need. They can provide information and support on all aspects of stroke from prevention to rehabilitation. The website contains lots of information about stroke, and includes a discussion board, Talkstroke, where people affected by stroke can share their experiences.

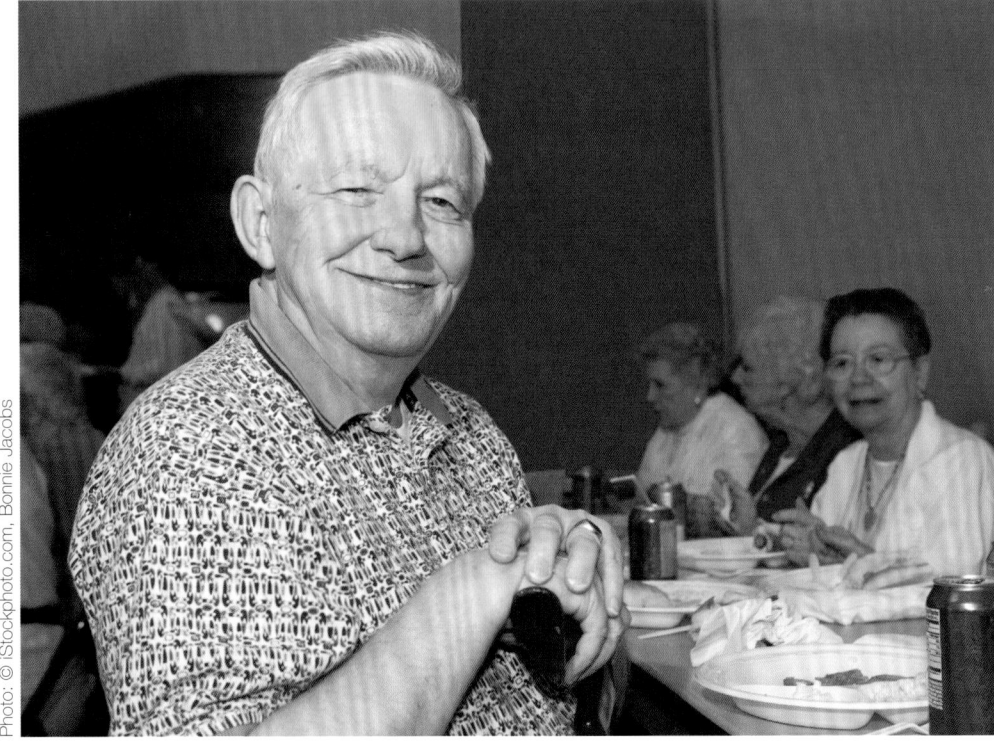

Photo: © iStockphoto.com, Bonnie Jacobs

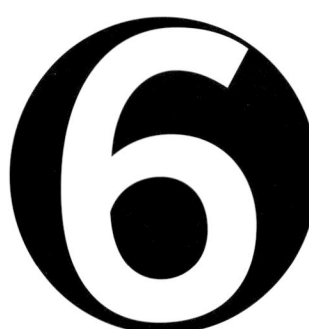

# Digestive system

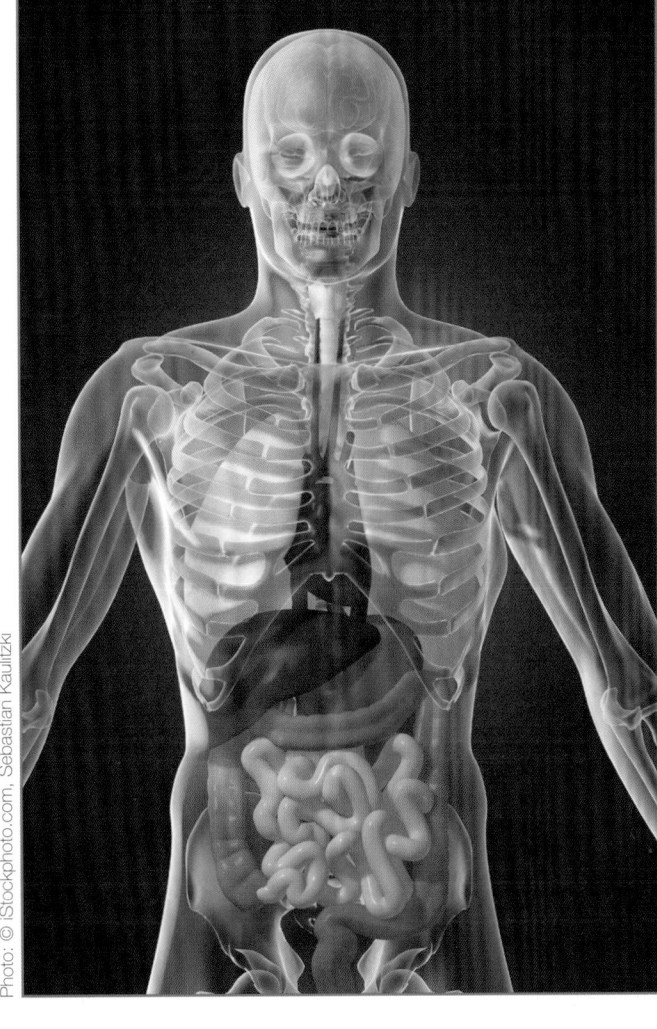

Photo: © iStockphoto.com, Sebastian Kaulitzki

# PART **6** Cirrhosis of the liver

## Introduction

Cirrhosis is the deterioration of the liver due to gradual internal scarring of its tissues. This destroys the ability of the liver to carry out its numerous and vital functions such as cleaning the blood. Many drugs and toxins such as alcohol are broken down in the liver. It also produces hormones and albumin to control body functions and maintain the right environment for tissues in the body. Very importantly it produces many of the clotting factors which stop bleeding.

## Symptoms

In the early stages there are only mild symptoms. These can develop into vomiting, weight loss, general malaise, indigestion and swelling of the abdomen. Bruising becomes easier to produce, with frequent nosebleeds and blood in the urine. Small red spider-like spots can appear on the upper chest arms and face. Later on, frank jaundice may occur with a yellow pigment in the skin and white of the eyes. Men lose their libido and develop female-shaped breasts.

## Causes

There are many causes which include chronic alcohol abuse, malnutrition, and infections such as hepatitis B.

## Prevention

Drink in moderation. Get vaccinated against hepatitis where appropriate.

## Complications

Unfortunately liver failure is often fatal. Liver transplantation is possible, and can save lives with a suitable donor, but this is a last resort.

## Self care

High-protein food challenges a liver already under stress from cirrhosis. Vitamin B complexes may help protect the liver but this is controversial.

## Action

Make an appointment to see your GP.

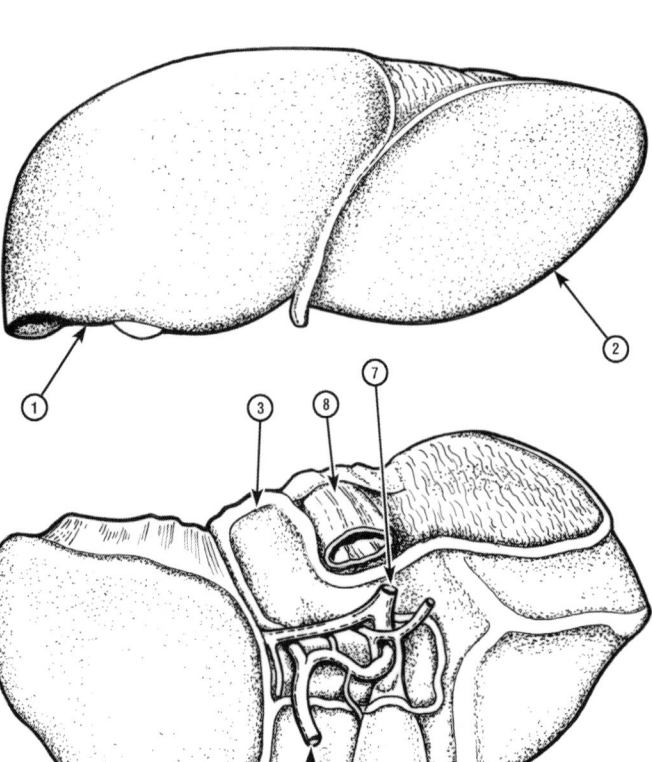

H32932

The liver

1 *Right lobe*
2 *Left lobe*
3 *Caudate lobe*
4 *Quadrate lobe*
5 *Hepatic artery*
6 *Gall bladder*
7 *Portal van*
8 *Inferior vena cava*

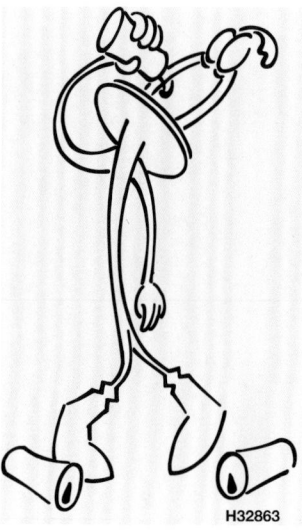

H32863

Too many soakings will cause your filters to block and corrode. Try to drink in moderation

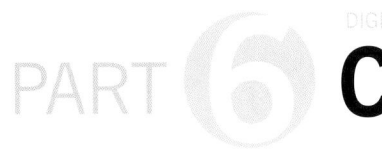

# Constipation

## Introduction

One of the great British obsessions is with passing a motion every day. If this doesn't happen we think we are constipated. In fact there is no 'normal' number of times you need to go to the toilet. What we do know is that putting it off for too long can cause constipation. Thankfully, the serious causes of constipation are relatively rare especially in people under 45 years old.

## Symptoms

A significant change in normal bowel movements with very irregular and difficult to pass motions. There may be abdominal pain and bloating.

## Causes

Perhaps the single greatest cause in older people is a lack of activity. This is particularly true if there is some disability. Not drinking enough non alcoholic fluids and a lack of fibre in the diet are also major factors.

Many people do not realise that over use of laxatives can cause a severe constipation, particularly once they are stopped. Some medicines, particularly pain killers containing codeine, are powerful constipating agents. Stress can cause constipation, not least because it can lead to poor diet, but also stress directly affects the bowel.

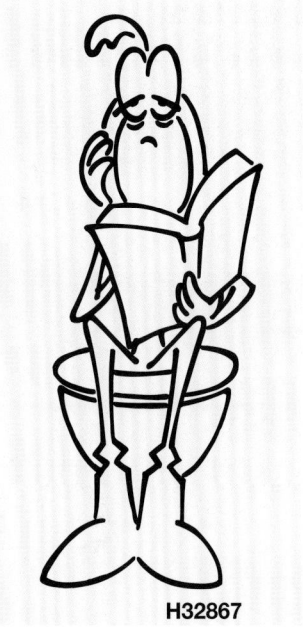

**H32867**

Faulty exhausts can usually be fixed quite easily

## Prevention

Most of the preventative measures are just sensible attention to the things that cause constipation such as:
- Increase your fluids, particularly pure fruit juices.
- Increase your activity.
- Wean yourself off laxatives.
- Eat more fibre and fruit.
- Ask your doctor about the medicines you are on at present.

## Complications

Although it feels terrible, constipation rarely causes any serious harm. The big danger is ignoring the warning signs of something more serious and not having it checked out soon enough.

## Action

See your pharmacist. Make an appointment with your doctor if:
- After a few days you begin to vomit as well.
- There is severe abdominal pain.
- You pass any blood in the motion.
- You are losing weight.
- The change in bowel habit happened without any good reason.

# PART 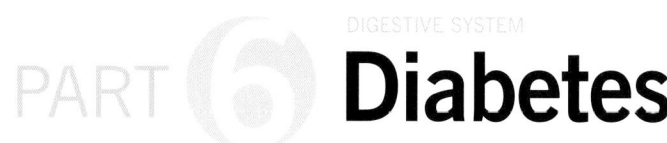 **Diabetes**

## Introduction

Sugar in the blood varies between certain fairly narrow limits. Because people with diabetes have little or no insulin (a hormone that breaks down sugar), there is a constant tendency for the blood sugar levels to rise. An excessive rise is associated with the over-production of dangerous acidic substances called 'ketones'.

Type I or insulin dependent diabetes, in which the man produces no insulin, affects about 1% of the population.

Type II diabetes, often called maturity-onset diabetes, is regarded as a condition in which the body cells don't react to insulin, or in which the amount of insulin produced by the pancreas is not enough for the body to function normally.

Type II diabetes can often be treated simply by diet and, if necessary, weight loss. This reduces the sugar demands but, possibly more important, it also makes lowered demands on the insulin supply. Other cases require oral anti-diabetic drugs which stimulate the pancreas to produce more insulin.

Diabetes UK estimate there are 1 million people in the UK with diabetes, and another 1 million as yet undiagnosed.

## Symptoms

Thirst, excessive urine and, in type I diabetes, weight loss are the major symptoms.

## Causes

Diabetes is caused by the failure of the specialised pancreas cells called islet cells to produce the hormone insulin. Insulin is essential for the building up of important large molecules, such as fats, proteins and glycogen, from small molecules such as glucose and amino acids and for the uptake of glucose for energy by cells such as muscle cells.

## Diagnosis

Diabetes is diagnosed by finding sugar in the urine, and by testing the levels of blood sugar at different times of day.

## Prevention

At present it is not possible to prevent type I diabetes.

The risk of type II diabetes can be greatly reduced by eating less so as to avoid obesity. Put simply, fat is not just a feminist issue, it's a diabetes issue.

## Complications

Hypoglycaemia is an abnormally low level of sugar (glucose) in the blood. This is a dangerous state as the brain is totally dependent on a constant supply of glucose as fuel. Hypoglycaemia occurs when there is a failure of balance between insulin dosage, food intake and energy expenditure

Hypoglycaemia can cause headache, mental confusion, slurred speech, abnormal behaviour, loss of memory, numbness,

double vision, temporary paralysis, fits, coma and death. The pulse is rapid, there is trembling, faintness and palpitations, and there may be profuse sweating.

The diabetic's behaviour is often irrational and disorderly and may be mistaken for drunkenness. The most common cause of hypoglycaemia is a relative overdose of insulin. The dose taken may be the same as normal but the carbohydrate intake may have been reduced or the amount of exertion increased so that fuel is used up faster than normal.

The immediate treatment is to take sugar and this will usually end an episode. Those with insulin dependent diabetes should always carry readily digested sugar or some other complex carbohydrate such as a biscuit, which takes longer to digest to prevent a sudden relapse. The drop in blood sugar can also be caused by over-dosage with oral hypoglycaemic drugs.

Glucagon is a protein hormone produced by the islet cells of the pancreas, which has an effect opposite to that of insulin. By causing glycogen, stored in the liver, to break down to glucose, it increases the amount of sugar in the bloodstream.

Poorly controlled diabetes can lead to eye, kidney and heart problems as well as erectile dysfunction. For example, diabetic retinopathy (a disorder, caused by diabetes, that affects the eyes) is the most common cause of blindness in the UK adult population.

## Treatment

Any form of diabetes can be effectively managed so it doesn't seriously affect your life. Look at Sir Steve Redgrave, having diabetes hasn't stopped him achieving his goals.

Type I diabetes is treated with insulin injections and diet and exercise control, all monitored by frequent checks of the blood sugar levels. Pancreatic or islet cell transplantation is still experimental but there have been major advances.

Type II diabetes is treated by weight loss, diet control, oral hypoglycaemic drugs and also insulin injections.

## Action

Make an appointment to see your GP.

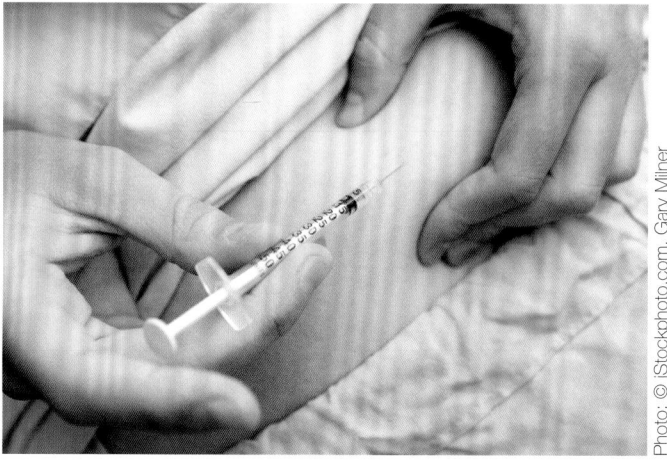

Photo: © iStockphoto.com, Gary Milner

PART 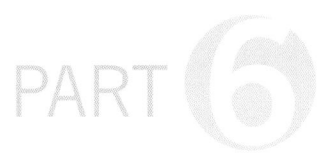 **6**

# Bowel cancer

*This section has been developed by the national charity Beating Bowel Cancer.*

## Breaking down taboos

To take a stereotype, the British man is well known for his reluctance to talk openly – let alone seek advice – about his own health. With so-called 'embarrassing' problems, the British stiff upper lip is even more tightly pursed. While toilet humour is an accepted form of banter in the office or over a drink, talking about any personal problems related to bottoms is a real no-no for many men – even with health professionals, close family or friends. Language is often a barrier for men trying to describe their symptoms, with words such as 'rectum' or 'diarrhoea' causing acute social embarrassment.

> Bowel cancer is more common in men than women, and more men will die from it as well. Part of the reason is later diagnosis.

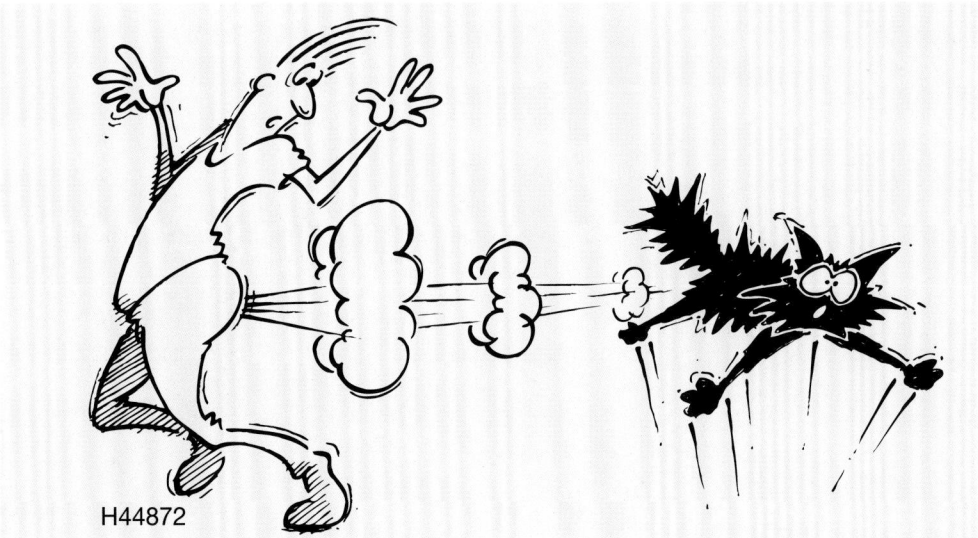

H44872

Bowel cancer is not caused by eating vindaloo

Although many people find it embarrassing to talk about symptoms of bowel problems, it is surprising how common they really are. There are lots of common conditions that could cause changes in the workings of the bowels, pain and bleeding from the bottom. In most cases, it won't be cancer.

## The scale of the problem

Bowel cancer is the second most deadly cancer in the UK – only lung cancer kills more people. Around 35,600 people are diagnosed with the disease each year and over 45% will die as a result. That means that it claims the lives of over 16,000 men and women in the UK each year.

However, bowel cancer is one of the most curable cancers if caught early enough. It is estimated that around 80% of cases could be treated successfully if caught at an early stage.

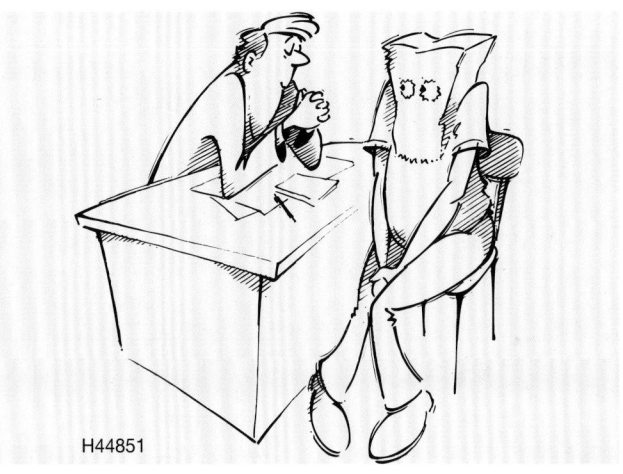

British man is well known for his reluctance to talk openly

H44851

115

## What is bowel cancer?

The large bowel is a question-mark-shaped tube of muscle – about four feet long – which runs from the appendix, via the colon, to the rectum. Bowel cancer is cancer of any part of this tube. If it is not treated, it will increase in size and may cause a blockage, or it can ulcerate, leading to blood loss and anaemia.

Most cancers start with wart-like growths known as polyps on the wall of the gut. Polyps are very common as we get older – one in ten people over 60 have them. However, most polyps do not turn into cancer. If potentially cancerous polyps can be found at an early stage, they can be removed painlessly without the need for a major operation.

## Don't sit on your symptoms

The most common symptoms are change of bowel habit and rectal bleeding. However, these are also common in people who don't have cancer. The facts show that:

- Nearly 20% of us experience bleeding from the bottom each year.
- Over a third of us experience constipation or diarrhoea at some point in our lives.

If you have any of the higher risk symptoms outlined below, it is safe to 'watch and wait' for up to six weeks. But if they persist, you should get advice from your GP and ask about the possibility of further investigation.

- Change of bowel habit (especially important if you also have bleeding) – a recent, persistent change of bowel habit to looser, more diarrhoea-like motions, going to the toilet or trying to 'go' more often.
- Rectal bleeding – look out for rectal bleeding that persists with no reason. For example, bleeding can be due to piles – but if so you will have other symptoms such as straining with hard stools, a sore bottom, lumps and itching. If you are over 60 piles could be hiding more serious symptoms, so it is especially important to get this investigated.

## Other high risk symptoms and signs

- Unexplained anaemia, found by your GP.
- A lump or mass in your abdomen, felt by your GP.
- Persistent, severe abdominal pain which has come on recently for the first time (especially in older people).

## What's wrong with me?

Most people with these symptoms do not have bowel cancer, but if they persist beyond the 6 week 'watch and wait' period it is very important to have further tests to rule it out.

Your symptoms could be caused by the following:

- Piles or haemorrhoids: soft swellings, a bit like spongy varicose veins, which usually have other symptoms such as pain and itching. Bright red bleeding found on the toilet paper or sudden large amounts of blood are almost always caused by piles. Your GP or pharmacist will be able to recommend a fast and effective over-the-counter treatment
- Polyps: wart-like growths on the bowel lining, which can sometimes cause bleeding. These can be removed painlessly without the need for an operation.
- Fissures: a split or tear in the lining of the gut, sometimes caused by constipation. Fissures can be treated with creams available from the pharmacist

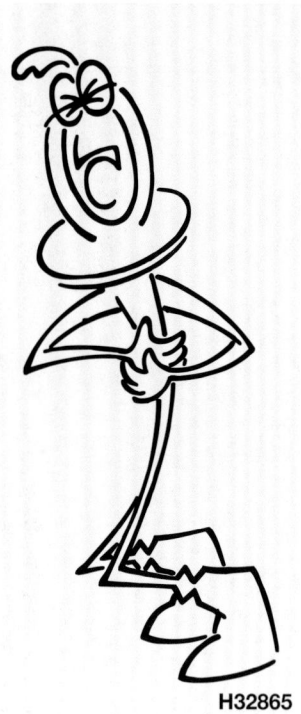

**H32865**

Corrosion in your fuel tank can be dangerous. Get it sorted out before you get a leak

Early detection gives the best protection, so know your bum, chum.

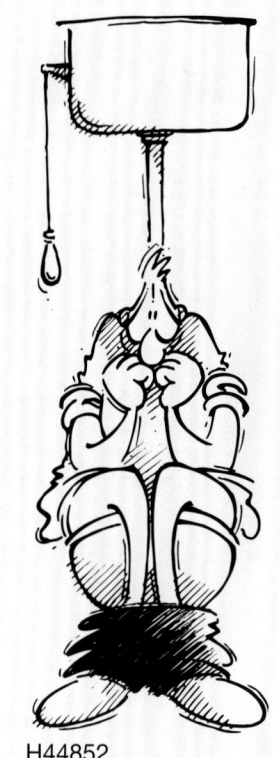

**H44852**

Don't sit on your symptoms

- Crohn's disease: Painful inflammation of the gut, which can put you more at risk of bowel cancer. If you suffer from the condition, you should ask your GP to be monitored regularly for bowel cancer.
- Ulcerative colitis: inflammation of the bowel which can cause bleeding and mucus. This condition can put you at a greater risk from bowel cancer and you should talk to your GP about being monitored.

In the league table of commonest male cancers, bowel cancer comes in at third place after cancer of skin and prostate.

## Family history
While bowel cancer can in some cases be put down to genetics, family history doesn't necessarily mean that you are going to get it. In general, the closer the relatives are to you (eg, brother, sister, mother, father, child) and the younger they were diagnosed, the more you need to get it checked out. The following is a guide to the action you may need to take depending on your family history:
- One close relative under 45 affected. Talk to your GP about screening in your area. It is usually recommended 10 years before the age at which your relative developed the disease.
- Two or more close relatives from the same side of the family. The younger those relatives, the more need there is for you to discuss screening with your GP.
- Less strong family history (such as a grandparent who died in their 70s). You are probably not at an increased risk. However, do talk to your GP if you are worried.

Screening for bowel cancer can help to detect polyps, which may be cancerous, at an early stage, and is usually carried out using a simple procedure called a colonoscopy. Alternatively, if you have been diagnosed with cancer, or you have a relative with bowel cancer who is willing to be tested, you might be offered genetic testing if your doctor thinks that your family is likely to have a genetic mutation in one of the known bowel cancer genes.

## Diet and lifestyle
In many cases bowel cancer occurs without any obvious cause. However, experts also suggest that a diet high in red meat and low in fibre, fruit and vegetables can increase the risk of bowel cancer. Obesity, high alcohol consumption and lack of physical exercise may also put you at risk.

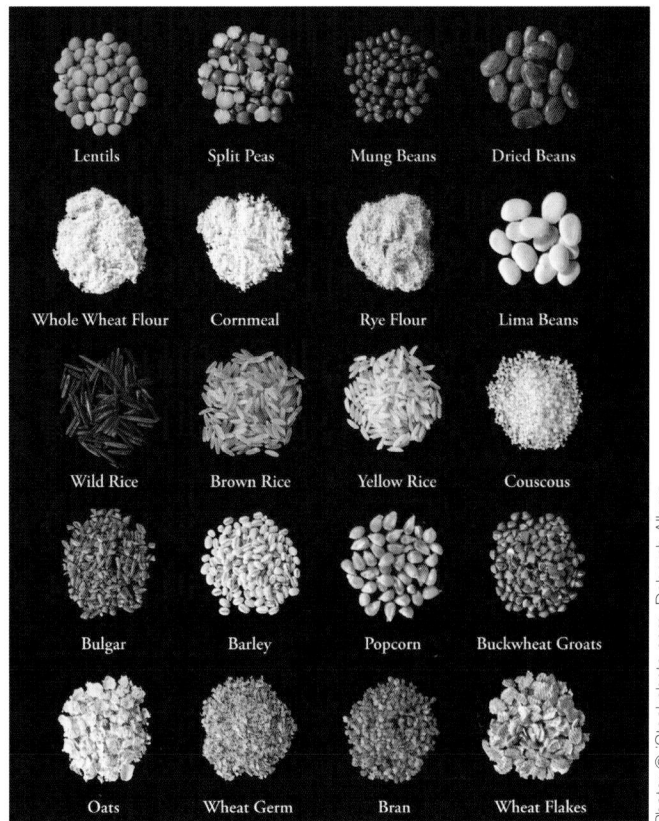

Lentils · Split Peas · Mung Beans · Dried Beans
Whole Wheat Flour · Cornmeal · Rye Flour · Lima Beans
Wild Rice · Brown Rice · Yellow Rice · Couscous
Bulgar · Barley · Popcorn · Buckwheat Groats
Oats · Wheat Germ · Bran · Wheat Flakes

Photo: © iStockphoto.com, Deborah Albers

## Eating healthily
A high fibre diet is particularly recognised for reducing the risk of constipation, irritable bowel syndrome and bowel cancer. Fibre is indigestible plant material such as cellulose, lignin and pectin which is found in fruits, vegetables, grains and beans. There are two types of fibre – soluble and insoluble. Fibre provides bulk to your food, helps it pass easily through the gut and also retains water (so making us feel full and therefore we eat less).

Reports suggest that we should be eating 18g of fibre each day – yet most of us probably eat much less (around 10-12g). To give a couple of examples, a banana contains 1.8g, as does 1 slice of wholemeal toast.

When increasing your fibre intake, start slowly and build up to the recommended level.

> Your risk increases if there is bowel cancer in the family, but diet and smoking are among the main culprits.

| High fibre food | Lower fibre food |
| --- | --- |
| Whole grain breads, eg, 100% whole wheat, cracked wheat, multigrain, pumpernickel or dark rye | White bread |
| Whole grain cereal containing bran, oatmeal, barley, bulgar, cracked wheat; also Shredded Wheat, multigrain or granola cereals Refined cereals | |
| Whole grain flours, eg, whole wheat, rye, graham (eg, biscuits, muffins) | Foods made with white flour |
| Whole grain pastas, brown rice or wild rice | Refined pastas, instant or polished rice |
| Fresh fruits and veg | Fruit juice |
| Salads (with variety of raw vegetables) | Plain lettuce salads |
| Baked beans, cooked lentils, split peas | Meat, fish, poultry |
| Nuts, popcorn, seeds, dried fruit | Crisps, other snacks |

# Exercise for life

Recent research has found compelling evidence that regular exercise could cut the risk of developing bowel cancer by 50%. The recommendation is that to help reduce the risk of cancer, people should aim for 30 minutes of moderate intensity physical activity at least three times a week.

# Being referred for hospital investigation

How you are investigated depends on what is available at your local hospital.

People with higher risk symptoms should be referred within two weeks for investigation. Most people with these symptoms do not have cancer, but it should be ruled out by special tests.

The results of the tests are received by the patient at the hospital. Waiting for the results can be worrying and frustrating – and going to the appointment for your news can be extremely nerve-wracking. If you are worried, talk to your family, friends or your GP.

If your results are negative, you may be diagnosed with another common gut condition (see *What's wrong with me?* above) and given appropriate treatment.

> Bowel cancer is not caused by sitting on hot radiators, eating vindaloo or even using newspaper for bog roll.

# After the diagnosis

After initial diagnosis, you will discuss the options open to you with your specialist who will put together a treatment plan (depending on the type and size of the cancer, what stage the cancer is at and your personal health and age) including:
● When and where treatment will take place.
● What drugs will be available.
● Who will be treating you.

The main forms of treatment for bowel cancer are as follows.

### Surgery

During the operation the piece of bowel that contains the cancer is removed and the two open ends are joined together. The lymph nodes near the bowel may also be removed because this is the first place to which the cancer may spread. Surgery can be used alone, or in combination with radiotherapy and/or chemotherapy.

### Chemotherapy

This treatment uses anti-cancer drugs to destroy the cancer cells and is often given after surgery to reduce the chances of the cancer coming back. It is also given when the cancer is advanced and has spread to other parts of the body.

Chemotherapy drugs cause different side effects in different people. Some people experience few side effects; even those who do will have them only temporarily during treatment. Some of the common side effects are tiredness, hair loss, mouth ulcers and nausea. Chemotherapy is sometimes given with radiotherapy before surgery.

### Radiotherapy

This treatment is normally used only to treat cancer of the rectum and can be given before or after surgery. Radiotherapy may also be given as a palliative treatment to relieve symptoms of the disease, eg, to reduce pain.

### Colostomy

Most people diagnosed with bowel cancer do not need a colostomy – also called a stoma. Some people may need a temporary stoma but this can often be reversed after a few months. Although people need to time to adjust to having a stoma, life can carry on as normal. Contact the British Colostomy Association for more information.

# Will the cancer come back?

After you have had treatment, you will need to have regular check-ups every few months to make sure that the cancer has not returned or spread. If the bowel cancer was diagnosed and treated early there is a very good chance that it will not recur after treatment.

Even if the cancer does recur it can be treated with a combination of further surgery, chemotherapy or radiotherapy. If the cancer has not returned after five years, you are considered clear.

# Emotional support

Remaining positive and strong for friends, family and children can be difficult when you are going through the trauma of diagnosis and treatment yourself. Talking to friends or partners can help – but you may also want to ask your doctor about specialist support available to you such as counsellors or nurses.

There are also many national and local charities, patient support groups and help lines which could offer you information, help and emotional support.

If you can't find the help you need – or want to try to help others – you may want to consider setting up your own local patient support group.

## Some things increase your risk
● A junk food diet (high in fats and sugars, low in fibre).
● Bowel cancer in the close family.
● Lack of activity.
● Being overweight.
● Smoking tobacco.
● A bowel condition called polyps or adenomatous polyposis significantly increases your risk, even in another member of your family. Trying to pronounce it can be pretty stressful too.

## The good news is you can reduce your risk
● Check out your diet. Reduce the amount of fat and sugars and boost fruit and vegetables.
● Regular physical activity and keeping your weight under control.
● Discuss any family history with your doctor, who may advise more frequent tests.
● Quit the weed!

# PART 6 Oesophageal (gullet) cancer

## Introduction

This particularly nasty cancer is unfortunately not rare, with about 1 in 50 of all new cases of cancer being that of the oesophagus. It is more common in people from Iran or China although their risk falls after a few generations in the UK. Men will suffer from this cancer almost twice as often as do women although this is set to change as men increasingly give up smoking, one of the main causes of oesophageal cancer.

Although predominantly a disease of old age, men of 45–50 years can develop it. As the symptoms tend to be confused with indigestion or heartburn, late presentation to the doctor is the norm rather than the exception.

## Cause

Drinking neat spirits and smoking come high on the list of suspects, but otherwise the causes are not really known. Pre-existing problems with the gullet such as strictures (narrowing) may increase your risk from cancer but it is by no means certain. Even so it is worth keeping an open mind and seeing your doctor if the symptoms become worse.

## Symptoms

Unfortunately there may be no symptoms until late in the course of the disease. Once established these can include:
- Pain and difficulty swallowing. This starts with solid food but later includes fluids as well.
- Undigested food being brought up after a meal. If the obstruction is large there can also be problems swallowing saliva until this food is brought back up.
- Persistent coughing as a result of food 'going the wrong way' when being brought back up.
- Weight loss and lack of appetite.

## Diagnosis

A barium swallow can help show any constriction. A radio opaque solution is swallowed while X-rays are taken; this will be followed by endoscopy using flexible telescope to take samples from any tumour seen. The big danger is from it spreading to other parts of the body and a CT or MRI scan may be used to check for these metastases.

## Treatment

More than with most other cancers a great deal depends on whether there has been any spread. A localised tumour can be removed, but distant spread is much more difficult to treat. Making swallowing easier by using radiotherapy or chemotherapy to reduce the size of the tumour can make remaining life much more bearable.

## Prevention

Diluting your drinks and taking them in moderation along with stopping smoking are the best ways of reducing your risk.

The digestive system

1  Tongue
2  Liver
3  Duodenum
4  Rectum
5  Caecum
6  Ascending colon
7  Oesophagus
8  Pancreas
9  Tranverve colon
10 Small intestine
11 Stomach
12 Descending colon

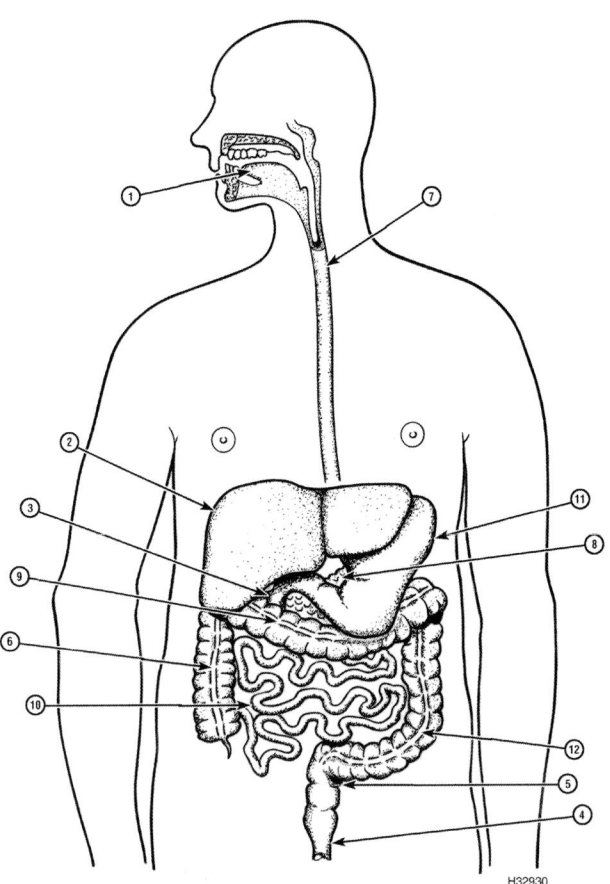

H32930

# PART 6 Cancer of the stomach

## Introduction

Stomach cancer is thankfully on the decline but is more common in men than in women, affecting about 1 in 7,000 each year. It is the sixth commonest of the potentially fatal cancers but rare under the age of 30, becoming commoner with increasing age.

There was great concern amongst some health professionals when ranitidine (Zantac), a treatment for reducing stomach acid production, was released from prescription only-status for sale across the pharmacist's counter. Fears that stomach cancer would go undiagnosed with a consequent increase in deaths were unfounded as, for reasons unknown, the reverse occurred.

## Symptoms

Stomach upsets are common, but stomach cancer is comparatively rare. Perhaps the most disturbing feature of stomach cancer is the difficulty in distinguishing it from the symptoms of stomach or duodenal ulcers. Most men complain of pain high in the abdomen in the angle between the ribs – follow your breast bone down to the soft bit – it is also often relieved by food. Unlike common stomach upsets, the pain refuses to go away on its own. Some men confuse it with angina, especially if they already suffer from a heart condition. The pain, however, is not helped by nitrate sprays or patches.

Late detection is the problem. The difficulty of early diagnosis means the cancer is often advanced by the time it is suspected and symptoms may also include swallowing difficulty, loss of weight, nausea and vomiting. Waiting and hoping it will go away is a bad idea.

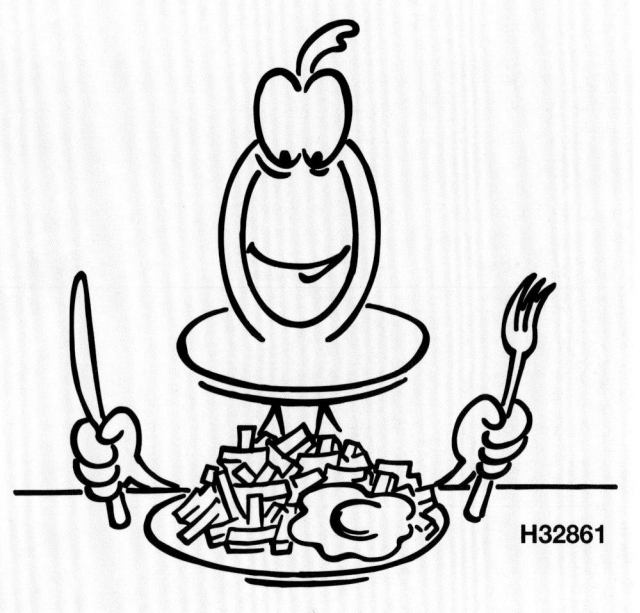

H32861

## Causes

Although a lack of fruit and vegetables in the diet may have a link, the jury is still out over foods causing stomach cancer. Things that irritate the stomach such as Helicobacter pylori bacteria may be linked with both stomach ulcers and stomach cancer. Similarly, alcohol and cigarette smoking may also increase your risk. Recent research suggests that too much salt in the diet may also be a factor.

As people with blood group A are more likely to develop stomach cancer there may be a genetic element in the causation. If there is stomach cancer in the family you should keep an open mind over stomach upsets or pain that refuses to go away. Even so, the fact that your mother, father, sister or brother developed stomach cancer is by no means an indication that you will as well. The number of men developing stomach cancer is falling anyway and this may be connected with the fall in cigarette smoking. Reducing your risks makes good sense whatever your blood group or family history.

## Diagnosis

Not surprisingly, diagnosis of stomach cancer can often be later rather than sooner. This is made all the worse by men's tendency to put off going to see their doctor. Clues come from the symptoms you describe to your doctor, and this is usually followed up with direct viewing through a flexible fibre optic instrument (gastroscope) which provides a view of the cancer and allows biopsies to be taken. A barium meal X-ray will show up stomach cancer in 90 per cent of cases. CT, MRI and ultrasound scanning can also be helpful, especially if there is any possibility of spread to other parts of the body.

## Prevention

Even though stomach cancer is on the decline you can reduce your risks further through common sense steps such as diluting and moderating your alcohol drinks, but most of all by stopping smoking.

If there is any family history of stomach cancer or you suffer from intermittent stomach pain, ask your GP to check for the Helicobacter pylori bacteria.

Most importantly, see your doctor early rather than later with any symptoms which refuse to go away or which are not helped by simple painkillers or antacids.

## Treatment

Treatment depends very much on how soon the cancer is diagnosed. Surgical removal of the tumour is possible if it is not too far advanced, and chemotherapy will generally be used to mop up any remaining tumour cells.

Keep you spark plugs in good working order and adjust your mixture to ensure appropriate fuel burning

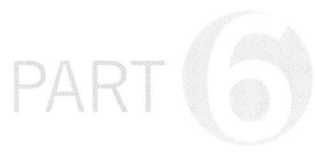

# Heartburn (reflux) or indigestion

Indigestion is more common in middle aged people, after heavy meals or alcohol consumption and is often worse at night.

Regurgitation or 'reflux' is painful although rarely dangerous. Stomach acid escapes into the gullet causing chest pain. It can be mistaken for a heart attack.

## Symptoms

Symptoms can appear in the following ways:
- Vague pain below the ribcage extending into the throat.
- Acid taste in the mouth.
- Excessive wind.

## Causes

- Classically after a heavy meal or drinking.
- 'Rich' food, often with a high fat content.
- Excessive smoking.
- A leaking valve at the neck of the stomach (Hiatus hernia).

## Prevention

- Avoid food which provokes an attack.
- Sleep with your upper body propped up with pillows.
- Avoid eating just before bed time.
- Eat small meals more often.
- Avoid aspirin and non-steroidal anti-inflammatory drugs.

## Complications

Most indigestion is harmless but annoying. The acid refluxing into the throat does not appear to cause any serious damage. The greatest danger is ignoring repeated attacks or confusing them with a heart attack. When in doubt seek medical help immediately.

## Self care

Your pharmacist will advise about indigestion remedies (antacids). Avoid taking large amounts of sodium bicarbonate (baking soda) as this is turned into salt in the body. A glass of milk before bed can help.

## Action

See your pharmacist or make an appointment to see your GP.

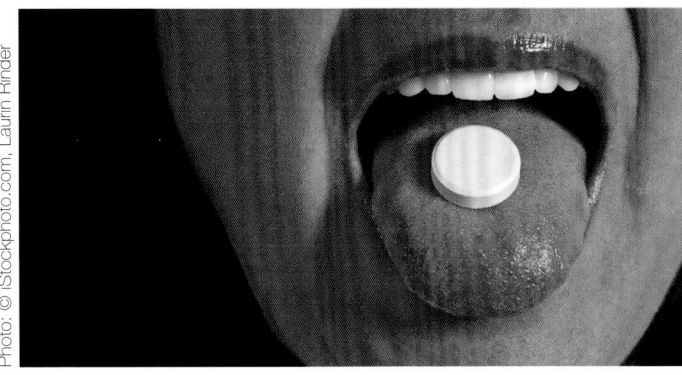

Photo: © iStockphoto.com, Laurin Rinder

# PART 6 Inguinal hernias (groin)

## Introduction

Muscle, fat, and skin generally keep the body contents where they should be. Occasionally, either through a muscle weakness, strain or congenital problem some part of the body will squeeze through a gap and find itself where it really shouldn't be.

The most common form of hernia involves a loop of bowel which is pushed though a weakness or defect in the muscle of the abdominal wall. They are rarely dangerous unless the bowel becomes trapped, swells and cuts off its own blood supply.

An inguinal hernia is usually a loop of bowel forced through a weakness in the abdominal wall at the groin. For anatomical reasons men suffer from inguinal hernias far more often than do women.

## Symptoms

Many men know when the rupture happened. Most describe a tearing sensation in the groin usually while lifting something heavy or even straining at the toilet. A small bulge appears at the crease between the thigh and abdomen. It can be felt better by standing up, placing two fingers along the crease of the groin and coughing. A light tap will be felt if there is a hernia.

This can get bigger as more bowel is pushed thorough the gap, extending even into the scrotum.

## Causes

While the male genitals are being formed a gap is formed in the abdominal wall to allow the testicles to travel from the abdomen into the scrotum. This leaves a potential weakness in the wall which may give way under strain.

Weak abdominal muscles and being generally unfit are said to increase your risk but not nearly as much as incorrectly lifting heavy weights.

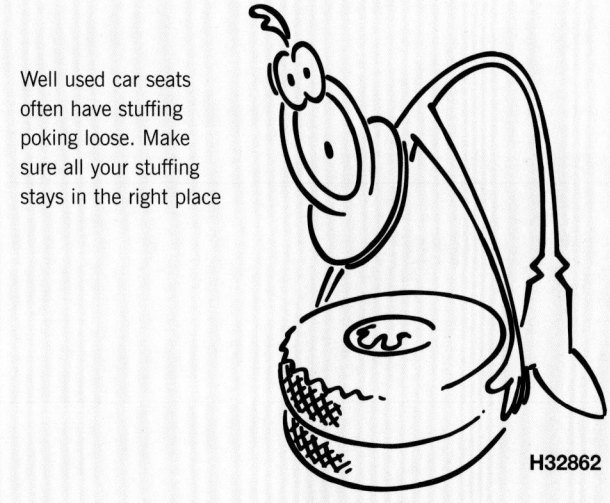

Well used car seats often have stuffing poking loose. Make sure all your stuffing stays in the right place

H32862

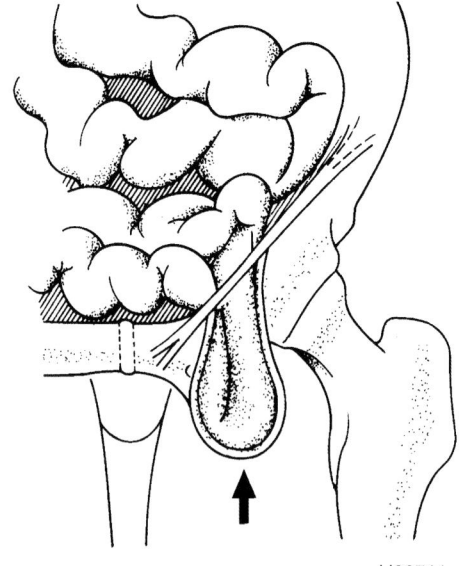

Formation of an inguinal hernia (arrowed)

H32711

## Prevention

Hernias are very common. Lifting is often a cause, so carrying heavy objects correctly is vital. If your work involves lifting heavy object or moving awkward things then ask for advice from your employers. Wearing a protective truss while lifting can also help, whilst keeping fit and maintaining muscle tone, especially the abdominal muscles, will help prevent a hernia.

## Complications

If the loop of bowel is blocked it will cause an obstruction, and you will experience pain. Your abdomen will swell and you may bring up foul smelling vomit.

This is an emergency not least because it can go on to become strangulated, cutting off its own blood supply. You will usually get some warning of this happening as the hernia becomes intensely itchy, painful, tender and hot.

## Self care

Protective girdles and trusses can prevent the hernia from protruding through the abdominal wall. Thousands of trusses are sold or prescribed every year and they do work well for some people.

Even so, modern surgery is now so quick and safe that it is probably better to have the hernia repaired than risk obstruction or strangulation later on in life. It can now be performed under a local anaesthetic so almost all age groups can be successfully and safely treated.

## Action

Make an appointment to see your GP.

PART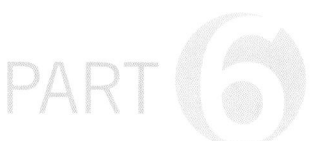

# Itchy anus (pruritus)

## Introduction

An itchy bottom is very common, and more common in adults than we like to admit in public. Children are less inhibited and make the problem clear for everyone to see. There are very few serious conditions which cause the itch although it can be embarrassing.

## Symptoms

A great deal depends on what is causing the itch. Threadworms lay their eggs in a ring around the anus at night which irritates the skin. The fine white worms can be seen in the motions. Piles, tears around the anus and irritation from excessive wiping after diarrhoea will make the anus itchy shortly after passing a motion.

## Causes

Other than those mentioned there is not always an obvious reason for itching although it is usually worse in warm weather.

## Prevention

- Wear loose cotton underwear.
- Eat a high fibre diet to prevent constipation causing small tears around the anus or piles.
- Use damp toilet paper first, then dry paper after passing a motion.
- Avoid harsh toilet paper and strong soaps.

## Complications

Constant itching can cause infection which only makes the itching worse.

## Self care

- Creams are available from your pharmacist to ease the itching.
- Check the motions for worms, particularly if there is a night time itch.
- Ask your pharmacist for a worming medicine.

## Action

See your pharmacist.

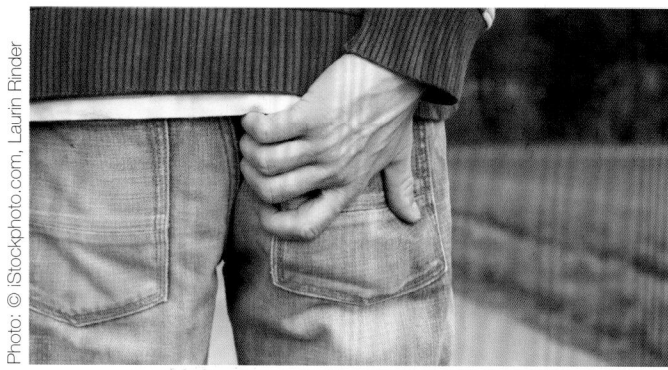

Photo: © iStockphoto.com, Laurin Rinder

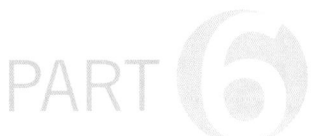

PART 6

# Metabolic syndrome

Forget what your maths teacher told you. Sometimes 2 plus 2 can equal five. If you have one risk factor for heart disease and then develop another, the risks don't just add together. For example, if you have hypertension your risk of suffering a heart attack is three times higher than someone with normal blood pressure. If you have both raised serum cholesterol and hypertension you are nine times more likely to develop heart disease than the average man. If you also smoke, your risk is 16 fold higher.

In 1988, an American researcher called Gerald Reaven recognised that having a large amount of visceral fat, in conjunction with other risk factors, dramatically increased the risk of developing heart disease and other conditions. Today, doctors call this cluster of risk factors the metabolic syndrome. If you have three or more at of the following you have the metabolic syndrome:

● Waist circumference of at least 40 inches (102 cm). This should not be measured where the waistband of your trousers sits but higher up around the level of your belly button where your waistline is at its largest.
● Triglycerides over 150 mg/dl (1.7 mmol/l). Triglycerides are a type of fat in your blood. Like the better known low-density lipoprotein (LDL; remember L for lethal) high levels of triglycerides increase your risk of developing heart disease.
● Levels of high-density lipoprotein (HDL) cholesterol under 40 mg/dl (1.0 mmol/l). HDL is the good fat – remember H for healthy. HDL carries cholesterol from your tissue to your liver, where it is destroyed.
● Blood pressure over 130/80 mmHg.
● A level of glucose in your blood while fasting over 110 mg/dl (6.11 mmol/l).

To find out your level of the last four in this list, you need to enlist the help of your GP. But if you've piled on the inches around the gut it is a good idea to get them checked.

Waist circumference should be measured around the level of your belly button where your waistline is at its largest

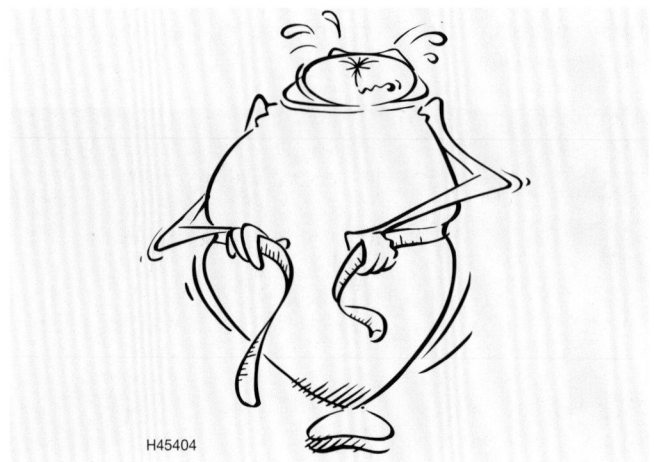

H45404

PART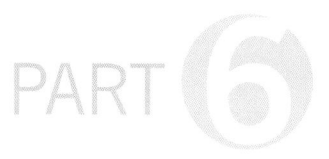

# Mouth ulcers

## Introduction
Ulcers in the mouth are very common. The vast majority are harmless and will clear on their own. Unfortunately some ulcers may be more serious and need the attention of your doctor. There are different types of ulcer the most common of which is the 'aphthous ulcer' seen more in teenagers. Teeth with jagged edges or badly fitting dentures will also cause ulcers, particularly on the gums and cheeks.

## Symptoms
Aphthous ulcers are small, white and usually less than pin head sized with a red border and despite being particularly painful will disappear within a week or so. They usually appear on the inside of the lower lip or inside the cheeks.

Drinking something hot or acidic like orange juice usually makes their presence known. Ulcers from teeth or dentures are usually larger and get bigger rather than disappear. Any ulcer which fails to get better within 2-3 weeks should be seen by your dentist or doctor.

## Causes
Aphthous ulcers appear spontaneously but more often during stress or being run down. Constant rubbing from a tooth, filling, dental plate or dentures will also cause an ulcer. Tongue and mouth cancer is extremely rare in young people.

## Prevention
Except for correct maintenance and checking of dentures there is no real prevention from mouth ulcers. Some doctors feel that vitamin C helps reduce mouth ulcers but the evidence is thin on the ground. Regular dental check ups will ensure any persistent ulcer is sorted out.

## Complications
Ulcers from teeth or dentures can become infected making eating even more painful.

## Self care
Aphthous ulcers may respond to salt water rinses. A mild cortisone cream will speed the recovery. Avoid antibacterial mouthwashes or lozenges which at best are useless and may even make matters worse. Make sure your dentures fit properly.

Avoid using gels which numb the pain as it will only disguise the extent of the problem. If the ulcer has not gone within 2–3 weeks, see your dentist or doctor.

## Action
See your pharmacist or dentist.

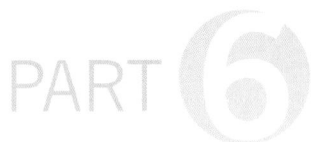

# Peptic ulcers

## Introduction

There are two main types of peptic ulcers, gastric and duodenal. Both affect the lining of the stomach and are more common in people over 40 years. Prolonged use of high doses of steroids, e.g. for asthma or rheumatic conditions, can cause a gastric ulcer. Even relatively small doses of anti-inflammatory drugs can lead to an ulcer in the stomach in people who are susceptible. Duodenal ulcers are more common in men. They heal more easily than the gastric variety and usually develop just at the beginning of the duodenum.

## Symptoms

The symptoms of peptic ulcers tend to overlap, but a fairly general pattern is recognised:

### Gastric ulcers

Constant pain or cramps can occur which are particularly bad after eating (eating tends to settle pain in a duodenal ulcer). Indigestion remedies (antacids) often settle the pain but it invariably returns. Belching is common and embarrassing. Vomiting can occur.

### Duodenal ulcers

Most people know they have developed a duodenal ulcer at around 2 am when they wake with a pain like a red hot poker just above the belly button. Drinking milk can help, but hot spicy foods make it much worse. Eating small amounts of food often relieves the pain.

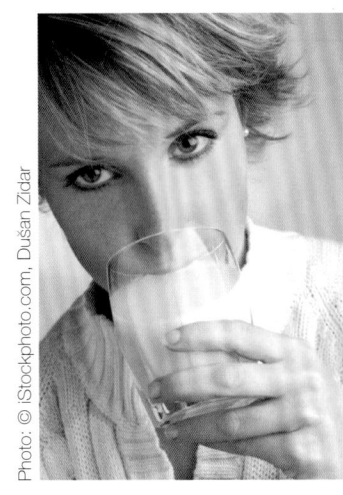

Photo: © iStockphoto.com, Dušan Zidar

## Causes

Ulcers may be caused by a bacterium called Helicobacter that lives in the stomach. Your doctor can check for this. Stress, smoking and alcohol abuse may also be causes.

## Prevention

Avoid smoking and excessive alcohol. Milk and indigestion remedies (antacids) do help but only give temporary relief.

## Complications

Call your doctor if there is:
- Red blood or brown soil-like blood in your vomit.
- Black tar-like blood or fresh red blood in your bowel motions.
- Severe pain just below the rib cage.
- Dizziness when standing up.
- A strong thirst.

## Self care

Most peptic ulcers will respond well to treatment with modern drugs which reduce the amount of stomach acid. You can also help ease the pain by using indigestion remedies or antacids.

### Note

If the pain has just started but is lasting more than a week, despite medicines from your pharmacist, call your GP.

# PART 6 Piles (haemorrhoids)

## Introduction
Although the constant butt of jokes, piles are painful and annoying. Thankfully they are rarely serious.

## Symptoms
Pain on walking or sitting along with bleeding from the anus are the commonest symptoms. The blood is often found on the toilet paper after passing a motion which can also be painful. External piles may be seen as small black grape like bodies just at the anus. Internal piles will sometimes descend through the anus only to return after passing a motion.

## Causes
Some people are more likely to develop piles than others. It has nothing to do with your preference of beer. Straining at the toilet, perhaps as a result of constipation, is well recognised. Standing for long periods may be a factor which is made worse by being overweight. Even lifting heavy weights has been suggested as a cause as it puts pressure on the veins in or near the anus. Contrary to what we were all told at school, sitting on hot radiator pipes does not appear to cause piles.

## Prevention
High fibre diets not only bulk up the motions, they may also help prevent cancer of the bowel. Similarly, taking plenty of fluids, especially fruit juices, increases the speed of the bowel.

Constipation is linked to inactivity so by increasing your activity you will reduce the likelihood of piles. Being overweight puts pressure on the veins near the anus in a similar way to pregnancy. Reduce weight.

## Complications
Bleeding can occur which is more embarrassing than dangerous. Piles can also thrombose (clot) causing even more pain and making it difficult to get them back inside the anus. Constipation can occur from not wanting to pass a motion because of the pain. This then makes passing a motion even worse. A vicious cycle.

## Self care
- Ice packs really do help.
- Use a small car tyre filled with cold water to sit on.
- Use a bulking laxative.
- Use soft toilet paper.
- Go to the toilet when you feel you need to, don't put it off.
- If passing a motion is really painful, use a lubricating, analgesic cream obtainable from your pharmacist an hour before you go to the toilet.

## Action
Make an appointment to see your GP. Although piles are far more common, some bowel cancers present late as they are ignored as piles.

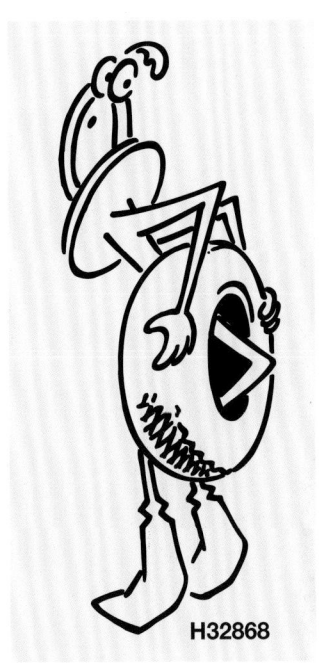

H32868

If you find yourself lost in Chalfont St Giles, go see your pharmacist for directions

Formation of piles

1 *Normal lining*
2 *Rectum*
3 *Internal pile*
4 *External pile*
5 *Anus*

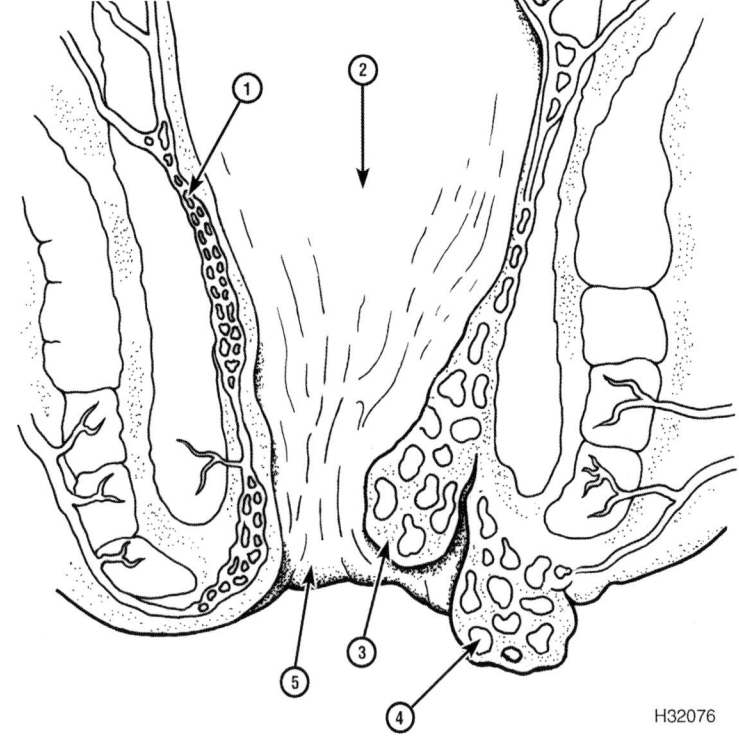

H32076

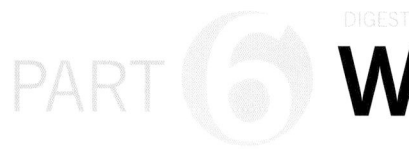

DIGESTIVE SYSTEM

# Worms

Although we don't like to talk about it, worms are actually very common, particularly in children. It is not a sign of poor hygiene or bad living. Thread worms are the most common. They are itchy, embarrassing but harmless. Round worms are larger but less common. It is possible to be infected with worms from dogs and cats. Thankfully not so common, these infections can cause blindness. Tape worms are virtually extinct in the UK.

## Symptoms

You may actually see them in your motions as tiny white/brown worms in the stool.

Itchy bottoms, particularly at night, are the trade mark. The female lays her eggs just at the anus at this time, causing the person to scratch, pick up the eggs, and pass them on or re-infect themselves.

## Causes

Infection with worms usually comes from contact with an infected person. They spread very quickly within a family and can remain in families for considerable periods of time without the family realising it.

## Prevention

● Wash your hands after going to the toilet or handling animals.
● Wash your hands before eating.

## Complications

Thread worms and round worms are not serious. Worms from dogs or cats can cause blindness, even in the unborn child if caught by a pregnant woman.

## Self care

You can buy a preparation from your pharmacist across the counter but otherwise you will need a prescription from your doctor.

## Action

See your pharmacist or practice nurse.

You should worm your pets regularly. Your pharmacist or vet will advise you.

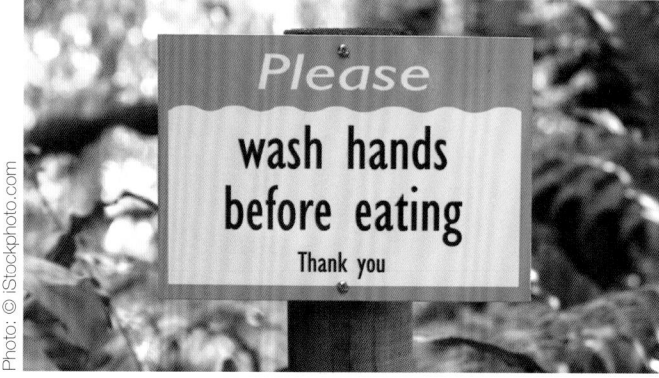

Photo: © iStockphoto.com

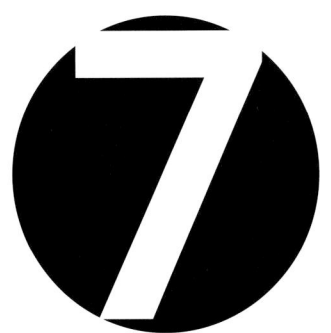

# Urogenital system

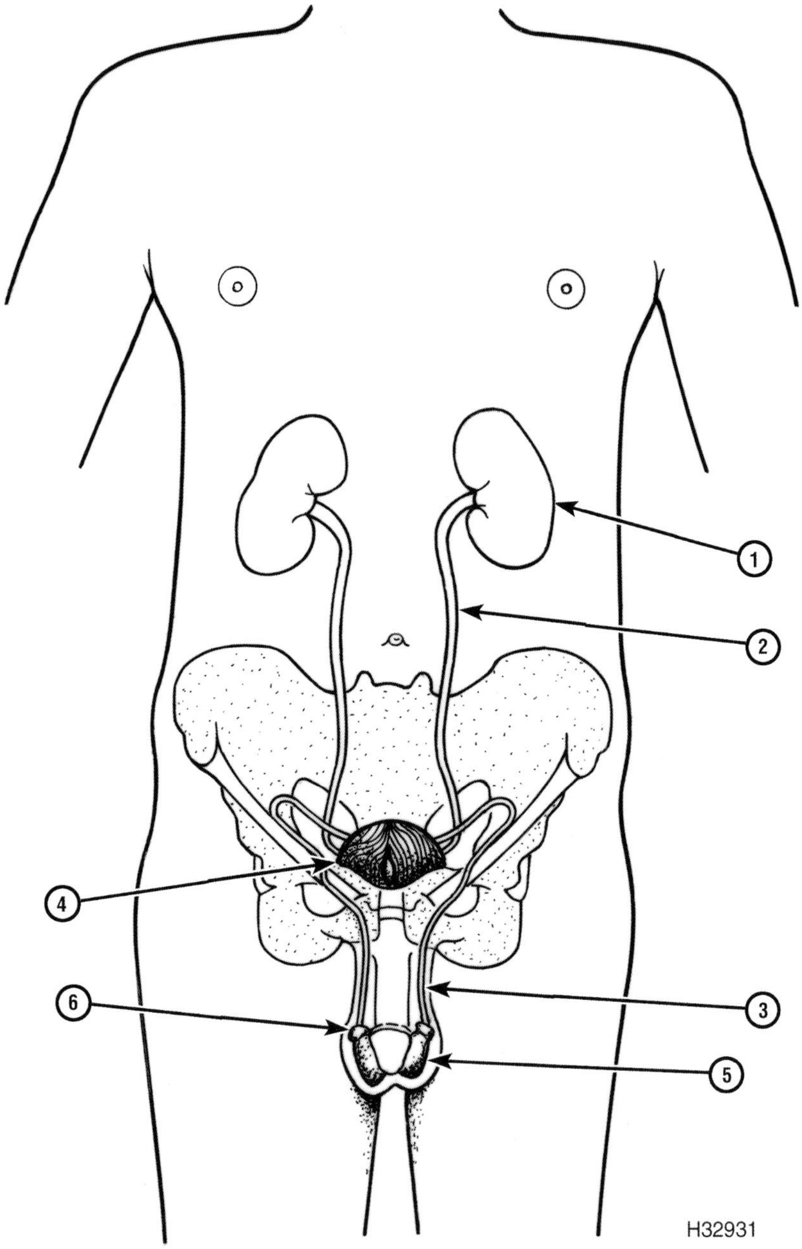

The urogenital system
1  *Kidney*
2  *Ureter*
3  *Vas deferens*
4  *Bladder*
5  *Testis*
6  *Epididymis*

H32931

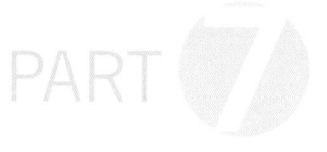

PART 7 # Benign Prostatic Hyperplasia

Imagine you are the owner of a classic Triumph Herald convertible. You are driving along when the engine splutters and dies. The fuel gauge says it all. No petrol. 'Ha' you grin, turning on the emergency tank in the boot to glide on. Two months later it happens again. But this time, no response from the emergency tank. On the polished teak dash board a bright blue bulb shines menacingly. Plenty of petrol but no oil. Rather worryingly it looks like a trip to the garage and a re-bore is on the cards. In a similar way a lot of men may worry about this sort of surgery which might be required as a consequence of their prostatic symptoms.

For men with enlarged prostates which have been diagnosed as Benign Prostatic Hyperplasia (BPH), there are two primary classes of drug available which may help avoid or delay the need for BPH-related surgery which some men have likened to a 're-bore'. They are called alpha-blockers and 5-alpha reductase inhibitors and many men have their condition effectively managed by one drug alone. For some men the use of both alpha-blockers and 5-alpha reductase inhibitors is a more effective treatment than single drug therapy.

It's important that a doctor is consulted early in all cases to make an accurate diagnosis. This Section aims to meet your information and educational needs so hopefully it will apply to any man who is the owner of an enlarged prostate that has been diagnosed as BPH.

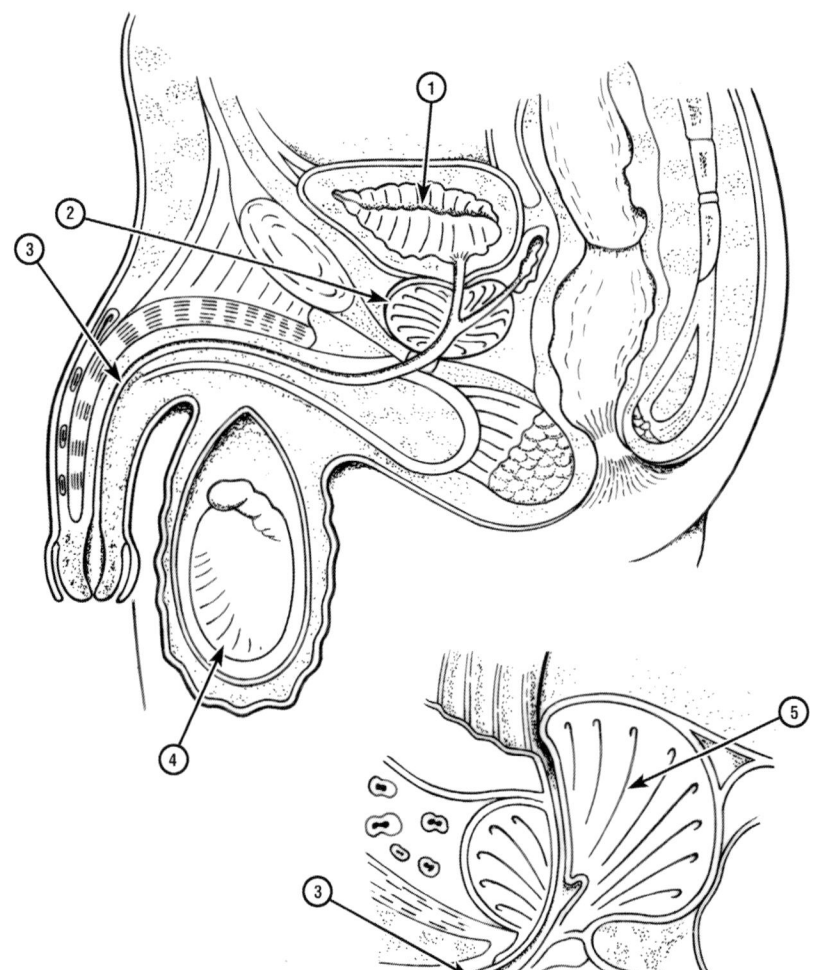

Normal and enlarged prostate gland
1  Bladder
2  Prostate (normal)
3  Urethra
4  Testis
5  Prostate (enlarged)

# Big prostate. Big problem?

An enlarged prostate is common, particularly in older age. It sits at the neck of the bladder, straddling the tube which carries urine and semen. Normally walnut sized, it provides nutrients and protection for the sperm about to make the long journey to the womb. Should it enlarge too much, there can be obstruction and even complete blockage of urine from the bladder to the penis. When caused by simple enlargement with no involvement of cancer, it is referred to as BPH. Unfortunately for the enlarged prostate owner, its impact can be far from benign.

Though the prostate continues to grow during most of a man's life, enlargement doesn't usually cause problems until later on. BPH rarely causes symptoms before age 40, but more than half of men in their sixties and as many as 90% in their seventies and eighties have some symptoms of BPH.

As the prostate enlarges, tissue layers surrounding it inhibit expansion. Inward pressure then constricts the urethra (the tube that carries urine from the bladder to the outside of the body) like a clamp on a garden hose. As a result, the bladder wall becomes thicker and irritable contracting even when it contains small amounts of urine, causing more frequent urination. Eventually, the bladder weakens and loses the ability to empty itself trapping urine inside. Narrowing of the urethra and partial emptying of the bladder cause many of the problems associated with BPH (see *Possible consequences of BPH*). Size generally does matter but it does not always determine how severe the obstruction or the symptoms will be.

Over 50% of men will have some problem with passing urine by the time they reach 60 years of age.

## Symptoms

Some of the most common symptoms of BPH include:
- Frequent trips to the toilet even during the night.
- A weaker urinary stream, so it takes longer to pass urine than it used to.
- Feeling of 'not quite emptying the bladder'.
- Need to push or strain to begin urination.
- Dribbling after passing urine.

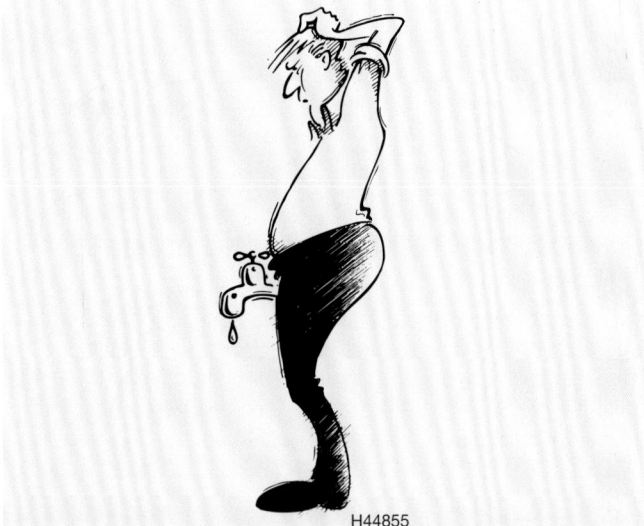

H44855

The symptoms are usually related to problems peeing

## Causes

We don't know why it enlarges but there are certain triggers:
- High levels of testosterone, the male sex hormone, and dihydrotestosterone (DHT).
- An imbalance between oestrogen and testosterone or DHT.
- Possibly, low protein, high carbohydrate diets, high fat diets.
- Western diets.

## Prevention

Even though we are not sure of the exact cause of benign prostatic enlargement, sensible protection would involve:
- Weight reduction if you are overweight. Oestrogen levels may be elevated in obese men.
- Limit animal fat intake, and reduce all fats anyway. It should represent about 25-30% of your energy needs.
- Eat at least half a kilo of fresh fruit per day.
- Increase your intake of antioxidants by eating carrots and citrus fruits.

## Diagnosis

### Digital Rectal Examination (DRE)

This examination is usually the first test done, often by your GP. The doctor inserts a gloved finger into the rectum and feels the part of the prostate next to the rectum. This gives the doctor a general idea of the size and condition of the gland. No one pretends it is not embarrassing but it is not painful and doctors perform this test all their working lives.

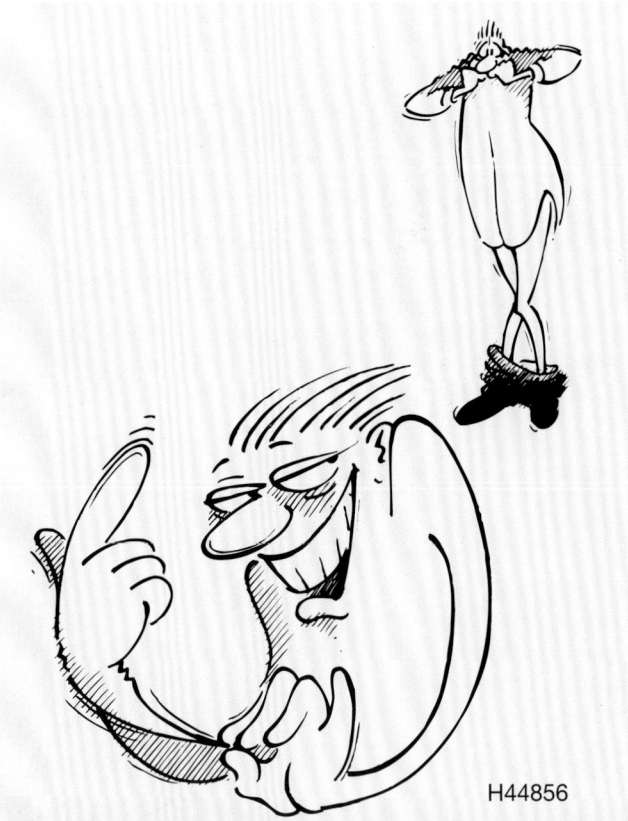

H44856

A digital rectal examination (DRE) is a simple test done by the GP

### Prostate Specific Antigen (PSA) blood test

PSA is a protein produced only by prostate cells. Frequently present at elevated levels in the blood of men who have prostate cancer, it is however, much more useful as an indicator of prostate size. Discuss with your urologist the best routes for action following your PSA test.

### Symptom score

Your doctor may give you a short questionnaire (called a symptom score or index) to fill out. The questionnaire does not positively identify the cause of symptoms, but is designed to measure their severity. The most commonly used questionnaire is the International Prostate Symptom Score (IPSS).

### Rectal ultrasound

In this procedure, a probe inserted in the rectum directs sound waves at the prostate forming an image of the prostate gland. It is painless and gives a very good indication of the problem's causes.

### Urine flow study

A reduced flow often suggests BPH.

### Cystoscopy

The inside of the bladder and the wall of the tube connecting it to the penis (urethra) can be examined using a thin tube, the cystoscope.

## Possible consequences of BPH

### Progressively bothersome urinary symptoms

Urination difficulties or LUTS (lower urinary tract symptoms) may get worse over time. Symptoms can include reduced stream, increased voiding pressure, and urinating at night.

### Acute urinary retention or AUR

Untreated BPH may lead to the sudden and painful inability to pass urine. This condition usually requires emergency medical attention. A tube (called a catheter) is passed via the penis to drain the bladder. In some cases, AUR may also lead to prostate surgery.

### Bladder damage and/or bladder stones

An obstructed urethra causes increased pressure in the bladder. This pressure may cause the bladder wall to thicken or to form pouches (called diverticulae). Bladder stones may also occur as a complication of untreated BPH, due to the difficulty in completely emptying the bladder.

### Urinary tract infection

Patients with BPH are at risk for developing infections in the urethra, bladder, ureters, or kidneys.

### Renal impairment

Prolonged BPH can lead to urine pressure on the kidneys. This causes abnormal kidney function and possible kidney damage.

### BPH-related surgery

The most common surgical procedure is TURP (Transurethral Resection of the Prostate). An instrument is inserted through the urethra and used to remove prostate tissue.

## Self care

- Avoid drinking before going to bed.
- Keep your weight down.
- Alcohol can increase night time trips to the loo as well as daytime.

## Drug therapy

In the community, medicines are the mainstay of treatment for the symptoms of an enlarged prostate. Some herbal remedies (eg, saw palmetto) are available but have limited clinical evidence. Medicines fall into two main groups.

### The alpha-blockers

These drugs block special sites called alpha receptors, on cells found in the muscles around blood vessels and in the sphincter muscle (valve) at the opening of the bladder into the urethra. The drugs work by relaxing the sphincter muscles, increasing urine flow. Alpha-blockers act quickly but can become less effective as the prostate continues to enlarge. Not surprisingly they are very popular with men suffering from the symptoms linked to an enlarged prostate. As some of these drugs were initially developed to treat high blood pressure it is not surprising that side effects can include slight dizziness in a small number of men.

### The 5-alpha reductase inhibitors (5-ARIs)

Keeping the symptoms at bay for the long term is the role of 5-ARIs, which help reduce the rate of prostate enlargement by blocking an enzyme called alpha reductase found in the testes and scalp, inhibiting production of the hormone DHT (dihydrotestosterone). The use of 5-ARIs may also reduce the likelihood that you will develop AUR or need BPH-related surgery. Side effects are few, but in a small number of cases include reduced penile erectile function (around 3-5 men in one hundred). These symptoms disappear if treatment is stopped.

### Combination therapy

Following a major research programme, the British Association of Urological Surgeons (BAUS) recommend that men with an enlarged prostate could be treated with both alpha-blockers and 5-ARIs. For some men the use of both therapies is more effective treatment than single-drug therapy.

## Surgery and minimally invasive therapy

Not all men will find sufficient relief using drugs alone and surgery or new treatments such as laser or microwave procedures may be required.

Most doctors recommend removal of the enlarged part of the prostate as the best long-term solution for patients with BPH. With surgery for BPH, only the enlarged tissue that is pressing against the urethra is removed; the rest of the inside tissue and the outside capsule are left intact. Surgery usually relieves the obstruction and incomplete emptying caused by BPH.

## Transurethral resection of the prostate (TURP)

This is still the most effective surgical treatment for BPH and is used in 90% of all cases. With TURP, an instrument called a resectoscope is inserted through the penis. During the 90-minute operation, the surgeon uses the resectoscope's wire loop to remove the obstructing tissue one piece at a time. The pieces of tissue are carried by the fluid into the bladder and then flushed out at the end of the operation.

Most doctors suggest using TURP whenever possible. Transurethral procedures are less traumatic than open forms of surgery and require a shorter recovery period.

# PART 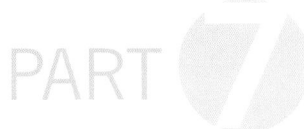 Kidney infections & stones

## Introduction

Kidneys are more than just filters, they also control blood pressure and stimulate the production of red blood cells. Their main role is to control the amount of fluid in the body and flush out toxins. If the body has too much water on board it becomes 'oedematous' and this can build up in the blood, damaging vital organs such as the brain. If there is too little water the body becomes dehydrated which can also damage vital organs, not least the kidney itself.

There are usually two kidneys, one on each side just beneath the back rib cage. They are connected to the bladder by long tubes (ureters). Sometimes there can be two ureters coming from the one kidney. In most cases this will not cause any problems but it can sometimes make infections more likely to occur. Kidney infections are relatively rare but can be serious. Kidney stones can form in the kidney and block the ureter which not only causes pain but may also make infection more likely.

## Symptoms

Infections can be painful with a heavy dragging sensation in the back. A high temperature is common and there may be blood clots in the urine. Tenderness over the muscles of the back can also occur. Vomiting is common.

Stones can form from calcium or oxalate (a form of acid) and can be a sign of a mineral imbalance in the blood. Renal colic is described as the worst pain known to man and often requires very powerful pain killers to control. The pain typically radiates down from the back to the groin. Small pieces of stone along with blood clots may be found in the urine.

## Causes

Infections can occur for no apparent reason but are also associated with congenital malformations of the kidney. Chronic dehydration is also a common factor. Reflux where the urine is forced back up the ureter is also a factor as is the presence of a stone.

## Prevention

Both infections and stones can be prevented by drinking plenty of plain water each day.

## Complications

Infections, dehydration and the back pressure from obstructions like stones can scar the kidney. If this happens repeatedly the kidney can cease to function and becomes a liability.

## Treatment

Antibiotics will treat the infection, although it does tend to recur if the underlying cause is not addressed. Stones can be removed by various methods such as ultrasound which disintegrates the stone. In some cases a long wire with a basket is used to pull the stone down the ureter.

In very severe cases it may be necessary to perform surgery and if the kidney has ceased to function it will need to be removed. Fortunately the remaining kidney is more than capable of performing all the required tasks. If both kidneys have failed dialysis is required until a suitable donor kidney can be found. Thousands of lives are saved every year by people having the good sense to carry a donor card with them at all times.

## Action

Make an appointment to see your GP.

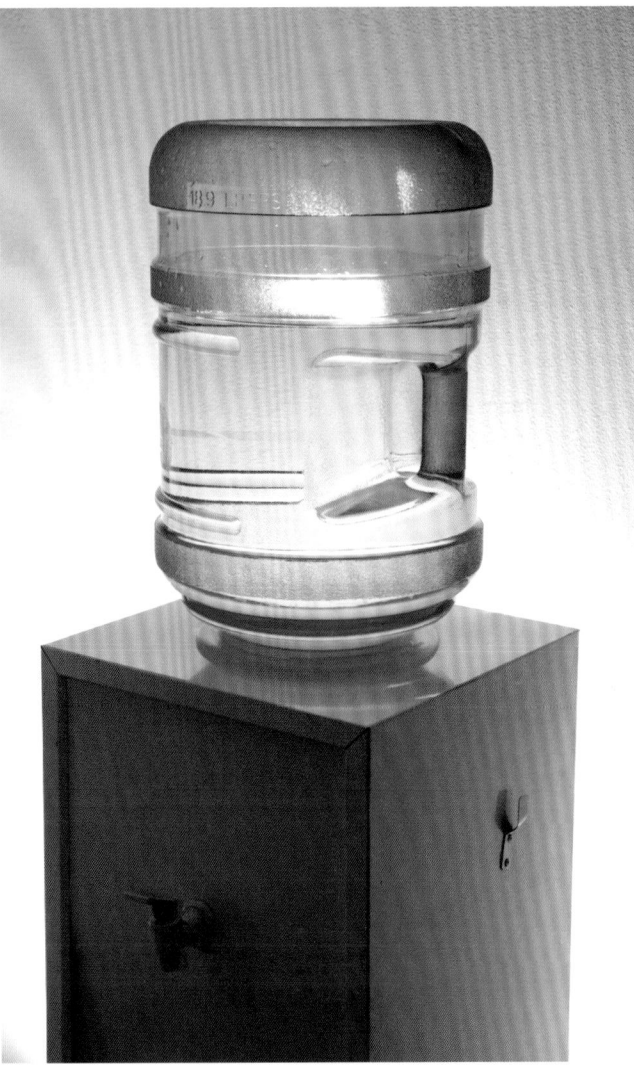

Photo: © iStockphoto.com, Don Bayley

PART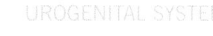

# Prostate cancer

### What is the prostate gland and what does it do?

Only men have a prostate gland. It's roundish and about the size of a golf ball. It is in the pelvis, hard up against the base of the bladder. The prostate surrounds the urethra – the tube that runs from your bladder inside your penis to the outside. You pee through it. Imagine the prostate as a fat rubber washer round a bit of tubing and you'll get the picture.

It grows to adult size at puberty, under the influence of hormones. In most men it also begins to enlarge again in early middle age. An enlarged prostate can cause problems for older men when they pee. These prostate problems are common.

The prostate's main job is to make prostatic fluid, one of four different fluids of the liquid part of semen. (Semen carries sperm and is what you ejaculate when you have an orgasm.) The prostate gland is, in fact, made up of a mass of smaller secretory glands which make prostatic fluid. It is also made of muscle, which contracts at orgasm expelling the fluid into the penis. This contraction contributes to some of the 'push' of ejaculation.

### When things go wrong

Problems with the prostate are common. Because of where the prostate is, peeing can become more difficult.

Some prostate problems are more serious than others. Prostatitis can affect men at any age and causes pain and discomfort due to inflammation and sometimes infection. BPH, or benign enlargement of the prostate, the most common prostate condition, affects older men (see *Benign Prostatic Hyperplasia* above). It can be quite uncomfortable. If you are an older man and have urinary symptoms this is the most likely cause. However, prostate cancer is a possibility.

If you are concerned about any symptoms you may have, visit your GP. He or she can examine you and decide whether you have no problem, an easily treated problem or a more serious one, like prostate cancer.

### What goes wrong?

Normally the growth of all cells in the body is carefully regulated. When cancer develops, the cells multiply and grow in an uncontrolled way and can spread elsewhere in the body.

Most commonly, prostate cancer is a slow-growing cancer and it can remain undetected because it never causes problems in a man's lifetime. But this is not true of all men. A few men will have aggressive cancers which spread quickly. Sometimes men have no hint that there is anything wrong until cancer cells move outside the gland and cause symptoms elsewhere in the body, often in bone.

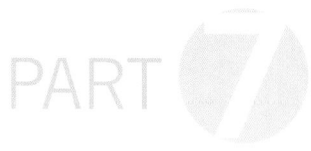

Your sleeping partner might not be. Sleeping, that is. Your frequent trips to the loo can be disruptive – you have the problem but unfortunately it's your partner who has seen the doctor and is taking the sleeping tablets to treat it.

Prostate cancer is not caused by vasectomy, injury, masturbation or reading the Kama Sutra under the bedclothes with a torch. Just as well or it could be teenagers suffering along with men predominately aged over 50.

Prostate cancer is catching up with skin cancer as the number one male cancer in the UK.

Men have roughly the same risk of developing prostate cancer as women have of breast cancer.

# Who gets prostate cancer?

Prostate cancer is diagnosed in more than 25,000 men every year in the UK and the number is rising as more cases are being detected due to the increased use of the PSA test. The majority of men diagnosed will be over sixty – commonly in their seventies. Men can be affected from the age of about 45 but this is rare. The risk of getting prostate cancer gets higher as men get older.

Older men of African or African Caribbean origin are at particular risk of getting prostate cancer. Men who have had a close male blood relative, particularly a brother, diagnosed with it seem also to have an increased risk of getting it themselves.

The Westernised diet of highly refined food with a high animal fat content also seems to increase the risk of developing prostate cancer. There is no firm evidence how to reduce the risk of prostate cancer but we know that adopting a healthy diet with more fruit and vegetables, less red meat and more fish is good for reducing the risks of other cancers and heart disease, and possibly prostate cancer.

# What are the symptoms?

It is important to be clear: Not all men get symptoms that show they have prostate cancer. In the men that do, not all men have exactly the same symptoms. You do not have to have all the symptoms on the list.

**The symptoms are usually related to problems peeing**
- Frequent need to urinate, especially at night.
- Rushing to the toilet.
- Difficulty starting to urinate.
- Straining to pass urine.
- Taking a long time.
- Having a weak flow.
- Getting the feeling that your bladder has no emptied properly when you have finished urinating.
- Dribbling after urination is complete.
- Pain or discomfort on passing urine.

**In addition, other symptoms can be**
- Lower back pain.
- Pain in the pelvis, hips or thighs.
- Impotence.
- Blood in the urine – but this is rarer.
- Pain on ejaculation.
- Pain in the genitals.

It is important to realise that any of these symptoms are also caused by problems which are nothing to do with prostate cancer. If you are concerned about any symptoms that you have, visit your GP.

# Diagnosis at the GP

When a GP thinks there might be a prostate problem he or she will do some tests. Common tests are:
- A blood test to measure the PSA level. Prostate Specific Antigen (PSA) is a protein that the prostate produces. It is normal for a man to have some PSA in the blood. If there is a problem with the prostate the levels of PSA in the blood can go up. The normal level is up to about 4 for a man of 60. It is slightly less for younger men and slightly more for older men. The PSA test is not a test for cancer, but it can show the GP that there is a problem with the prostate. The PSA test result may show that other tests in hospital are needed.

You may be able to reduce your risk by taking selenium and vitamin E supplements along with the occasional Bloody Mary, preferably with less Mary. Tomatoes reportedly reduce your risk.

Photo: © iStockphoto.com

- A physical examination called a DRE. A digital rectal examination (DRE) is a simple test done by the GP. The doctor feels your prostate through your rectum, either while you lie on your side or bend over a chair. Some men find a DRE uncomfortable or embarrassing, but it is over quickly. Your doctor may feel an irregularity on the surface of the prostate that makes him suspect cancer. An area may feel harder than the rest, or perhaps knobbly.

If he or she has concerns because of the PSA and DRE and any symptoms that you are having he or she will suggest that you go to the hospital for other tests.

# Tests in hospital

The doctor looks at the prostate with an ultrasound probe. The doctor uses the images to guide the sampling needles into the prostate, then removes a small amount of tissue from the gland with the needles (a biopsy). The pathologist (lab specialist) looks at the sample under the microscope. A report of the findings is sent to your urologist. If there is a cancer, the report will say whether it is slow growing, moderately aggressive or aggressive. The doctor may mention the Gleason score; two is the least aggressive and ten the most aggressive. It is important for the specialist to know how aggressive the cancer is, because this can affect the treatment options.

Other tests may be done. The doctors need to check whether the cancer has moved outside the gland. Like your Gleason score, the results of these tests may change your treatment options.
- The specialist may suggest a CT scan. CT is a way of using X-rays to take images like slices through the body. This allows the doctors to see the prostate, surrounding tissues and lymph nodes.
- Magnetic Resonance Imaging (MRI) is another way of looking inside the body but does not use X-ray. Powerful magnets are used to make the images.
- You may also need a bone scan. This depends on your other results. If the prostate cancer has spread some distance, bone is the most likely place to find it.

# Treatment

Prostate cancer is treated in several different ways. It depends on how aggressive the cancer is, where the cancer is in your body and how old you are. Your general state of health may make a difference.

Your urologist will discuss different options with you. You may see some other specialists such as a medical oncologist or a radiotherapist, often called a clinical oncologist, who treats cancer using radiation therapy.

## Localised cancer

If the cancer is localised, that is, only present inside the gland, it can be treated by radiotherapy, brachytherapy or surgery – see below. Your specialist may also discuss the 'no treatment' option – monitoring or active surveillance – with you.

All the treatments have side effects. You need to consider these when choosing treatments. Active surveillance, as explained later, avoids these side effects and might be an option open to you. Impotence and incontinence are the side effects which cause most concern.

### Radiotherapy

External beam radiotherapy is widely available and most units will now be offering the modern 3D conformal option. A course of treatment lasts five days a week, for 5–7 weeks. Possible side effects to discuss with a specialist include pain on passing urine, incontinence, bowel problems and impotence. You may be offered additional hormone therapy to help improve your body's response to radiotherapy.

Brachytherapy is an internal radiotherapy treatment where radioactive seeds are implanted into the prostate. This is done under anaesthetic and involves an overnight stay in hospital, but only at selected centres. Brachytherapy is not suitable for all men. If you are a good candidate for surgery it is also likely that you are a good candidate for brachytherapy. Side effects are mostly urinary problems. Impotence can occur as a longer term effect of this treatment.

### Surgery

The prostate can also be surgically removed in an operation called a radical prostatectomy. Surgery is not suitable for all men. For example it is not usually offered as an option for men over 70. If you are over 70 and choose radical treatment you are more likely to be offered radiotherapy. Impotence and incontinence are significant risks of this kind of operation. Ask your surgeon for details of how they may affect you later on. Recently radical prostatectomy has become available as a 'keyhole' operation from a few surgeons.

### Cryotherapy

This is a new treatment. It is not available in every area at the moment, but increasing numbers of centres are offering it. Doctors who do prostate cryotherapy use it for men who have already had radiotherapy as a 'first choice' treatment, but where the prostate cancer has recurred in the same area. Like some other treatments, incontinence is a possible side effect.

### Monitoring

As many prostate cancers are slow growing and non aggressive your specialist may suggest active monitoring or surveillance for you. Your PSA level will be cheeked regularly and you may have occasional repeat biopsies. Thus the cancer is monitored rather than treated. This is a good way of avoiding the side effects of treatment when the cancer is causing no physical problems. This option is most commonly recommended for older men. There may be good reasons for you taking this option, especially when your cancer is slow growing.

## Advanced prostate cancer

If the cancer has moved beyond the gland, your options are different. The cancer may be locally advanced – that is, in the tissues surrounding the prostate; or advanced – that is, affecting distant parts of your body. An operation to remove the prostate would still leave cancer behind so that is not a choice that will be offered to you. Your doctors may offer you radiotherapy and additional hormone therapy if you have a locally advanced cancer. You may be offered hormone therapy alone. It depends on each individual case.

## Hormone therapy

Prostate cancer needs the male hormone testosterone to grow and continue spreading. By depriving the cancer of testosterone, hormone therapy can cause the cancer to shrink . It will usually make the PSA levels drop too, to immeasurable levels in some men. Hormone therapy is good for relieving symptoms of the cancer, particularly bone pain and urinary problems. But it is not without side effects itself.

Hormone therapy does not cure the cancer but there is an excellent chance that it will keep the cancer in check for several years. It works wherever the cancer is in your body.

Drug treatments are commonly used as hormone therapy. This means you will be given monthly or three monthly injections, or daily tablets, or a combination of both. Your doctors will help you decide which treatment is best for you.

There is also a surgical from of hormone therapy. The testicles can be removed. With the improved modern drugs which are equally effective, these operations are much less common. It sounds alarming but for some men this is a good option. Such surgery is never performed without your fully informed consent. You do not have to choose this option if you are unhappy with it.

Common side effects of all forms of hormone therapy are: hot flushes, problems getting and maintaining erections and loss of interest in sex. Breast tenderness or swelling may also occur.

Hormone therapy eventually becomes ineffective against the cancer. Chemotherapy may then be offered. It is not used earlier because all the other treatments outlined here work better. However, at the later stages of prostate cancer chemotherapy works well in keeping the cancer at bay. It will not cure the cancer but should improve quality of life.

## Making choices

More than with many other conditions, there is no clear 'best treatment' for prostate cancer. Your doctor will explain the options to you, but you have to make the choice. This is not easy when you are having to come to terms with a diagnosis of cancer, so making choices also depends on having the right support around you. Your GP will help you. Your specialists, too – and their teams often includes specialist nurses whose job it is to support and inform you. Your family and friends will also be on your side.

# PART 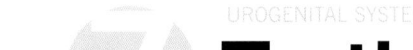 Testicular cancer

## Introduction

Thankfully testicular problems are relatively rare. Testicular cancer is the most serious. It represents only 1% of all cancers in men, but it is the single biggest cause of cancer related death in men aged between 18 and 35 years although it can develop in boys as young as 15. Currently about 1500 men a year develop the disease. Unfortunately the number of cases has doubled in the last 20 years and is still rising.

## Symptoms

- A lump on one testicle.
- Pain and tenderness in either testicle.
- Discharge (pus or smelly goo) from the penis.
- Blood in the sperm at ejaculation.
- A build up of fluid inside the scrotum.
- A heavy dragging feeling in the groin or scrotum.
- An increase in size of the testicle. (It is normal for one testicle to be larger then the other, but the sizes and shape should remain more or less the same.)
- An enlargement of the breasts, with or without tenderness.

## Causes

The causes of the increase are unknown. Exposure to female hormones in the environment, in water (possibly from the oral contraceptive pill in water supplies), or in baby milk have been suggested. In Spain and most Asian countries there has been no significant increase but we do not know why. At the same time sperm counts are falling across Europe and this may be part of the picture. Undescended testicles are a major factor (where the testicle stays inside the body after birth and will not sit in the scrotum). Men with one or two undescended testes have a greatly increased risk – one in 44. The condition can be corrected surgically, but must be done before the age of 10.

Your risk increases if your father or brother suffered from testicular cancer.

## Prevention

For once men are positively encouraged to feel themselves, but this time to do more than 'check they're still there'. Self examination is the name of the game. Check your tackle monthly like this:

- Do it lying in a warm bath or while having a long shower, as this makes the skin of the scrotum softer and easier therefore, to feel the testicles inside.
- Cradle the scrotum in the palm of your hand. Feel the difference between the testicles. You will almost definitely feel that one is larger and lying lower. This is completely normal.

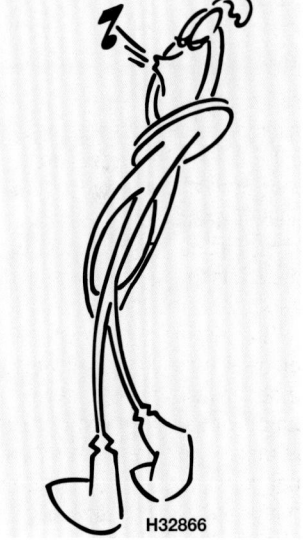

H32866

- Examine each one in turn, and then compare them with each other. Use both hands and gently roll each testicle between thumb and forefinger. Check for any lumps or swellings as they should both be smooth. Remember that the duct carrying sperm to the penis, the epididymis, normally feels bumpy. It lies along the top and back of the testis.

## Complications

Many types of testicular cancer can be cured in around 96% of cases if caught at an early stage. Even when these tumours spread, they can still be cured in 80% of cases, and large volume tumours can be cured in 60% of cases. Even so, late diagnosis increases the risk of a poorer response to treatment.

One testicle may need to be removed, but a prosthesis (false one) disguises the fact almost completely.

Treatment with radiotherapy or radiography may affect your ability to father children, but in many cases fertility is not affected. It is also possible to store sperm before treatment.

## Self care

Too frequent self examination can actually make it more difficult to notice any difference and may cause unnecessary worry.

Testis and scrotum
1  Vein
2  Artery
3  Vas deferens
4  Epididymis
5  Fascia
6  Testis
7  Muscle
8  Tunica vaginalis
9  Skin

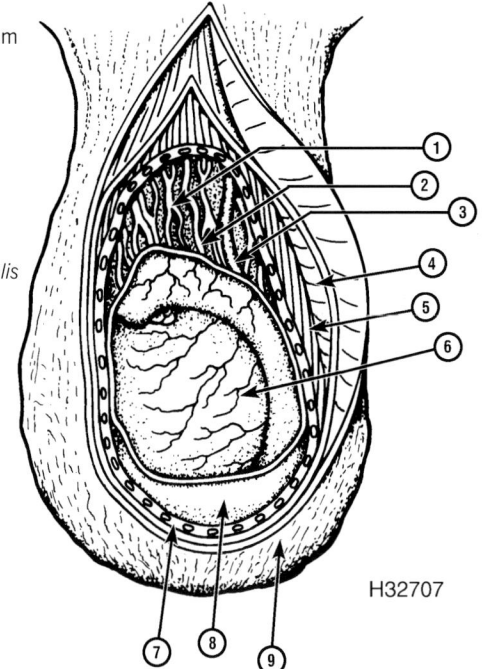

H32707

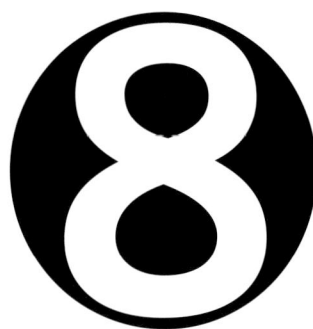

# 8

# Sex and reproduction

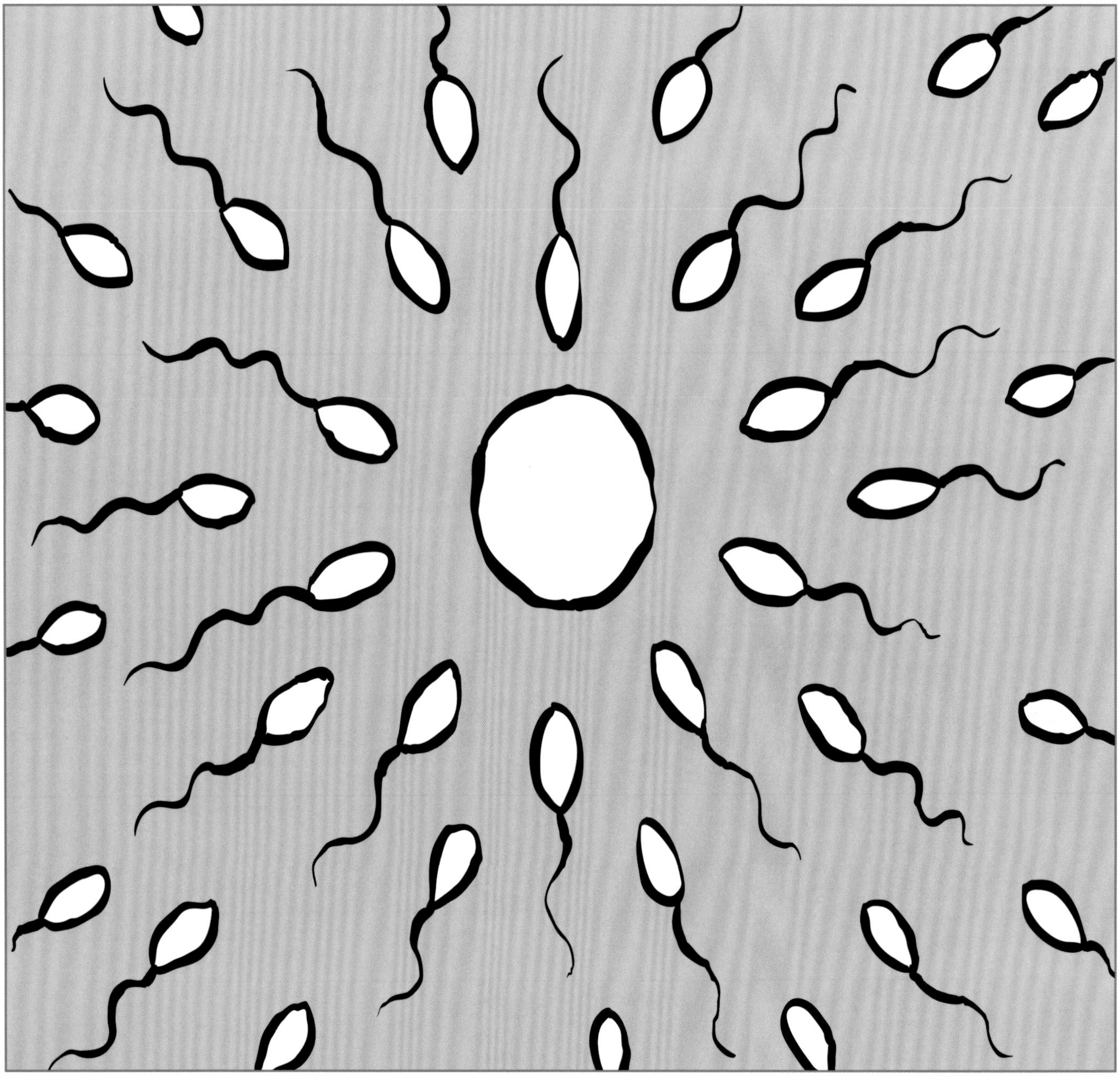

Photo: © iStockphoto.com, Brett Lamb

# PART 8 Timing is everything

## Introduction

Choosing the time of being a dad may not always be in your control, but if it is, there are advantages and disadvantages for young dad versus old dad.

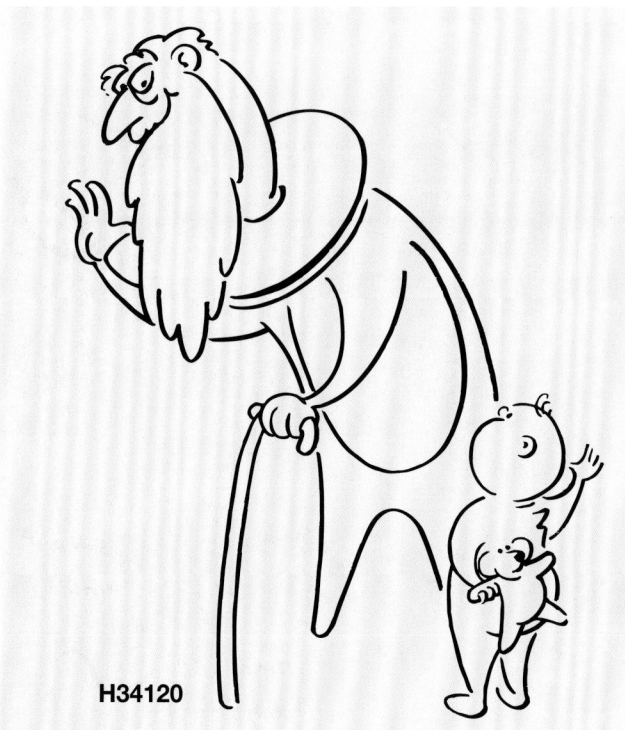

**H34120**

The older dad

### Can semen give you cancer?

There is no evidence that semen causes cancer. From an evolutionary point of view, it wouldn't really make much sense if all the females of a species promptly died a horrible death every time they tried to procreate. A sort of 'go forth and divide'. For many years a battle ranged over whether sex with uncircumcised men caused cervical cancer. It was noted that virgin women never contracted cervical cancer and that Jewish women in Israel had a lower incidence than women in, say, the UK. Obviously, the scientists thought, it's all down to the foreskin. When all the statistics are examined more fully it appears that promiscuity is a greater factor and that the presence or absence of the foreskin is of relatively little consequence.

It is worth noting that one organism suspected of causing cervical cancer is Human Papilloma Virus (HPV). This is transmitted by unprotected sex with a carrier of the virus; as ever, condoms provide more or less total protection.

## Teenage dad

Becoming a parent in your teens is generally best avoided if possible. Research shows that teenage mothers are significantly disadvantaged with regard to their standard of living later in life; teenage dads probably aren't much better off.

## Young dad

You are going to need all the youth you can muster, especially in the first few weeks when the jet lag from the lack of sleep starts to kick in. On the other hand you will be able to take part in their games as they get older without snapping your Achilles tendon and be young enough to enjoy regained independence once they leave home. You are also less likely to employ a crowbar to lever the remaining son out of the family home. Before you shout 'brace yourself darling' just a word in your ear. You may be losing the best years of your life. Along comes responsibility, a whole new look at car maintenance for necessity not fun, lost mates, especially the car maintenance variety, financial commitments when your earning power is at its lowest and of course that haunting fragrance of damp nappy.

## Middle-aged dad

It's easy to see the advantages of kids while you are in your thirties with more earning power, a good taste of the free unfettered youth, and your parents still around to do all the baby sitting while you swan off to breakaway holidays in the Antipodes but wait a second, mate. Work pressure is at its highest during your middle age especially with jobs under pressure from women. The life long-post is no more. Keeping on track with your career might be difficult with a few kids in the equation. Paradoxically you might spend more time securing their future than actually being with them.

## Older dad

We value age as a source of wisdom and patience and of course it is theoretically possible to become a dad no matter how old you are. You don't even need to worry about the sweaty bit either, even if masturbation is not possible through erectile dysfunction. Prostatic massage can often produce sufficient ejaculate for assisted insemination. Finance is also usually less of a problem and your decision to have kids is less likely to be based on an irrational red haze. Smaller family size is also more likely, increasing personal contact and lessening the burden of responsibility.

Just a thought however before dispensing with the Zimmer for a few vital moments. Death, the grim reaper, is more likely to rob your children of your presence at an earlier age. You are less likely to take part in their activities and conception may be more difficult. There is also an increased risk of genetic malformation. Even so, average life expectancy is increasing and the older dad of the industrial revolution with a life expectancy of less than 40 years, is the middle-aged father of today.

Perhaps not having too much control over the matter is better in the end.

# PART 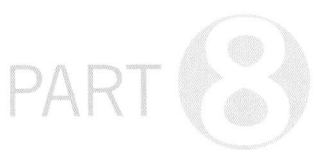 Getting started

## Is it possible to get stuck when making love?

Cramp is a dreadful invention. It always affects your calf just when you really don't want it to happen. Simply wiggling your little toe produces a pain equalled only by a meaningful relationship with Vlad the Impaler. Vaginismus is a cramp-like spasm which contracts the vagina. It is not so painful but it can be embarrassing. Some women even experience it when having a cervical smear performed. It can also occur during intercourse but the chances of endlessly doing the lambada with your trapped partner round and round the kitchen are extremely small. More important is the discomfort it can cause for both of you. Extended foreplay, which does not mean asking, 'Are you awake Sheila?' can do the trick. That and a sense of humour along with a relaxed atmosphere. But not too relaxed, you don't want to fall asleep, Sheila.

## Introduction

Ovulation usually occurs somewhere between 12 and 16 days before the start of the next menstrual period. This is known as the fertile period and it is during this time that the egg can be fertilised. If your partner has regular periods, this point can be worked out with reasonable accuracy by calculating backwards from when the next period is expected. Ovulation can be detected by a change in body temperature but this indicator is usually used when trying to avoid a pregnancy as it tells you that ovulation has already occurred. A change in the degree of stickiness of the mucus on the cervix is a better indicator that ovulation is about to take place. There are self-test ovulation kits available from your pharmacist that determine when ovulation is likely to happen. These are expensive and there is little evidence that they actually increase the chance of becoming pregnant any sooner then it would happen normally. Luckily, pinpointing the exact fertile period is not necessary for most people as sperm have the ability to stay alive inside the woman for several days. Therefore sex 2-3 times a week throughout the cycle will maximise the chance of achieving a pregnancy by ensuring that sperm are ready and waiting for when the egg is released.

Ovulation time

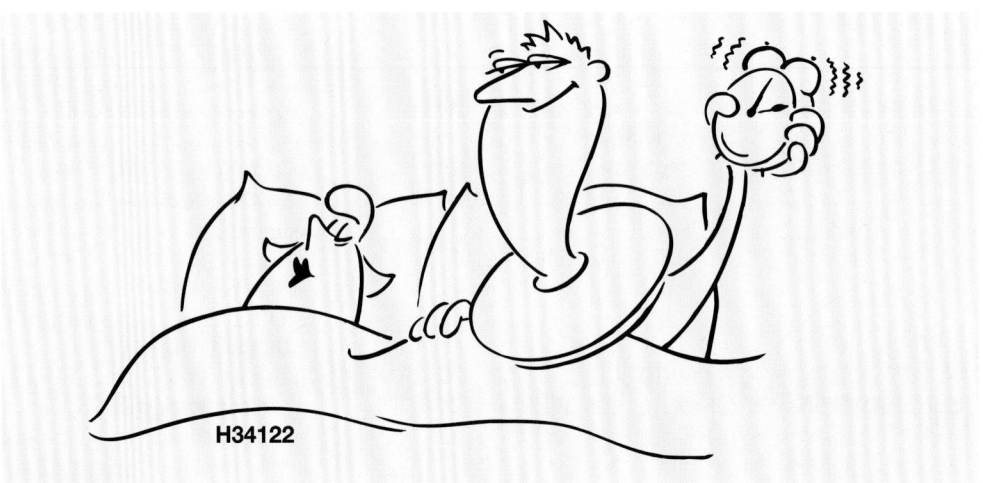

H34122

## Self help

There are some things you and your partner can do to help you be fit and healthy for pregnancy. Rubella infection in pregnancy can harm a developing baby, so your partner should check with her doctor to see if she needs a vaccination before you try for a pregnancy.

Women planning a baby should take 400 micrograms (0.4 mg) of folic acid every day from the time they stop using contraception until the 12th week of pregnancy, as folic acid reduces the risk of a baby having neural tube defects, such as spina bifida. (Those who have previously had a child with spina bifida or those who are taking drugs for epilepsy need to take bigger doses. Ask your doctor.) You can get folic acid from pharmacies.

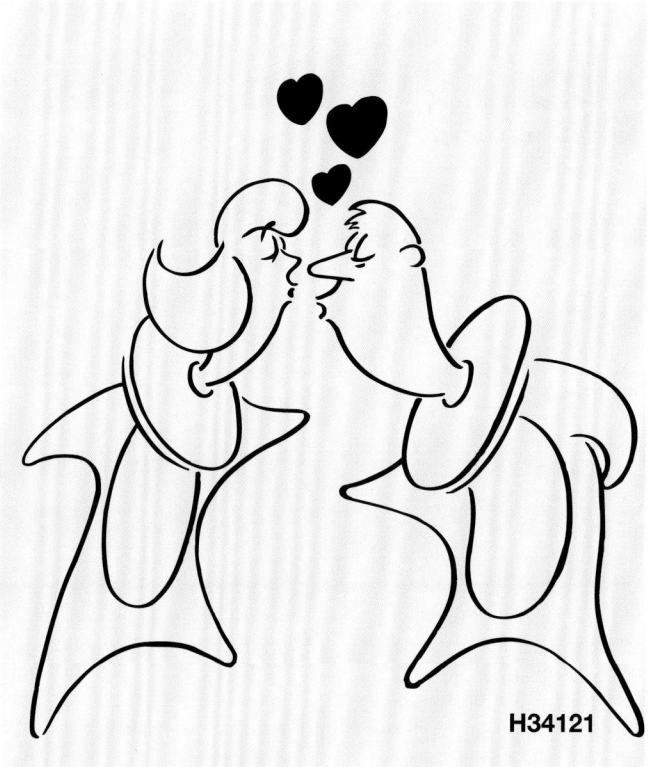

Getting started

A balanced diet with as much fresh food as possible will ensure enough vitamins and minerals are eaten. Soft cheeses, pâtés, soft-boiled eggs, cold prepared meats and cook-chilled foods should be avoided as there is a small risk of them being contaminated with listeria which can cause birth defects. Too much Vitamin A can be harmful to a developing baby, so pregnant women are advised not to eat liver or take Vitamin A tablets.

Both you and your partner should try to give up smoking, as smoking is known to carry risks for the developing baby and also to newborn babies. This is just as important for men, as smokers tend to produce fewer sperm and have more damaged sperm. Quit can give you both help and advice on how to give up smoking.

## Is it safe to have only one testicle?

This is a trick myth. Yes it is safe if you actually had the other one removed for whatever reason. An unremoved, undescended testicle increases your chances of cancer by at least four times. In terms of conferring immunity from becoming a father you are most definitely not safe. Each testis produces more than enough sperm to produce a chip off the old block. Similarly, your levels of testosterone will remain normal. The pituitary, a gland in the brain, controls the circulating amounts of sex hormone and simply prods the testicle into more action should levels fall.

## Is there something wrong with masturbating when you are having regular sex?

Masturbation is subtly different from sex. First it is almost one hundred per cent safe except when performed in zero gravity. Spacemen use the term Roger as a form of relief. Most men and women in stable, happy relationships also masturbate. This is where fantasy plays its part. Many people masturbate after sex to prolong the pleasure. This is particularly noted in couples where one or other of them falls fast asleep with the final gasp with little time to ask whether the earth moved for their partner also.

Heavy or frequent drinking can harm the baby's development. Alcohol should therefore be limited to no more than one or two units of alcohol once or twice a week. If you need advice on drinking phone NHS Direct or Drinkline.

Weight can affect fertility by interfering with ovulation. Women who are very underweight or overweight might want to talk to NHS Direct or their practice nurse.

Some sexually-transmitted infections (eg, chlamydia) can cause fertility problems, some can be passed to the baby during the pregnancy or at birth (eg, HIV) and some are thought to be linked with miscarriage or premature birth (eg, trichomonas and syphilis). Many of the infections have no symptoms so if you or your partner are worried that you may have caught a sexually-transmitted infection either recently or in the past, go to a genito-urinary medicine (GUM) clinic or sexual health clinic. The service is completely free and confidential. Most large hospitals have a GUM clinic – phone Sexual Health Direct or NHS Direct for details of your nearest clinic.

Women should avoid changing cat litter, wear gloves when gardening, and wash hands thoroughly after handling cooked meat. This prevents infection with a parasite (toxoplasmosis) which can harm a developing baby. It is also best to avoid X-rays and taking medication when you are pregnant or trying for a baby. Ask your doctor or a pharmacist if you need to do either of these.

Reducing the number of times you have sex to 'build up' a reservoir of sperm is not necessary. Sperm are produced constantly and each ejaculation contains many millions of sperm – more than enough to fertilise an egg. It is also not necessary to have sex every day, 2-3 times a week is plenty to achieve a pregnancy.

Not all couples achieve a pregnancy straight away so don't panic if it doesn't happen quickly as most couples get there within a year or so. Best just to try and be relaxed and enjoy not having worry about contraception for a while.

## Results

Testing for pregnancy is simple and accurate.

All pregnancies are followed by careful monitoring through regular visits to the doctor or midwife, ultrasound and a range of other tests where necessary, so the chances of serious problems with the birth or the baby are low.

# PART 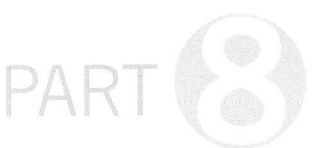 Contraception

Photo: © iStockphoto.com, Pederk

## Can you re-use a condom by turning it inside out?

Desperation is truly a terrible thing. The short answer to this question is yes, but your choice of sexual acquaintances may be severely restricted afterwards. You could also be a daddy as sperm can survive for a short space of time in the air. Additionally you may also contract just about any sexually transmitted disease going. But yes, you can re-use a condom by turning it inside out just like you can wear three day old socks by the same manoeuvre. On the other hand, it is probably best to shell out for another packet or have a cold shower. Both are a good deal cheaper in the long run.

## Introduction

There are numerous methods of contraception, most of which, it has to be said, depend more on the woman than the man. Not only is there a difference in the way the methods work and are used, but there is a significant difference in the protection each method provides.

## The male condom

Society is increasingly accepting the condom as one of the normal requirements of modern life. This has led to their wider availability and condoms can now readily be obtained – in supermarkets, from garages, by mail order, through slot machines, as well as in pharmacies. They are free from all family planning clinics and genito-urinary medicine clinics. Colours, flavours and new materials, like plastic, make interesting options. Condoms now come in different shapes and sizes, and it is often necessary to try a few different types before the right one is found. If used correctly condoms are 98 per cent effective at preventing pregnancy and they have the added advantage of providing good protection against many sexually transmitted infections. Hermetically sealed, the modern condom will remain usable for a long time (look for the expiry date); good quality condoms will also have the CE mark and the kitemark. Once the seal is broken they should be used quite soon as the rubber will perish on exposure to the air and the lubricant will dry, making it difficult to put on.

### Use of condoms

Using a condom correctly is essential for it to be effective. It should be put on before any contact between the penis and the vagina or genital area, and rolled on the correct way round. Air should be excluded from the end of the condom as it can cause

## Can you get pregnant while you are breast-feeding?

This question is usually asked by the father of twelve children. Although there may be a prolonged delay in the resumption of periods, and thus ovulation, there is no way of knowing just when it is going to start. Obviously an egg has to be released for a period to follow. If unprotected intercourse takes place at this time there will be an even more prolonged delay. Getting pregnant is another excellent way of stopping periods.

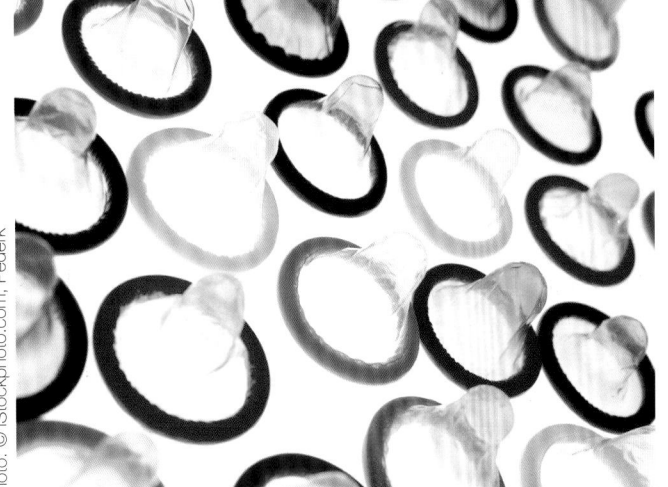

The condom

## Is butter or margarine a good lubricant when using a condom?

No to both, even if you would never know it wasn't butter. Oil-based lubricants dissolve latex condoms. Butter, margarine, cooking oil or even WD40 will produce a slippery slope towards a drippy willy not to mention unwanted fatherhood. Use only water-based lubricants.

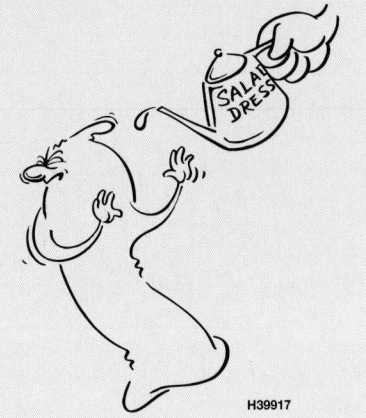

H39917

it to burst or slip off. Sharp finger nails, rings and teeth are a hazard. Only the soft finger pulps should be used to unroll the condom on to the penis. If extra lubrication is needed then only a water based one should be used with rubber condoms. There is a need to withdraw and remove the condom while the penis is still erect to avoid semen leaking out as the penis shrinks in size.

### Spontaneity

Perhaps the single biggest stated reason for not using condoms is the widely held belief that they inhibit spontaneous sex. Foreplay is an important part of enjoyable sexual activity and partners can involve the condom in this. Fears that they reduce the sensitivity of sexual experience have not been supported by research. Most of the problem is with the psychological inhibition some men have over their use but without doubt lots of foreplay does help.

## The female condom

The condom for women is relatively new, but regular users report favourably and many men prefer them to the male condom. Made of plastic it is larger in diameter than the male condom and has a flexible ring at each end. The smaller ring fits inside the vagina while the outer, larger, ring remains on the outside of the vagina. After ejaculation this outer ring should be twisted to prevent escape of the sperm and the condom gently withdrawn. Female condoms are 95 per cent effective, and also have the advantage of providing protection against many sexually transmitted infections.

## Oral contraception (the Pill)

The combined pill contains two hormones which inhibit the release of the hormones which stimulate the final development and release of ova (eggs) from the ovary. This partly mimics a pregnancy, which explains why some women suffer the milder symptoms of being pregnant when using this pill.

The combined pill is convenient, over 99 per cent effective when taken correctly, and has many advantages (including protection against cancer of the womb and the ovary). Like all drugs, there are health risks associated with its use. A very small number of women will develop a blood clot which can be life-threatening. Women who take the pill are also more at risk of being diagnosed with breast cancer or cervical cancer. However, for the vast majority of women the advantages of taking the pill greatly outweigh the risks.

The progestogen-only pill contains only one hormone and stops sperm from getting anywhere near the egg by maintaining the natural plug of mucus in the neck of the womb. It also makes the lining of the womb thinner. It is highly effective (99 per cent) and it is particularly useful for women who cannot use

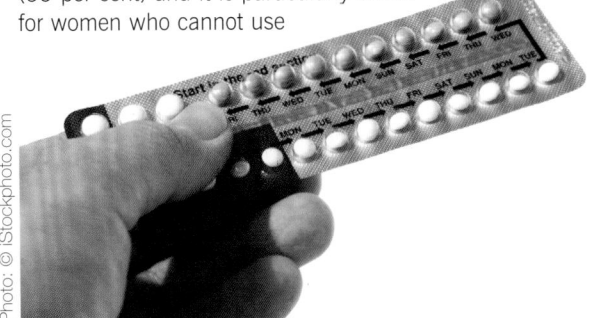

Photo: © iStockphoto.com

The Pill

### If the man does not actually ejaculate can the woman get pregnant?

This is part of the, 'You can trust me, I'm in complete control' approach favoured by men who mistakenly put their money into the chewing-gum machine instead of the condom dispenser. As this fundamental error was caused by fifteen pints of lager you have some idea about just exactly how much control he will have over his bodily functions. If you like a bit of a flutter on the Grand National you might want to take your chance on the lager reaching those places three of sand and two of cement cannot reach. It will not, however, make any difference to your risk of picking up a nasty sexually transmitted disease such as HIV.

In terms of 'fates worse than death', men produce a pre-ejaculatory fluid designed to smooth the troubled waters for the following sperm. Even without ejaculation this fluid may contain sperm sitting in the pipeline from an earlier more successful mission. If any man asks you to accept this 'guarantee' you should first check whether he can chew the gum he bought and walk at the same time. Accepting his assurances entitles you to free chewing gum. Sit down while you eat as you might trip over your feet.

the combined pill, and those who are breast-feeding. It has, however, to be taken regularly at the same time each day, and can have the disadvantage of causing irregular bleeding.

## Intrauterine contraceptive device (IUD)

These small plastic and copper devices are inserted into the womb by GPs, or by doctors or nurses at family planning clinics. They prevent pregnancy by stopping the sperm and egg meeting; they also make the lining of the womb unsuitable for implantation should fertilisation occur. They are over 99 per cent effective, can be left in place for up to eight years, and can be used by women both before and after having children. They are not suitable for women who are at risk of getting a sexually transmitted infection, and can make periods longer and heavier. To minimise the risk of infection, tests are done before the IUD is put in. The IUD is removed very easily by a doctor or nurse and has no effect upon sensation during intercourse.

## Intrauterine contraceptive system (IUS)

These small plastic T-shaped devices contain the hormone progestogen. They are inserted into the womb by GPs, or by doctors or nurses at family planning clinics. They prevent pregnancy in the same way as the progestogen-only pill. They are over 99 per cent effective, can be left in place for up to five years, and can be used by women both before and after having children. Initial side-effects can include irregular bleeding, but periods then tend to become lighter and shorter, or stop altogether; period pain is also reduced. Like the IUD, the IUS is removed very easily by a doctor or nurse and has no effect upon sensation during intercourse.

## Hormone implant (for women)

One small rod containing progestogen is inserted under the skin in the arm, usually using a local anaesthetic. It works like

## How long after sex can you take the morning after pill?

The so-called emergency contraceptive pill is simply a very high dose of sex hormones. It prevents a fertilised egg from implanting on the uterine wall. One dose is taken immediately followed 12 hours later by another. After 48 hours the chances of preventing pregnancy begin to decline. If left too long there is a theoretical danger of damaging the developing foetus without stopping the pregnancy. You will need a pregnancy test performed three weeks afterwards.

It is very effective but not in the same league as the oral contraceptive pill itself. You need a doctor's advice if you suffer from high blood pressure or have ever had a problem with blood clots.

the progestogen-only pill and lasts for three years. The main disadvantage is that it can cause irregular bleeding for several months. It is over 99 per cent effective and is easily removed in a minute or two.

## Hormone injection (for women)

The hormone progestogen is given as an injection every 8 or 12 weeks, depending on the type used. It is over 99 per cent effective and works by stopping the ovaries producing eggs. It shares many of the advantages of the combined pill, but can cause irregular bleeding and weight gain. Once the injections stop it can take a year or more for periods to return.

## The male Pill

The day when a male pill will be available slowly gets nearer. There have been successful human trials in the UK, and in the next decade we should see a male hormonal method of contraception. At the moment it is unclear whether this will be in the form of a pill, an implant or an injection.

## Female sterilisation

This is a permanent method of contraception in which the fallopian tubes are either cut, sealed or blocked so that eggs cannot pass down them to the uterus (womb). It has a failure rate of 1 in 200, making it 99.5 per cent effective – as good as other long-term reversible methods. Should it fail, it carries a greater risk of the egg implanting in the fallopian tube (ectopic pregnancy). As a general anaesthetic is required and the operation is more invasive it is a more complicated and risky procedure than vasectomy. It is possible to reverse the operation but with limited success, and with an increased risk of ectopic pregnancy.

## Emergency contraception

'Emergency' contraception is a safe and effective way of preventing pregnancy. It involves either taking tablets containing progestogen (which are used within 72 hours of sex but are more effective the sooner they are taken) or inserting an IUD. Emergency methods can be used when no contraception was used or when regular contraception has failed. Emergency pills are safe to take and have no lasting effects on future fertility. Emergency contraception is available free from GPs and family planning clinics. In addition, emergency pills are free from NHS Walk-in centres and can be bought from pharmacies by women over 16.

## Natural methods

It is only possible for your partner to conceive within 24 hours of ovulation. However, because sperm can live for several days, sex that happens up to seven days before ovulation can result in pregnancy (this sex can even be during a period). It is possible to estimate the fertile period by noting certain changes in the body. Using a fertility thermometer and a chart it is possible to detect the sudden rise in temperature of around 0.2 degrees Celsius which occurs at ovulation. Monitoring changes in the cervical mucus help identify the time before and after ovulation. The mucus becomes thin, watery and clearer before ovulation, and afterwards returns to being thicker, stickier and whiter.

When practised according to instruction, natural family planning is 98 per cent effective, although it does take a while to learn it as a method and requires commitment from both partners.

## Does masturbation make you deaf?

Given the horrendous hours junior doctors work, asking any casualty officer this question will invariably prompt a reply of 'Pardon?' In truth masturbation doesn't affect your hearing. Worse still it has no such effect on your mother's hearing either, who invariably rushed into your bedroom thinking you were being attacked by a Doberman with a stutter. Woody Allen knows a good thing when he experiences it. 'Don't knock it' he said in the film *Annie Hall*, 'it's sex with someone you love'. The Talmud states categorically, 'Thou shalt not masturbate either with hand or foot'. Yes, masturbation may not make you deaf but catching a genital verucca off your own foot really is the pits.

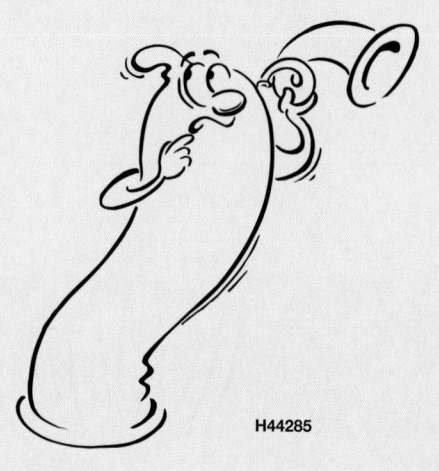

H44285

## Is petroleum jelly the best lubricant?

Yes, is the answer if you are talking about a baby's bum, but for use with a condom you would be wiser using sandpaper. At least you would feel the condom falling to pieces. Petroleum based lubricants will dissolve most condoms, particularly the ultra-thin varieties. Always use water-based lubricants; they are also a less of a fire risk during burning passion.

# Can you use a tampon to prevent pregnancy?

There is a doctor in England who uses tampons to stop severe nose bleeds. Walking around with a tampon up your nose has not yet hit the television advertisements. I suspect you might not feel quite so free if you walked into the local transport cafe in this nasally disadvantaged state. Tampons are a marvellous invention for soaking up blood such as the menses, or a nose bleed for that matter. Unfortunately they are not quite so good at stopping little genetic torpedoes hell bent on being the first successful headbanger. Not only will they not prevent pregnancy, they have even less protection against sexually transmitted diseases.

Part of a casualty officer's life is taken up by removing these machines after being rammed home in a fashion not unlike loading a cannon. Worse still they can be forgotten and fresh tampons used for the rest of the period. Removing them can then be hazardous as the tampon becomes saturated with offensive bugs a lot worse than headbangers. Septic shock is no joke and lives have been lost, so de-tampon before the fun with your ramrod, if you follow my drift.

# Vasectomy (male sterilisation)

Vasectomy is a simple and permanent method of contraception. You don't need permission from your partner but obviously it makes good sense. Fortunately there is no reported effect on enjoying sex. The testicles continue to produce sperm but rather than being ejaculated with the semen the sperm are reabsorbed in each testicle. Sperm therefore doesn't build up inside the testicles. As with any surgical procedure you will have to sign a consent form.

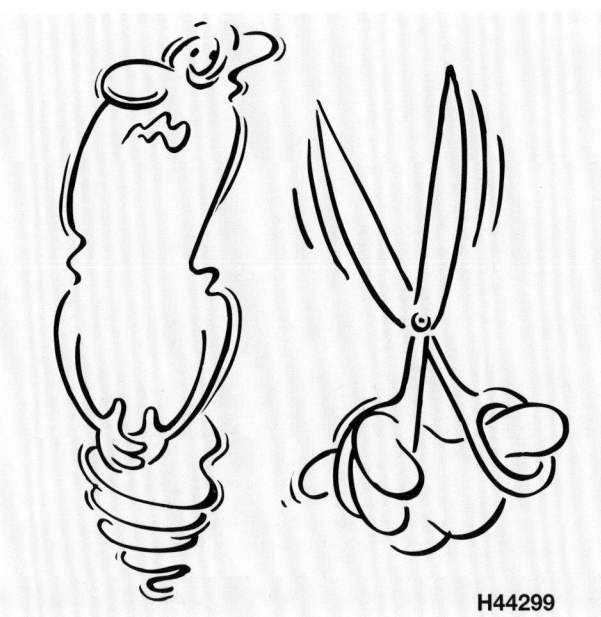

H44299

Vasectomy

## When it should be done

Although there is no lower age limit for vasectomy, young, childless men need to consider this method carefully to avoid later regret. It should therefore only be chosen by men who, for whatever reason, are sure that they do not want children in the future. Counselling is recommended so that other contraception options can be discussed and the procedure fully understood. A vasectomy immediately following a birth, miscarriage, abortion or family or relationship crisis is a usually a bad idea.

## How it is performed

You can ask for a general anaesthetic but it is generally performed under a local anaesthetic. A small section of each vas deferens – the tubes carrying the sperm from the testes – is removed through small cuts on either side of the scrotum. The ends of the tubes are then cut or blocked. Stitches are rarely required on the scrotum. It is a simple and safe operation lasting around 10-15 minutes, and can be done in a clinic, hospital outpatient department or doctor's surgery.

## Recovery

Discomfort and swelling lasting for a few days is normal but this settles quickly with no other problems. Simple pain-killers help. Occasionally this can last longer and needs your doctor's attention. Strenuous activity should be avoided for a week but you can return to work immediately and have sex as soon as it is comfortable. As the testicles continue to produce testosterone your feelings, sex drive, ability to have an erection and climax won't be affected. Despite numerous scares in the popular media, there are no known long-term risks from a vasectomy.

## Effectiveness

After a vasectomy it can take a few months for all the sperm to disappear from your semen. You need to use another method of contraception until you have had two consecutive semen tests which show that you have no sperm. While vasectomy is highly effective failures are still possible (1 in 2000). The failure rate should be discussed before the operation and it should be pointed out on the consent form. While vasectomy is excellent in preventing pregnancy it will not protect against sexually-transmitted infections. Using a condom is the best protection for this.

## Future prospects

Reversal operations are possible but not always successful and will depend upon how and when the vasectomy was done. Reversals are not easily available either privately or on the NHS.

# Is cling film a suitable alternative to a condom in an emergency?

Obviously the word emergency means different things to different people. Cling film, or rubber gloves for that matter, are not a suitable alternative to anything except pockets full of tuna and cucumber, and smelly fingernails. Despite its name, cling film slips off very easily once wet. Similarly with rubber gloves unless you choose the fingers very carefully and with a fair degree of prescience. Worse still, phthalates present in plastic food wrappings may make the whole thing an academic exercise through chemical emasculation.

# PART 8 Impotence (erectile dysfunction)

## Introduction

Even in these enlightened times there is still confusion over erectile dysfunction (ED/impotence) and infertility. A man can father children without being able to have an erection. Problems with erections are common. At least one in 10 British men have had some sort of erectile dysfunction at some stage in their lives. Furthermore, around one man in twenty has permanent erectile dysfunction problems. This is not helped by most men's reluctance to discuss these problems, despite the fact that virtually all of them can be overcome by relatively simple treatments.

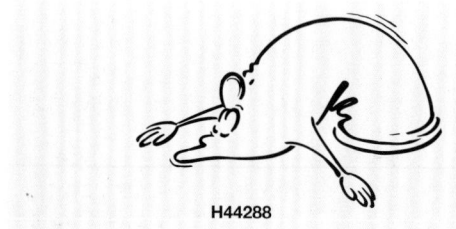

**H44288**

The penis works by hydrostatic pressure

As the penis works by hydrostatic pressure allowing blood into the spongy tissues of the penis but restricting its outflow, anything which affects the blood vessels or nerves which bring this about will influence the ability to have an erection. Unfortunately there are a large number of things which will interfere with this process, not least medicines prescribed for totally different reasons.

At one time, what was going on between a man's ears was considered the major factor for ED. We now know that around one third of all cases will be purely psychological, and will often respond well to non-clinical treatments such as sex counselling. Generally speaking, if you have erections at any other time other than during attempted intercourse then you have a psychological rather than physiological problem. Successful erections during television programmes, sexy videos or self-masturbation bode well for the future, although it is not a 100 per cent test.

## When the flesh needs convincing

While there is great variation in the actual size of the penis throughout the animal kingdom, humans come top of the list in their group, the primates. (However, unlike some of the other primates we do not have prehensile tails.) For all primates the penis appears to have a disproportionate influence over the

Almost half the penile structure is hidden within the pelvis
1 Erectile tissue
2 Urethra
3 Scrotum
4 Testis
5 Prostate
6 Seminal vesicle
7 Bladder

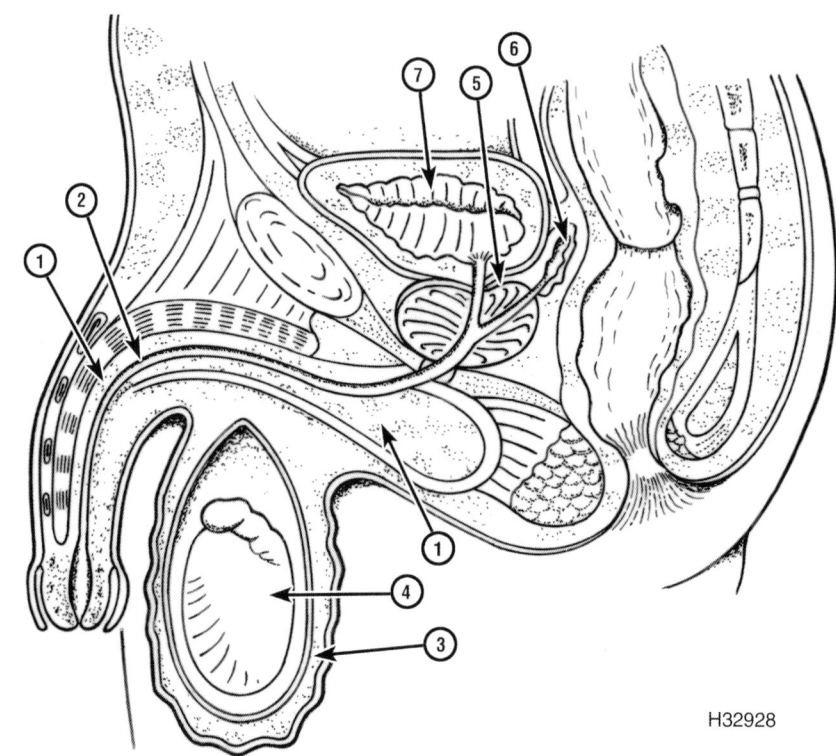

H32928

everyday life of the species; few other animals give sex, as distinct from reproduction, the same level of priority. Similarly, the role of the human penis is complex and extends beyond a means of transferring sperm to the female or even passing urine. Society places a certain importance on the size of a man's penis. It is said that the CIA seriously considered supplying over-sized condoms to villagers during the Vietnam/Cambodian war to enhance the 'prowess' of American troops in the eyes of the enemy.

### Hydraulic system

There is no bone in the penis. Its function depends upon a hydraulic system which Citroën owners will readily understand. Just as a balloon filled with water is more rigid than one without, the erect penis uses the same principle, using blood rather than water as the stiffening medium. By allowing blood into spongy tissue within the penis, but restricting its exit, the penis can enlarge by around 2 inches during an erection.

While valuable for placing sperm well into the vagina, an erection hinders the passing of urine. Indeed there is a one-way valve at the base of the penis which prevents urine being passed at the same time as sperm. Urine or sperm travel down the penis from the bladder or testes in a thin tube called the urethra.

The thin skin of the penis is covered in small bumps which may be important in stimulation of the sexual partner. Unfortunately they also cause a disproportionate amount of concern, particularly amongst young men. These are the sweat glands and hair follicles that are not normally felt on thicker skin. They are even more noticeable during an erection because the skin is stretched much thinner.

### Average sizes

While men are prone to exaggerate, the average size of the human penis is around three-and-a-half to seven inches. There are operations which lengthen the penis by up to 50 per cent as almost half the penile structure is hidden within the pelvis. By cutting the ligaments which tether the penis to the pubic bones, the true length is exposed. The only serious side effect is the alteration in the angle of dangle. Instead of the erect penis standing to attention, it tends to take a more horizontal position. This is not said to adversely affect sexual pleasure. Numerous studies, however, have shown that penile length is not the main factor for sexual pleasure in the female or male partner.

A more effective and far less traumatic way of increasing penis length is to lose any excess weight.

# Erectile Dysfunction (ED)

### Age: the great escape

If ever there was a universal scapegoat for things that go wrong with the human body, particularly sexual activity, it has to be 'too many birthdays'. Thankfully we are realising that sex is not just for the young and the enjoyment of sex can go on indefinitely. Expressions such as 'dirty old man' are becoming less common as we all live longer and older people predominate in our society.

Age-related problems do exist, but they are by no mean the major cause. Some important facts have emerged with recent studies:

- There is a gradual decline in testosterone levels and levels of this hormone can have an effect on target organs such as the penis.

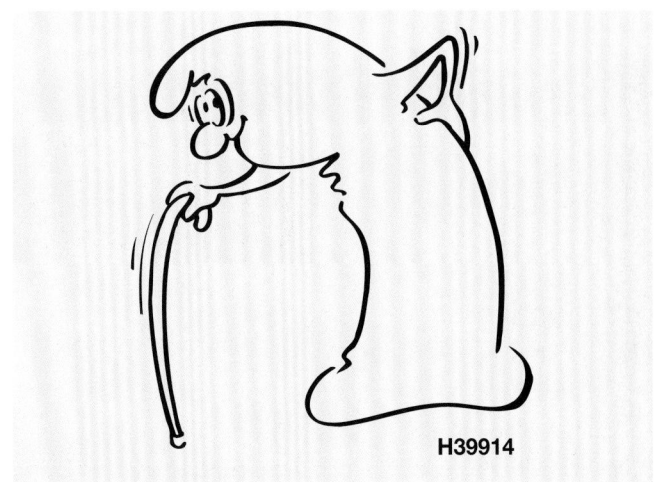

With age, erections take longer to develop and may require more tactile stimulation

- Erections take longer to develop and may require more tactile stimulation. Yes, the old Bentley may take longer to start than the new Porsche but it will give you a more comfortable ride. Might not run out of petrol so soon either.
- Self image and concerns over sexual activity tend to be problems in later life. Men are notoriously bad at confronting these problems and will often let age take the blame.
- Physical illnesses take their toll on sexual activity, not least because of the drugs which are commonly prescribed by way of treatment. We do tend to accumulate chronic conditions as we age.
- Gaps in sexual activity can be important, if only the toll they can take on sexual confidence. Bereavement, illness of the partner or divorce are good examples.
- Men are slow to admit depression to their doctors, older men even more so. Depression is a major factor for erectile dysfunction.

### Common medicines and alcohol

Some medicines are known to cause problems with erections:
- Some anti-depressants are paradoxically capable of making erectile dysfunction even worse. On the other hand, some can delay premature ejaculation, which can be helpful. Talk to your doctor.
- Some anti-hypertensive drugs for high blood pressure are common culprits. ACE inhibitors, alpha and beta blockers, and calcium channel blockers can all cause problems for certain individuals. You can change your medicine to help. Talk to your doctor.
- Alcohol is a common cause. Obviously binge drinking has an immediate effect but chronic alcohol abuse can lead to permanent problems with erectile dysfunction. Small amounts of alcohol in the blood (up to 25 mg per 100 ml, or a couple of drinks in plain English) make erections easier. Any more can cause the dreaded 'droop'.
- Tobacco has an immediate short-term effect but is a much worse long-term factor. You can't have an erection when you're dead.

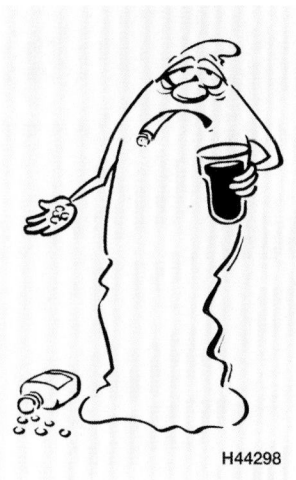

Medicines and alcohol can be a factor

## Common disease culprits

Diseases which affect the nerves or blood supply can also cause problems:

- Multiple sclerosis is the commonest spinal cord disease causing erectile dysfunction. There can also be bladder problems.
- Diabetes can cause a peripheral nerve problem which affects the ability to have an erection and tends to go undiagnosed for many years.
- Vascular (blood circulation) problems account for around 25 per cent of erectile dysfunction in men. They usually have an insidious onset and are made worse by taking even small amounts of alcohol.

## Diagnosis

A proper medical check-up is needed to look for any underlying cause of erectile dysfunction.

Your history will be the most important tool for diagnosis, but various tests on hormone levels are often performed.

Some diseases which travel in families, such as diabetes, hypertension or depression can also be an important clue to diagnosis. Details of drinking habits (remember brewer's droop?), smoking, diet and exercise can all be important.

## Examination

A number of tests can be performed to exclude physiological causes. These include tests for:

- Diabetes.
- Anaemia.
- Liver problems.
- Thyroid deficiency (the thyroid is a gland in the neck which acts as a sort of thermostat for body metabolism. If it is set 'too low' then everything slows down, including erections).
- Testosterone, prolactin and leutenising hormone levels. The balance between all three show if you are producing the right levels of hormone to make erections possible in the first place.

Your doctor will also check:

- Blood circulation. Poor blood flow thorough arteries in your legs can also mean the same thing for your penis. Your legs use bone to stay straight, your penis can only use the pressure of blood.
- Loss of facial hair, large breasts or small testes. These all indicate a hormone problem.

## Prevention

Avoiding excessive alcohol and tobacco are the obvious first lines of attack. Check with your doctor whether any drugs you are taking could be part of the problem.

## Treatment

Herbal and traditional remedies are freely available but there is little evidence for their effectiveness.

Some simple treatments require a sense of humour, not least vacuum devices which have been around for over 70 years. They work by drawing blood into the penis under a gentle vacuum produced by a sheath placed over the penis and evacuated with a small pump. By restricting the blood from leaving with a tight rubber band at the base of the penis, a respectable erection can be produced. It makes sense to remove the band after 30 minutes or so to avoid problems with blood clotting. They can be used in men with vascular problems.

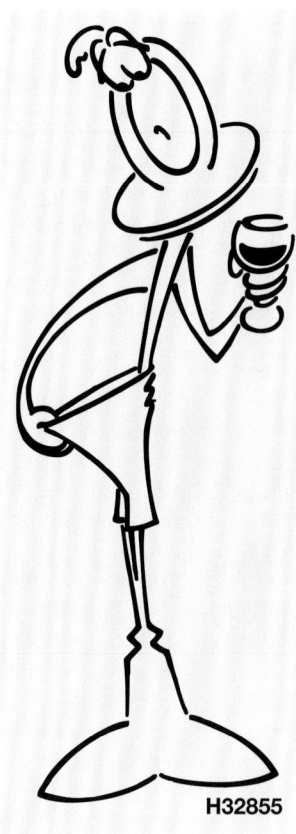

It is a golden opportunity to have a proper medical check for any underlying cause of erectile dysfunction

## Psychological causes

The treatment of psychological impotence depends on education, the use of methods such as the temporary prohibition of sexual intercourse, the encouragement of touching and sensual massage (sensate focus technique) and sexual counselling.

You will need to be honest with yourself and your counsellor. They will want to know a number of important things:

- Childhood experiences and your attitude to sexuality. This may well include the attitudes of your partner.
- Your sexual experience during adolescence.
- Your own body image and how you feel about your genitals.
- How content you are with your sexual relationships.
- 'Bad trips'. Have you had some painful experiences which are flavouring your appreciation of sex.
- Your feelings about sexual arousal. What is 'normal' or 'acceptable' practice.
- How you rate yourself as a sexual being.

After looking into these areas they will want to know if these problems came on suddenly, and what preceded them. Psychological problems tend to come on quite abruptly whereas physiological causes tend to be more insidious. Your medical history will be examined. Some drugs (medicinal and recreational) can cause erectile problems. Even homeopathic treatments can be a factor.

## Oral treatments

The great leap forward came with oral preparations which are increasing in number, mode of action, duration of action and safety. They allow as near as possible 'normal' sex but still require stimulation and arousal as they are not aphrodisiacs.

Although around 80% of men will be able to get an erection adequate for intercourse with drug support, probably less than half will continue with therapy in the longer term. The likely reason for this is that both doctors and their male patients tend to focus on erection and genital function rather than on sexual satisfaction, and this is a very personal factor. A rigid erection alone will not necessarily help you talk comfortably and openly about your sexual fantasies and ideas, particularly if you have not had sex for a long time.

Couples using drug therapies need ongoing support and encouragement until they are satisfied with the outcome of treatment. It is important that you understand how to use the drugs properly as nearly one third of men who failed to get adequate erections with a drug could do so when re-instructed on its proper use.

Another important issue is that, whether using drug therapy or not, older men take longer to get an erection and often require direct genital stimulation to do so. Some men believe that their inability to get an erection through fantasy or visual stimulation alone is abnormal, whereas it should really be expected with ageing. Variety really can be quite literally the spice of life here and more variety in sexual behaviour can be helpful. Cuddling, play and talking are all part of the sex act which will have gone as well so needs to be put back into practice.

## Injections

Hormone injections straight into the penis may be a better option. The needle is so fine it is virtually painless but you need to inject into different places to stop any scarring.

Injections of drugs straight into the spongy tissue of the penis can mimic the way the nerves work by restricting the blood flow out of the penis, thus producing an erection in men with these problems. It is surprisingly free of pain, although most men cross their legs just thinking about it.

These treatments can be effective in men who have not responded to oral therapies, but they may not always be acceptable to men or their partners. Unlike oral therapies, they provoke erection directly without the need for external stimulation.

## Penile implants

If there is no response to injections, a penile prosthesis may be the answer. Before you go down this road both you and your partner need to understand what is involved. There is a certain sacrifice of dignity which both of you will need to come to terms with. Having said that, many couples find the release of sexual frustration far outweighs the temporary embarrassment.

There are three versions of implantable devices:

- Semi-rigid rods, made of silicone, sometimes covered with stainless steel braiding, are inserted into the spongy tissue of the penis.
- Two self-contained cylinder pumps are inserted into the penis and filled by squeezing a reservoir in the base of the penis.
- Inflatable penis prostheses consist of a pair of inflatable silicone cylinders implanted in the penis which can be filled by squeezing a pump implanted in the scrotum.

They all work. But as the old saying goes, 'it's not the size, it's what you do with it that counts'. Foreplay, sexual experimentation, avoidance of routine and being honest with each other is just as important as having a functional erection. Oh yes, and a healthy dollop of a sense of humour too. Sex after all is not only enjoyable, it can be good fun as well.

## Does having sex on an aeroplane make your testicles blow up?

Fortunately not. Otherwise it would give terrorists a whole new dimension to plane hijacks. Members of the Mile High Club, an exclusive group of underweight individuals who loiter around airborne toilets, are particularly happy. 'You are aware of something which doesn't happen on the ground' one leading member who wishes to remain anonymous told me, 'perhaps it is the reduced cabin pressure'. More likely the cabin crew adjusting the video camera for the next office party. If you take a plastic mineral water bottle on board it will fizz far more on opening as the cabin pressure is maintained as the equivalent of that at a few thousand feet. This has no effect on the internal organs, or the external ones for that matter. Newton's law states, however, that to every action there is an equal and opposite reaction so you might like to tell your Mile High Partner to adopt the brace position.

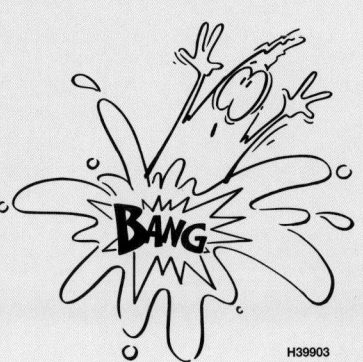

H39903

# PART 8 Artificial insemination and IVF

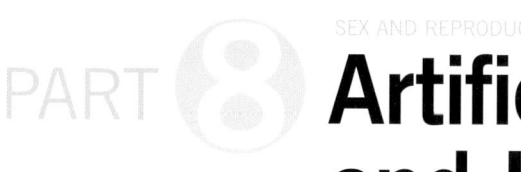

The term artificial insemination sounds daunting and cold. Some fertility clinics call it intra-uterine insemination for this very reason. Whatever it is called, it is actually a simple way of becoming pregnant if it is very difficult or impossible to manage it through sexual intercourse. If that does not work, more sophisticated treatments are available.

Note that impotence (erectile dysfunction/ED) and infertility are not the same thing. A man can be unable to have an erection yet be perfectly capable of having children by treating the erectile dysfunction (see *Impotence*) or by using assisted methods of conception. Sub-fertility, where there are too few sperm in the semen, or they are not able to swim correctly, does not necessarily mean that you cannot have children.

In cases of erectile dysfunction, seminal fluid can often be obtained by masturbation or by massaging the prostate under an anaesthetic. This is called AIP (artificial insemination by partner). With reduced fertility (sub-fertility) pregnancy can sometimes be achieved by placing the semen directly into the cervix. With severely reduced fertility, semen can be provided by another man. This is called AID (artificial insemination by donor). Most donors remain anonymous although the law is being pressed on this issue should your child wish to know their 'natural' father. You need to discuss this fully with your partner and medical staff.

Of course any form of artificial insemination carries connotations and must always be second best, but it is relatively easy, quick and results in the vast majority of cases in a perfectly normal baby.

## Is there a problem?

Out of every ten couples trying for children eight achieve pregnancy within a year, one couple will conceive within two years and the remaining couple will need medical help. Many doctors will not consider referring a couple for infertility investigations until they have been trying for around two years (one year if the couple are over 35 years old).

How long you should spend trying for pregnancy before seeking help depends to some extent on the medical histories and age of you and your partner. Consult your GP or attend a family planning clinic for women if your partner:
- Has irregular periods, or the menstrual cycle is shorter than 21 or longer than 35 days.
- Finds intercourse painful.
- Has a history of pelvic inflammatory disease.
- Has had any abdominal surgery.
- Has a history of chlamydia or another sexually transmitted infection.
- Is underweight or overweight.
- Is aged over 35.

Consult your GP or attend a family planning clinic for men if you:
- Have had an operation on the testes, or had treatment for testicular cancer or an undescended testicle.
- Have a history of chlamydia or another sexually transmitted infection.
- Have a history of mumps after puberty.
- Are very overweight.
  Be prepared to discuss questions such as:
- Your general medical health.
- Your partner's menstrual cycle.
- Previous methods of contraception.
- Any previous pregnancies/miscarriages/abortions.
- Any infections, including sexually transmitted infections.
- How often you have intercourse.

## Causes of infertility and possible treatments

A woman who has difficulty in ovulating may need a course of drugs.

A woman not producing eggs may need another woman to donate eggs (this is not routinely offered).

A woman with blocked fallopian tubes may need surgery or assisted conception.

A man with a low count and/or poor quality of sperm may need assisted conception to aid fertilisation using his own sperm. Alternatively, sperm from a donor may be needed.

There may be other, less common, causes and a couple may have a combination of problems, so investigations need to be completed even if one problem is found at an early stage. Most problems can be helped, with varying degrees of success. Sometimes, even after full investigations, the reason for infertility cannot be found but assisted conception treatment may still be successful.

Visiting your GP gives you and your partner the opportunity to ask about the possible investigations and treatments, waiting lists and any costs. You can then decide if you want to go ahead with tests and/or treatment. You will want to know what treatments are offered locally on the NHS and, if you wish to consider

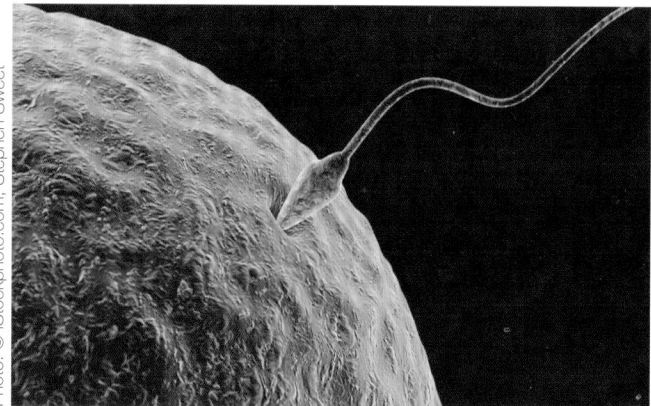

Photo: © iStockphoto.com, Stephen Sweet

paying for private treatment, what private treatments are available locally. You should also find out whether the NHS will meet the costs of any prescribed drugs or if you will have to pay for them.

While GPs can do some preliminary investigations, you may need to be referred to a specialist fertility clinic. If so, you will need a referral letter from your GP. The provision of specialist services within the NHS is limited in some areas and waiting lists vary for certain types of treatment, so try to find out how long you are likely have to wait for an appointment.

## Eligibility for NHS treatment

The type of treatment you can receive on the NHS depends on a number of factors, including what infertility services local health services decide they will purchase.

Some patients will be investigated and treated at their local hospital, others may be referred on to a specialist unit. There is often a limit on the amount of treatment you can receive.

While most tests and investigations are carried out on the NHS, around 80 per cent of in-vitro fertilisation (IVF) treatment is carried out privately. You need to find out what the funding and selection criteria are to see if you will be eligible for NHS treatment. You could also contact the Human Fertilisation and Embryology Authority (HFEA) for a copy of its Patients' Guide to clinics. The reputations and success rates of different fertility clinics vary widely. If venturing outside the NHS, be wary of fraudulent practitioners – check on the HFEA website.

## Fertility tests

A specialist clinic will be able to carry out many different kinds of tests to see what the problem is and to find out which treatments will be best for you.

Clinics offer different types of treatment, and no single clinic is going to be best for everyone. Practical factors such as the opening times, the costs, the length of the clinic's waiting list and the travelling involved are also important.

The kind of tests that are done vary from clinic to clinic. Once you have a diagnosis, fairly simple treatment or surgery may be all that is needed. Not all of the following tests may be necessary, but they include:

- **Semen analysis** to look at the number, shape and size of sperm and how well they move. More than one test should be carried out.
- **Blood or urine tests** to check hormone levels.
- **X-rays/scans** to find blockages or check blood supply to the testes.
- **Blood, urine and cervical mucus checks** to verify hormone levels or detect ovulation.
- **Ultrasound scans** to check if a follicle, which should contain an egg, is being produced. Treatment for ovulation problems usually involves drugs by tablets, injections or nasal inhalations – and has a high success rate if the correct diagnosis has been established.
- **Sperm mucus crossover** – this checks if the woman's cervical mucus allows her partner's sperm through.
- **Endometrial biopsy** – a tiny sample of womb lining (endometrium) is removed to check that it is free from infection and that ovulation has occurred.
- **Hysterosalpingogram** where dye is passed through the fallopian tubes to check that they are open and clear of obstruction.
- **Laparoscopy** (usually under general anaesthetic) uses a thin telescope-like instrument to view the female reproductive organs through a small cut below the navel. It checks for scar tissue, endometriosis, fibroids or any abnormality in the shape or position of the womb, ovaries or fallopian tubes. At the same time a dye may be passed through the fallopian tubes to see if they are open and clear.

## Assisted conception

Assisted conception techniques have been used successfully for many years and a range of techniques is available. It is now possible for some men with very low sperm counts or even with no sperm in their semen to have their own genetic children. A specialist clinic will be able to advise you on which treatment will be best for you.

The most well-known treatment is in-vitro fertilisation (IVF) in which eggs are removed from the woman, fertilised in the laboratory and the embryo is then placed into her womb. Others include:

- **Donor Insemination (DI)** uses sperm from anonymous donor, where there are severe problems with the man's sperm.
- **Gamete Intra-Fallopian Transfer (GIFT)** uses a couple's own eggs and sperm, or those of donors, which are mixed together and placed in the woman's fallopian tubes where they fertilise.
- **Intra-Cytoplasmic Sperm Injection (ICSI)** uses a single sperm injected into the woman's egg which is then transferred to the womb after fertilisation.

These are not miracle solutions. The age of your partner is very important. A woman aged under 35 has a much better chance of a successful pregnancy than one over 40.

## Donor insemination (DI) of sperm and donor eggs

If a man produces no or few normal sperm, carries an inherited disease, or has had a vasectomy, then insemination using sperm from an anonymous donor may be considered. Egg donation may be an option if a woman is not producing eggs or has a genetic problem. The decision to use donor sperm or eggs can be a difficult one. You can get help in making this decision from a counsellor or support group.

Clinics which offer this service have to send information about donors, recipients and the outcome of treatment to the HFEA. Donors have to meet extensive screening criteria, including HIV testing. A man may not usually donate sperm after ten live births have resulted from his semen donations. Donors do not have to be anonymous and most clinics will accept a donor who a couple have found for themselves.

## Counselling and support

Couples report that the many hospital visits needed and the time spent waiting between treatments to learn if each stage has worked is stressful. All units providing IVF and other licensed conception techniques have a legal responsibility to offer counselling. Counselling can allow you to talk through what the treatment entails and how you feel about it, and can give support during the process and if the treatment fails.

If you don't want to see a counsellor at the clinic you are attending, the British Infertility Counsellors Association can put you in touch with your nearest infertility counsellor. Some people find being in contact with others in a similar situation or with a support group helps them through infertility.

# PART 8 Sexuality

**Women appear to come to terms with their sexuality far better than do men. More to the point they are able to talk to other women far easier than men can talk about being gay to other men. Some men agonise for ages before opening the closet door. Few are sorry they ever did.**

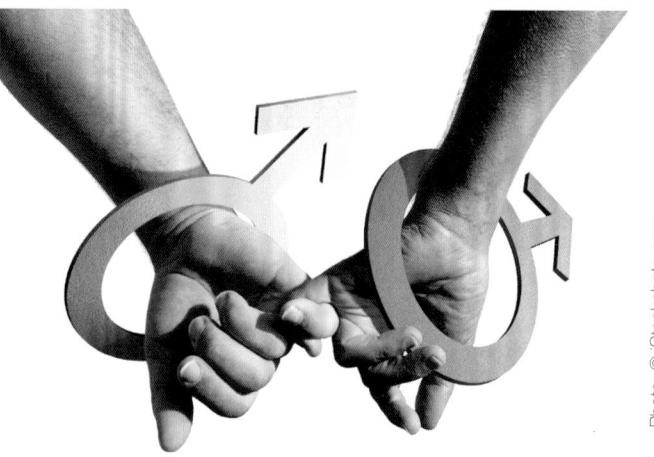

Photo: © iStockphoto.com

Sexuality is a broad spectrum and it is possible, indeed common, for heterosexual men and women to be attracted to members of their own sex. This increases in certain situations where only the one sex is present. This does not make it right or wrong, it is simply an expression of human sexuality. In the rest of the animal kingdom such behaviour is also common. Whales in particular are known to have sexual play with members of their own sex. As the penis of the blue whale is at least six feet long this may explain that great spout of water which comes out of their heads. There is nothing to be ashamed of in investigating and examining your own sexuality. But be careful. Use safer sex and get in touch with a lesbian or gay helpline for some good advice. No matter how attractive you find Willie the killer-whale do not attempt under any circumstances to approach him without a 6 ft condom.

Thanks to all the pressures from society, parents and the law, people will try to rationalise their sexuality in bizarre ways. Instead of simply saying to themselves, 'I just so happen to like people of the same sex and find them sexually attractive' they will make up 'reasonable explanations'. This is also true of parents and society who will jump to conclusions such as upbringing or dressing the person as a baby in the wrong colour. Men try these mental contortions more than women, but both sexes produce some pretty weird interpretations of reality.

So otherwise where is the problem? The problem is with other people, girlfriends, parents, etc. Many men and women who eventually come out are pleasantly surprised at the reaction of their girlfriend/boyfriend when they tell them. They probably suspect anyway and may be attracted for exactly this reason. Parents generally go through a fairly predictable grief reaction. Disbelief, anger, guilt (did they make you gay?) and then coming to terms with the reality. Many parents not only continue to love their gay or lesbian children, they become fiercely supportive. There are some very famous bisexual people around. In truth for every famous bisexual person there are countless thousands of perfectly ordinary bisexual men and women living everyday lives.

Many women, like some men, find that they can still love someone without 'normal' sexual play. This tends to become more like sisterly love rather than that of true lovers in the sexual sense. Unfortunately for some women they confuse this with what is expected from a relationship without realising just how much they are missing. Awareness can then come gradually and not like a blinding flash of light. Recognising habit for what it is can be important for future happiness and fulfilment.

Men are generally aware of their sexuality fairly shortly after puberty and certainly by around 16 years of age. Men will bow to pressure from family and friends and go through heterosexual relationships just to 'fit in'. They may even marry and have a family. For some women this can take longer and many find themselves married, with children sometimes, before they understand their true sexual persuasion. Man or woman, it can be devastating for a marriage and cause pain on all sides. Lesbianism is not abnormal, nor is being a gay man. They are both parts of the spectrum of human sexuality which simply make us richer in our human resource for love.

## Dressed to impress

Many people find this particular aspect of sexual enjoyment and personal fulfilment very attractive. Yet society can still be very harsh on people who commit the terrible crime of simply wanting to be who they are. If you feel more comfortable when you are dressed in the opposite sex's clothes then it gives a good insight into your personality and you should not suppress it unless it brings you into conflict with people who are less understanding than your friends. Being honest really is the best policy.

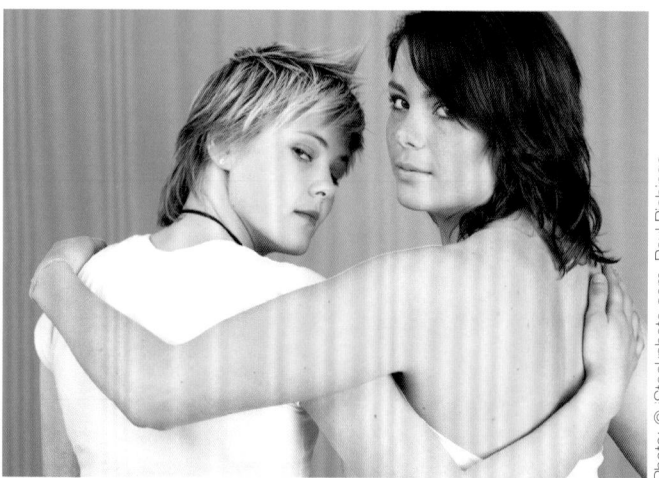

Photo: © iStockphoto.com, Paul Plebinga

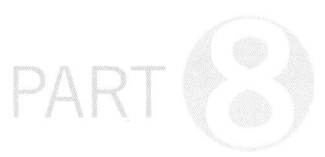

# PART 8

# Sexually Transmitted Infections

## Can you only catch HIV if you are gay?

So far as scary myths go, this has to be the mother of them all. The virus which causes HIV is not politically correct. It has no preferences for any particular sex or the way they choose to make love. It is true that in the UK more gay than straight men have developed the disease but things are changing. We have a had a breathing space of a sort because the 'UK' virus strain is not as virulent as we first thought. There has not been the major epidemic once predicted. Enter a nasty variation on a theme. Some parts of the world have been devastated by the HIV virus, hitting men and women, gay and straight. Once this virus gets going in the UK there will be no second chances. Even with our present variety, unprotected casual sex, gay or straight, is near suicidal. A condom provides almost 100 per cent protection and beats the hell out of half a lemon. Some of them even taste better too, so I am told.

## Introduction

Just one tip for preventing sexually transmitted infections, always practise safer sex. No ifs or buts. Use a condom whenever you have sex, because to be honest sexually transmitted infections (STIs) are a great leveller. They can affect you at any age, whether you're straight or gay, in a long-term relationship or with a casual partner. Symptoms don't always show up immediately, so you could have been infected recently or a long time ago. If you haven't practised safe sex or are at all worried, you can have a confidential check-up, and treatment if needed, at a genitourinary medicine (GUM) or STI clinic. Call NHS Direct for details of your nearest clinic.

## Chlamydia

Non-specific urethritis (an inflammation or infection of the urethra) is a term which includes infection by chlamydia. Men suffering from this infection may complain of an intense burning sensation when passing water. There may also be a white discharge. It actually causes few problems for men, but can be disastrous if passed on to women. It is not only the single biggest cause of infection of the fallopian tubes, leading to infertility and ectopic pregnancy (a potentially lethal condition where the baby attaches to the wall of the fallopian tube instead of the womb), but can cause blindness and pneumonia in a child born to an infected woman. Condoms provide almost total protection.

### Treatment
Chlamydia is treatable with antibiotics.

### Action
Make an appointment with your GP or your local Genito-urinary (GU) clinic.

## Hepatitis B

Hepatitis B is one of the more deadly sexually transmitted diseases, but a vaccine exists which prevent it. Even so, roughly 700 men each year are infected, and the numbers are growing steadily. It can cause as little as a flu-like illness, or as much as total destruction of the liver. Typically, it will cause varying degrees of jaundice (yellowing of the skin and the whites of the eyes). This is caused by the build-up of a pigment which is normally broken down by the liver.

Obviously, most people will not require immunisation, but depending upon your lifestyle it may be wise. It is transmitted via bodily fluids, and only requires a tiny fraction of blood to transmit the disease. The virus can survive a week or more in the dried state and so can be picked up from, for instance, a razor. There is no way

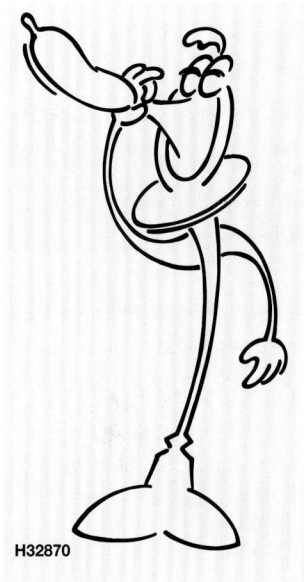

H32870

If you are going to have a bang, make sure you use your own airbag protection

## Does taking the Pill protect you from STIs?

STI stands for Sexually Transmitted Infection. The Pill most definitely does not stop you picking up fellow travellers. Condoms on the other hand will protect you from almost all nether region nasties *and* prevent unwanted pregnancies. Unfortunately men will often leave contraception all up to the woman. Vaginal condoms are now available which really do protect a woman from a fate worse than death, in fact just death.

of knowing if the person with whom you are having sex harbours the infection. The incubation period (how long it takes before the illness manifests itself) is six months from infection. Some people can even 'carry' the virus and not exhibit the condition.

## Genital Herpes

This is the third most common STI, and is currently uncurable. Herpes Simplex Virus (HSV) comes in two forms, HSV I and HSV II. Both infect parts of the body where two types of skin meet together, such as the corners of the mouth, and the outer parts of the genital areas. The virus causes crusted blisters, and then

---

### Can you can catch sexually transmitted diseases off a toilet seat?

This is the standard question from people who treat British bogs like some of those you find in French camp-sites. For the enlightenment of those of you who always caravan instead, you stand over a small hole while attending to nature. This teaches you two things:

- If God was French he would have put eyes in our bums.
- French men prefer trousers without turn-ups.

On the plus side, your rear end never actually touches those parts that other people's rear ends have touched. At least not until you pull the chain and it flushes the entire loo area before you have a chance to get out of the door, slipping in the process.

Even so, sexually transmitted diseases are so called because that is how they are transmitted. Otherwise they would be called 'toilet transmitted diseases' and there would be no such things as turn-ups. Viruses such as the one which causes HIV cannot survive for any significant amount of time in the open air. Similarly bacteria and other small organisms responsible for these infections need body fluids to survive. This immunity does not extend to larger creepy crawlies like lice or crabs which can survive for a while, particularly their eggs which are laid on the pubic hairs. Mind you, telling your doctor that you picked up your itchy little hitch-hikers from a public loo may raise an eyebrow, but the treatment will be the same.

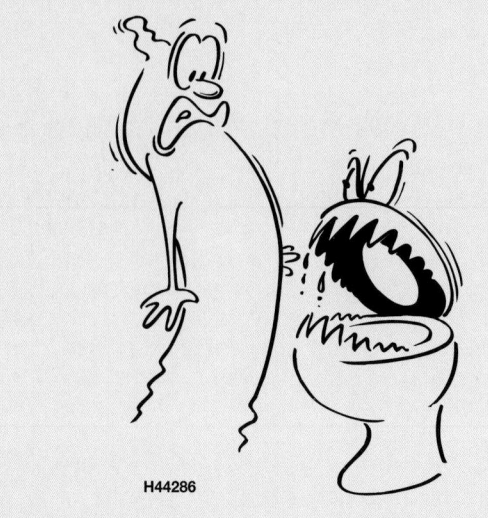

H44286

---

ulcers that weep a thin, watery substance. This substance is highly infectious, since it contains the Herpes virus. Coming in attacks which can last for months and then disappear for years, or even never return. You are definitely infectious during the presence of the sores, but it is possible to catch the virus even when the sores are not present. Stress and other illness can bring on attacks.

### Treatment
Anti-viral drugs can be applied directly to the affected skin or taken orally. They are most effective if used before the sores break out. This is signalled by a tingling, itchy, painful sensation in the affected area. Condoms with a spermicide appear to offer greater protection than those without. You need to arrange your sex life around the condition if you are having an attack as this means you are highly infectious. Otherwise, the use of condoms gives maximum protection for your partner.

### Action
Make an appointment with your GP or your local Genito-urinary (GU) clinic.

## Genital warts

Papilloma viruses, which cause warts, can affect any part of the skin. The virus can be transmitted by physical contact including sexual intercourse. Like the warts commonly seen on people's hands, they can vary in size from tiny skin tags to large masses. One in eight people attending GUM clinics has genital warts. Around 100,000 people are treated for genital warts each year in the UK

### Treatment
There are drugs which can be applied directly to warts which will cause them to disappear. Genital warts usually cause little discomfort, although they are often itchy and may bleed with scratching. Use a condom to prevent catching or transmitting them in the first place.

## Syphilis

Over the past 50 years syphilis has been rare in the UK, but now, along with most other sexually transmitted infections cases are rising. It is caused by a microscopic parasite, which is highly infectious. Most people are unaware of the infection, but if it is not treated it can develop over a number of years into a condition which can affect the brain. Women show few signs of the infection in the early stages except for small ulcers around the vagina so it can go unnoticed by the woman or by their partner during intercourse. The parasite cannot pass through a condom, so this will give almost 100% protection.

### Treatment
An injection of antibiotics will cure the condition if it is caught in the early stages.

## Trichomoniasis

Causing a yellow/green discharge from the penis and vagina, this microscopic parasite lives in the urinary tract and usually causes pain when passing water.

### Treatment
The parasite is sensitive to antibiotics.

## Gonorrhoea

Caused by a bacterium, this disease often gives few symptoms, leading to common misdiagnosed. It is commonly known as the clap from the French word *clapoir* meaning sexual sore but is not rare. It can cause a yellow/white discharge from the penis, along with pain on passing water. Most of the symptoms of infection start within 5 days of infection and include a vague ache of the joints and muscles. Although these disappear after a further 10 or so days, the person remains infectious. It can cause reduced fertility if not treated.

### Treatment

Antibiotics are usually effective. Condoms provide almost 100% protection from infection.

## HIV & AIDS

Following infection with the human Immunodeficiency virus (HIV) there are less white blood cells called CD4, thus lowering the body's resistance to infection. Although the virus only appeared in the UK in 1982 there are over 4,000 new cases reported each year with perhaps 10 times this number unrecognised.

Early stages of infection generally go unnoticed and it needs an antibody test from a blood or saliva sample to confirm the presence of the virus. A vague non-specific illness similar to flu sometimes follows the infection at around 6 to 7 weeks later. A variable period of time, years even, can then pass completely symptom free. The occurrence of oral thrush, persistent herpes (cold sores) or strange chest infections which clear only slowly with treatment are ominous signs of the body's declining ability to fight off other infections.

Body fluids are often cited as the carrier of the virus. Actually this can be narrowed down to blood, semen and saliva. Although the risk of infection from saliva is extremely small it makes sense to avoid obvious risks such as oral sex without adequate protection. The main routes of infection are:

- Sexual transmission via blood from small cuts either in the mouth (oral sex), vagina, anus or penis. Sexual orientation is not exclusive, everyone is at risk.
- Blood transfusion in countries with poor medical resources is still a risk. You can buy a travel kit from your GP.
- Sharing dirty needles or even razor blades.

According to the World Health Organisation (WHO) up to 90 per cent of those people infected in the world contracted HIV through heterosexual sex. Dental dams and male and female condoms, particularly those containing spermicide, give a high degree of protection both to you and to your partner.

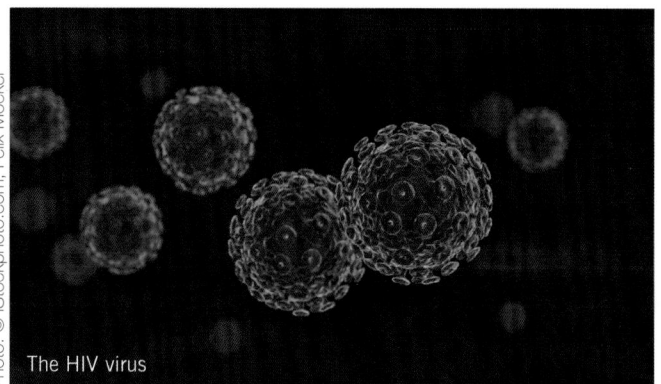

The HIV virus

Photo: © iStockphoto.com, Felix Möckel

---

## Can semen make you fat?

Semen is a mixture of fructose (the same sugar as honey), an acid neutralising substance, minerals, lubrication fluid and tiny amounts of sperm. It has a calorific value similar to honey from very lazy bees. (Expert opinion varies – there's a surprise – but a figure of between 5 and 15 calories per average ejaculate seems to be the consensus.)

As far as oral sex is concerned, then, whether the semen is swallowed or spat out doesn't really make much difference in terms of making the recipient fat. (There is a risk of passing on STIs though. If in doubt, use a condom.)

Absorption of semen in the vagina is poor and contributes little if anything in the way of energy. On the other hand the effort involved in getting it there is the equivalent of a five mile jog. On balance, therefore, semen definitely does not make you fat.

Although extra lubrication is often required, do not use oil-based lubricants such as petroleum jelly or baby oil. They will damage the condom. There are water-based lubricants available. If you are not sure, ask the chemist; they will not be embarrassed to give advice.

### Treatment

It is not all doom and gloom. New treatments are significantly extending life expectancy. Even so, the name of the game is prevention.

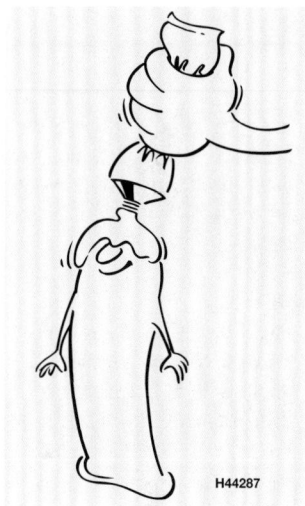

H44287

### Action

You can attend either your own doctor or the local genitourinary medical clinic (GUM), which is located at one of the major hospitals in your area. Confidentiality is all-important at these clinics but you will need to be honest with the doctor. You can give a false name or remain anonymous if you feel more comfortable.

## Can you get HIV from mouth to mouth resuscitation?

As most of the teenage population appear to be performing this life saving procedure on each other every Friday night, the answer is probably no. There is a theoretical risk from saliva which may contain infinitely tiny amounts of the virus, but this risk is so small as to be non existent. If the resuscitee is bleeding from the mouth this increases the risk but it is still relatively small. Blowing through a perforated piece of plastic barrier film further reduces the risk. At the end of the day you have to decide whether the small risk is worth it. The chances of meeting someone needing this attention who has HIV out of a population of 58 million is extremely small.

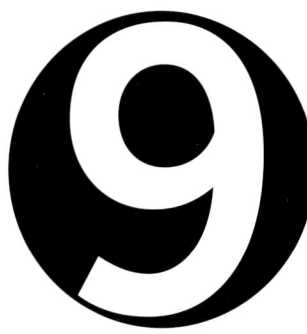

# Skin, bone and muscles

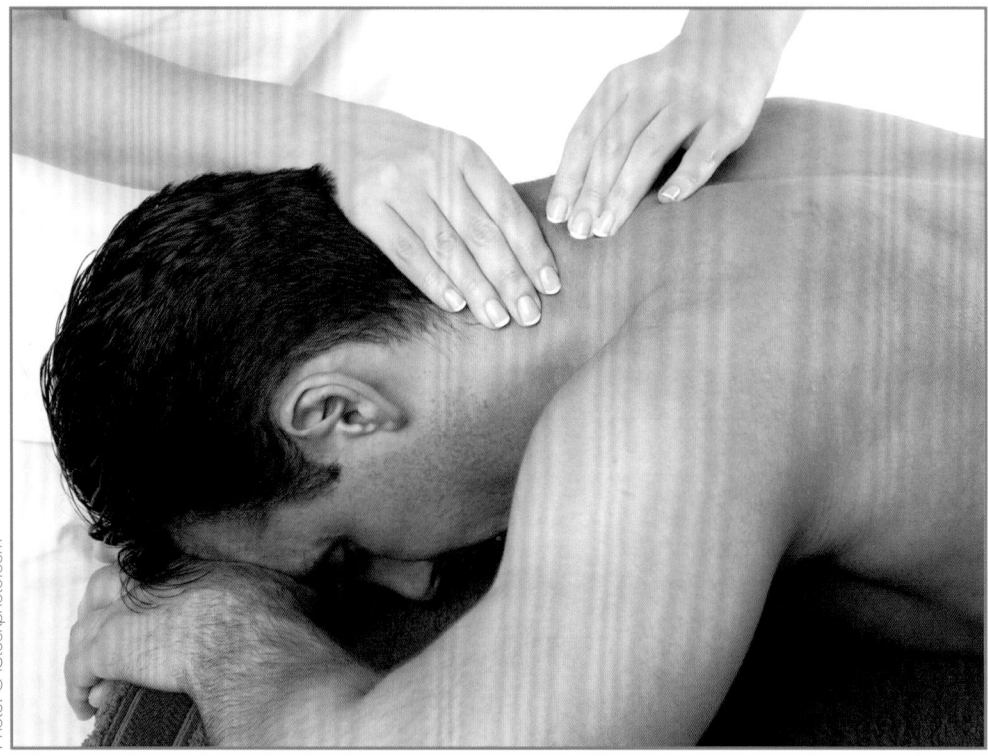

Photo: © iStockphoto.com

# PART 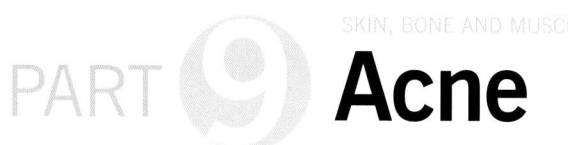 Acne

## Introduction

Although mainly seen in teenage men, acne can also affect older men and women. Thankfully, most people will be free of acne after the age of 20 but it can persist even longer. With early recognition, acne can be effectively treated avoiding disfiguring scars. Some people are affected much worse than others but the way a spot develops is basically the same. Small glands in the skin (sebaceous glands) produce a oily/wax substance called sebum which helps protect skin and hair. The opening to these glands on the skin surface (pores) can block with a mixture of dead skin and sebum leading the way for infection. Pus builds up behind the blockage and the gland swells. Eventually the pressure forces the pus out of the pore.

Permanent scarring may happen with prolonged infection of a number of glands which are close together.

## Symptoms

Blackheads, whiteheads and larger spots appear mainly on the face and less often on the neck, upper chest, back and upper arms. There is a cycle with spots healing while others appear.

## Causes

Contrary to popular myths, diet has little if any effect on acne. Eating 'too much chocolate' is not a cause. Masturbation, blamed for just about every ill, is not a factor.

Dirty skin is also not a cause. In fact, washing too often, particularly with strong soaps can make things worse.

Changes in hormone levels around puberty are probably the most important cause.

We are increasingly aware of stress either causing or making acne worse. General ill health and being 'run down' undoubtedly affect the skin making acne worse and may even trigger it in the first place.

## Prevention

- Avoid harsh soap but keep your skin clean with fresh water.
- Try not use products containing alcohol.

## Complications

- Scarring from infected spots.
- Lack of self confidence in company.

## Self care

- Use a paper towel to dry if possible.
- Don't squeeze spots. Simply wash well.
- Lotions containing benzoyl peroxide can help if you are not allergic to it.

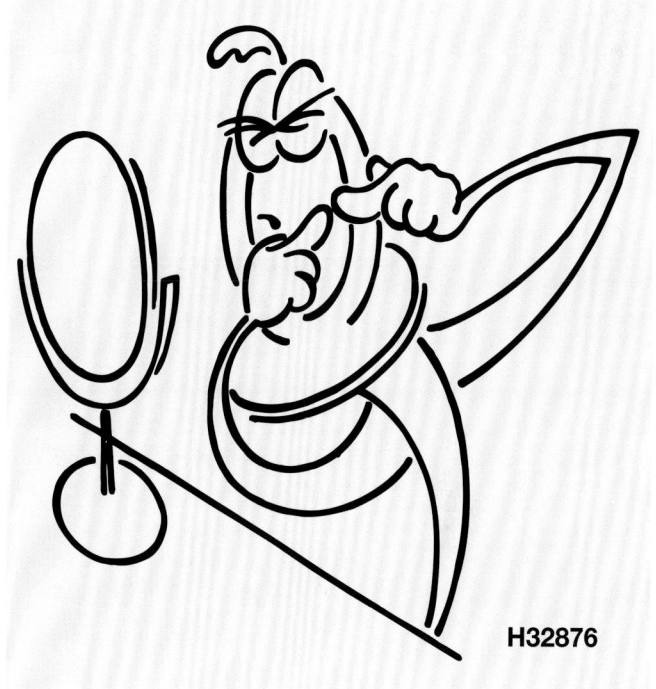

H32876

## Action

Initially, see your pharmacist.

Make an appointment to see your doctor if:
- It is spreading.
- The spots are getting larger and are infected.
- The spots are leaving scars.

There are treatments available which really do help but are available only through your doctor.

In severe cases your doctor can prescribe a long term course of antibiotics.

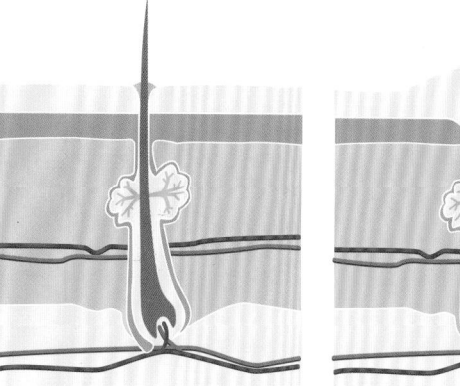

Acne vulgaris

Photo: © iStockphoto.com, Terrainscan

PART 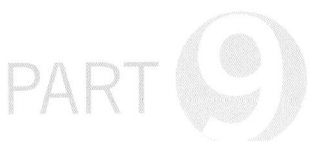 9

# Athlete's foot

## Introduction
Areas of broken skin especially between the toes are a sure sign of the fungus 'tinea'. It can actually develop in many other places on the body where it is called 'ringworm'. It prefers warm damp areas and is infectious but not as much as we once thought.

## Symptoms
- Red, itchy broken skin between the toes which can become white and boggy when damp.
- A strong smell may be present, particularly after wearing shoes for a while.
- Pain on bending toes, or tenderness over the toes.

## Causes
Tinea Is a fungus which can be picked up from swimming pools, baths or even wet floors. Sharing towels can transfer the fungus between people. Wearing trainers without socks makes it easier for infection to take hold.

## Prevention
- Keep your feet dry and well ventilated.
- Wash your feet every morning and evening. Take care to dry them well, especially between the toes. Never use talcum powder.
- Wool or cotton socks are better than man-made fibres.
- Footwear with plenty of ventilation is essential.
- Let your feet see daylight as often as possible.
- Try not to wear trainers without socks.

## Complications
Loss of skin can be extensive causing severe pain.

The infection can spread into the nails causing disfigurement and discolouration. The nails can become incredibly thick which can be painful as well as unsightly.

## Self care
Simply keeping your feet dry for an extended period can help but you will usually need to use an antifungal cream or powder.

Antifungal creams and powders can now be bought across the counter without prescription. Don't stop using until after a couple of weeks of fungus-free feet.

Toe nail infections require prolonged courses (around 4-6 weeks) of antifungal drugs available only on prescription.

## Action
See your pharmacist.

# PART 9 Boils & styes

## Introduction

Boils generally form from infected hair follicles. If this is on the eye lid it is called a stye. When the body fights the most common cause of boils (the bacterium Staphylococcus) it builds a protective wall around the infection preventing it from spreading. Unfortunately this also impedes the body's natural defences from attacking the bacteria and a cyst or boil develops. After a certain length of time the skin lying over the boil will breakdown releasing the pus. Carbuncles are just collections of boils very close together and are thankfully not seen very often.

## Symptoms

It's hard to miss a boil. A painful red lump appears on the skin which gradually gets larger and more painful. The area around the boil is also very tender and slightly inflamed. After a few days a white/yellow 'head' forms which means the boil is about to burst through the skin to release the pus and ease the pain. Some boils will disappear without actually releasing the pus through the skin.

## Causes

Being 'run down' or suffering from some illness which lowers your body's defence against infection can increase your risk from boils. 'Dirty' skin is not a cause of boils. Over washing with antiseptic soaps may even increase your risk.

## Prevention

There is no real prevention against boils but if you are suffering from them often you should see your doctor.

## Complications

Some boils can persist and come back again in the same place. This may leave a scar.

### Note

Staphylococcus also causes a particularly nasty food poisoning which comes on quite soon after eating infected food. If you are handling food at home you should cover the boil, wash your hands and make sure there is no contact with your cooking. You are not allowed to work in any capacity with the preparation or serving of food for public consumption if there is a danger of contamination from a boil.

## Self care

Once the head has formed you can encourage the boil to break by using warm water compresses. Soak some cotton wool in warm water mixed with a couple of spoonfuls of salt. Press it against the boil gently squeezing at the same time. Do not use the highly dangerous method of putting the mouth of a heated bottle to the boil then cooling the bottle to 'draw' the pus. It can cause infection in the bloodstream and may leave a scar.

## More information

Persistent boils can occur if your body's defences against infection are affected by conditions such as diabetes or HIV. Long courses of steroids can also lower your resistance to infection. Some doctors will prescribe antibiotics but others feel that this may delay the natural eruption of the boil through the skin. Once the head is formed some doctors will lance the boil by cutting into the head and breaking down all the layers within the boil allowing it to drain freely.

## Action

Ask your pharmacist for advice.

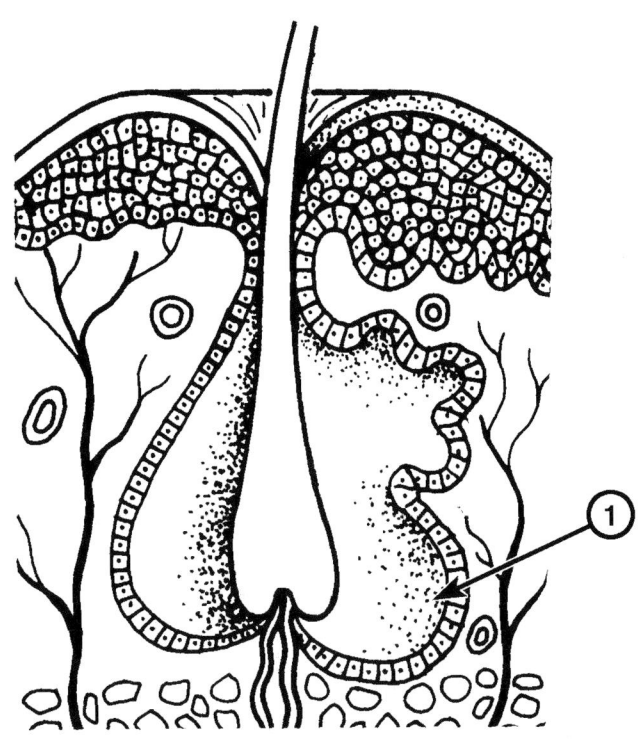

H32714

A boil generally forms from a pus-filled hair follicle (1)

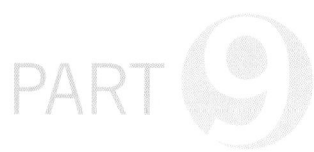

PART 9 **Bone metastases**

## Introduction

The process of metastasis is when cancer, which has developed in one area of the body, spreads and invades another area. Bone is a common site of metastasis for several types of cancers including: prostate, kidney, lung, breast and thyroid cancers, and multiple myeloma.

Cancerous cells, once present in the bone, can cause damage which gives rise to the uncomfortable symptoms often experienced by cancer patients with bone metastases. These bone complications are often referred to as skeletal related events (SREs). Bone metastases are treated by preventing SREs.

## The bone

Bone is a type of connective tissue made up of minerals, such as calcium and phosphate, and the protein collagen. The outer layer of the bone is called the cortex and the spongy centre of the bone is called bone marrow. Bone tissue is porous and alive, with blood vessels running through it.

Like any other part of the body, the bone has to be broken down and replaced to keep its structural integrity. Healthy adult bone is continuously reshaped in response to stresses and strains (remodelled) through a process of bone resorbtion and bone formation. Two kinds of cells are involved in this process: osteoblasts (bone-forming cells) and osteoclasts (cells that break down, or resorb, bone).

Bones carry out a number of functions in the body:
- The skeleton provides structural support for the body.
- Bones store and release minerals that the body needs to function.
- Bone marrow produces and stores blood cells.

## How does cancer spread to the bone?

When cancer cells break away from a cancerous tumour (a primary tumour), they can travel to other parts of the body through the bloodstream or the lymph vessels moving through the bloodstream or lymphatic system. Cancer cells can then lodge in an organ at a distant location and establish a new (secondary) tumour.

Treatments for bone metastases include physical therapy

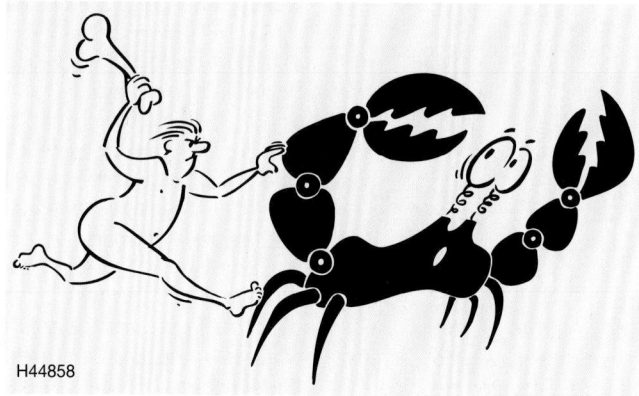

H44858

Secondary tumours that spread to bone (bone metastases) are not the same as primary bone cancer that starts in the bone (sarcoma). A tumour that has metastasised to bone is made up of abnormal cancer cells from the original tumour site and not of bone cells.

When cancer cells spread to the bone, they commonly lodge in the spine, rib cage, pelvis, limbs, and skull.

In cancer, the normal bone remodelling process is disturbed. Once cancerous cells are present in the bone, they cause abnormal 'dissolving' or wearing away of portions of the bone. This dissolving activity leaves holes called 'osteolytic lesions'. Bones are left fragile and weak so that they break or are prone to fracture.

In prostate cancer the tumour may stimulate bone to form and build up abnormally and the areas of bone resorbtion are therefore not filled. These areas of new bone are known as 'osteosclerotic lesions'. There is not the appropriate coupling between bone breakdown and bone formation, so the bone gets worn away and thinned. The result is fragile bone that can easily fracture or collapse.

# What are the symptoms of bone metastases?

### Bone pain
Pain is the most common symptom of bone metastases and is usually the first symptom that people notice. At first the pain may come and go and tends to be worse at night or with bed rest. Eventually the pain may increase and become severe. Obviously, not all pain indicates bone metastases. Your doctor can help distinguish between pain from metastases and aches and pains from other sources.

### Fractures
Bone metastases can weaken bones, putting them at risk of fractures. In some cases, a fracture is the first sign of bone metastases. The long bones of the arms and legs and the bones of the spine are the most common sites of fracture.

### Spinal cord compression
When cancer metastasises to the spine, it can squeeze the spinal cord. The pressure on the spinal cord may not only cause pain, it may cause numbness or weakness in the legs, problems with the bowels or bladder, or numbness in the abdominal area.

### High blood calcium levels
High levels of calcium in the blood (hypercalcaemia) can be caused when calcium is released from the bones during the remodelling process. High calcium levels may cause nausea, thirst, constipation, tiredness, confusion and/or reduce your appetite, part of the reason for weight loss, another feature of cancer. If untreated, it may cause a coma or abnormal heart rhythm.

### Other symptoms
If bone metastases affect the function of its bone marrow, other symptoms may be experienced depending on the type of blood cell affected. Red blood levels may drop, causing anaemia that leads to symptoms of tiredness, weakness, and shortness of breath. If white blood cells are affected, the person may develop infections that cause fevers, chills, fatigue or pain. If the number of platelets – a special cell involved in blood clotting – drops, abnormal bleeding may occur, a common first sign. It is usually noticed after brushing your teeth or by a small cut refusing to stop bleeding.

# How are bone metastases diagnosed?

### X-rays
Radiographic examination (X-rays) can provide information about what part of the skeleton the cancer has spread to, as well as the general size and shape of the tumour or tumours.

The damaged areas usually show up as dark spots on the X-ray film. But bone metastases often do not show up on X-rays unless the cancer is well-advanced.

### Bone scan
Bone scans can detect bone metastases earlier than X-rays can. They also allow the doctor to monitor the health of all the bones in the body, including how they are responding to treatment.

In a bone scan, the person is given an injection of a low amount of radioactive material. The radioactive substance is attracted to diseased bone cells throughout the body. Diseased bone appears on the bone scan image as darker, dense areas.

### Computerised tomography (CT) scan
The CT scan provides X-ray images to look at cross-sections of organs and bones in the body. Rather than provide one image as a conventional X-ray does, the CT scanner takes many pictures as it rotates around the body. A computer combines the images into one picture to show if cancer has spread to the bones. It is particularly helpful in showing osteolytic metastases that may be missed with the bone scan.

### Magnetic resonance imaging (MRI)
MRI scans use radio waves and strong magnets instead of X-rays to provide pictures of bones and tissues. They are particularly useful in looking at the spine.

### Laboratory tests
Bone metastases can cause a number of substances, such as calcium and alkaline phosphatase, to be released into the blood in amounts that are higher than normal. Blood tests for these substances can help diagnose bone metastases.

# How can bone metastases be treated?
The two main aims in the treatment of bone metastases are, firstly, to relieve the symptoms experienced by the patient and to ensure they are made more comfortable, and secondly, to reduce the number of cancer cells in the primary tumour and bone where possible.

### Radiotherapy
Radiotherapy is the term used to describe the use of high-energy beams, often X-rays, to destroy cancer cells. An accelerator generates the beams, or alternatively, radioactive isotopes are used.

For bone metastases radiotherapy can be extremely effective at relieving pain and controlling the growth of tumour cells in the area of the bone metastases. It may also be used to prevent a fracture or as a treatment for spinal cord compression.

Typical radiotherapy treatment is administered once a day in 10 treatments over a two-week period, full effects of the treatment may take 2–3 weeks to occur. However, the reduction in bone pain may begin to occur between 7 and 10 days. During this time, patients are still advised to take painkillers prescribed by their doctor. This type of radiotherapy, which targets the area of bone affected, can cause some side effects. They include skin changes in the area being treated and a temporary increase in the symptoms of bone metastases.

### Bisphosphonates

Bisphosphonates are drugs that restrict the action of the osteoclasts. They are not a treatment for the cancer itself but may help to reduce the breakdown of the bone and so reduce the risk of fracture and discomfort.

Intravenous (IV) bisphosphonates are the standard treatment for tumour-induced hypercalcaemia (TIH) and have become an integral part of the current treatment of skeletal metastases, reducing the incidence of skeletal complications and the need for radiotherapy treatment and surgery to bone. They are generally administered in the outpatient department or, where facilities allow, in the patient's own home or at the GP's surgery, once every 3–6 weeks. Some bisphosphonates can be taken by mouth as tablets but these must be taken on an empty stomach an hour before food.

### Radioisotopes

Radioisotopes are another method used to treat the symptoms experienced by patients with bone metastases. They are mildly radioactive substances (such as strontium-89) and are injected into a vein, usually in the arm. The radioisotope travels through the bloodstream to the bones, where it injures or destroys active cancer cells in the bone, relieving symptoms.

A swelling around the tumour area ('tumour flare') in the days following treatment may occur. Therefore, the patient may experience a temporary increase in pain.

### Chemotherapy and hormone therapy

Chemotherapy drugs are used to kill cancer cells throughout the body. They may be taken orally or given intravenously.

Hormones are substances that occur naturally in the body and they control the activity and growth of normal cells. However in the cases of cancers such as prostate and breast, hormones can trigger the growth of those cancerous cells.

Hormonal therapy uses drugs to prevent hormones from forming or acting on cells to promote cancer growth. There are many different types of hormonal therapy and they all work in slightly different ways; in some cases several types of hormonal therapy may be given together. The therapy is administered either orally in the form of tablets or with injections.

Hot flushes and sweats are reported side effects. In most cases they are quite mild but on occasion some can be fairly severe.

The goals of chemotherapy and hormone therapy in patients with bone metastases are to control the tumour's growth, reduce pain, and reduce the risk of skeletal fractures.

### Surgery

Very occasionally, when tests show that an area of bone is affected, the diseased bone is removed under anaesthetic and replaced with a pin or a replacement part. Tumours that have developed next to a joint such as the hip are also generally removed during an operation and then the joint is replaced.

### Other therapies

Other treatments for bone metastases and their symptoms include physical therapy and drug and non-drug approaches to control pain. Many different drugs or combinations of drugs can be used to treat pain from bone metastases. Non-drug approaches to managing pain include the use of heat and cold, relaxation techniques and therapeutic beds or mattresses.

# PART 9 Corns and calluses

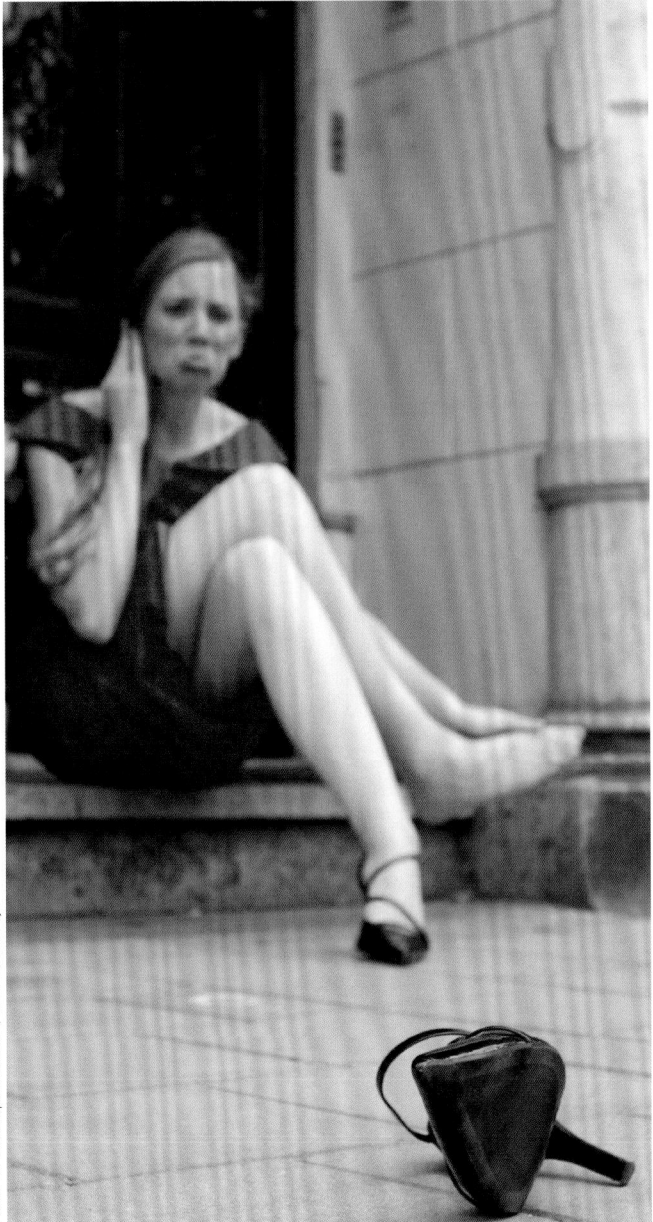

Photo: © iStockphoto.com, Michel de Nijs

## Introduction

People who always walk barefoot do not develop corns, simply thick skin on the soles of their feet. Localised skin thickening occurs over areas which are under constant pressure or rubbing. Classically they will form over the back of the toes or where the toes join the foot. Corns will also form over the ball of the foot. Calluses are also simply thick skin often seen on the hands of people performing heavy manual labour.

## Symptoms

Thick skin itself is not painful. It is the pressure it exerts when pressed on by the shoe which causes bruising and pain. Calluses on the hands reduce sensitivity.

## Causes

The most common cause of corns is badly fitting shoes.

## Prevention

Buy shoes that fit properly and try to walk around the house barefoot.

## Complications

Constant bruising can cause a deep ulcer beneath the corn. People with diabetes should beware of this as they may not feel the pain and allow the ulcer to grow and become infected.

## Self care

Wearing well fitting shoes will make the corn disappear. You can buy corn removal pastes from your pharmacist but the corn will reappear if you continue to wear badly fitting shoes. Pumice stones and sandpaper files can be used to reduce the size of the corn but over zealous attacks on the thick skin can cause bleeding and infection. Soft rubber cushion pads can reduce the friction but may actually increase the pressure making things worse.

## Action

See your pharmacist or chiropodist.

# PART 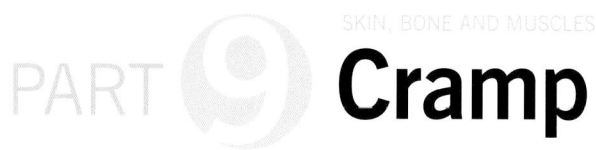 Cramp

## Introduction

Most of us will suffer cramp at some time. Muscle spasm which lasts for a few minutes most often occurs in the lower legs and feet. Lack of oxygen may be a factor but in most cases there appears to be no real reason although it happens more often while lying in bed.

Unfortunately there are some serious conditions which will cause repeated attacks of cramp particularly when walking.

## Symptoms

There is a warning tightness of the muscle with a small degree of pain. Movement at this point seems to trigger a full blown attack and the muscles tighten into a hard ball involuntarily. Indeed trying to move it only makes the pain and tightening worse.

Eventually the pain and tightness subsides but here is a feeling that another movement would trigger a fresh attack.

## Causes

Over exertion, sitting for prolonged periods, for example on a plane journey, over-heating, dehydration and exercising with a full stomach are all proposed causes of cramp.

In each of these cases the common factor is poor blood supply or over exertion. 'Normal' cramp can happen without any of these factors being present.

## Prevention

Avoiding each of the causes shown above is the only real prevention. Warm up exercises before strenuous activity such as running or swimming will not only help avoid cramp, they will also prevent tendon injury.

## Complications

Forcing a limb, foot or toe to move against the cramp can tear the muscle or its ligaments.

## Self care

Cramp will eventually disappear on its own but can be helped by gentle massage of the affected muscle and gradual movement of the affected limb.

## Action

If you are regularly suffering from cramp in any muscle you should make an appointment with your doctor.

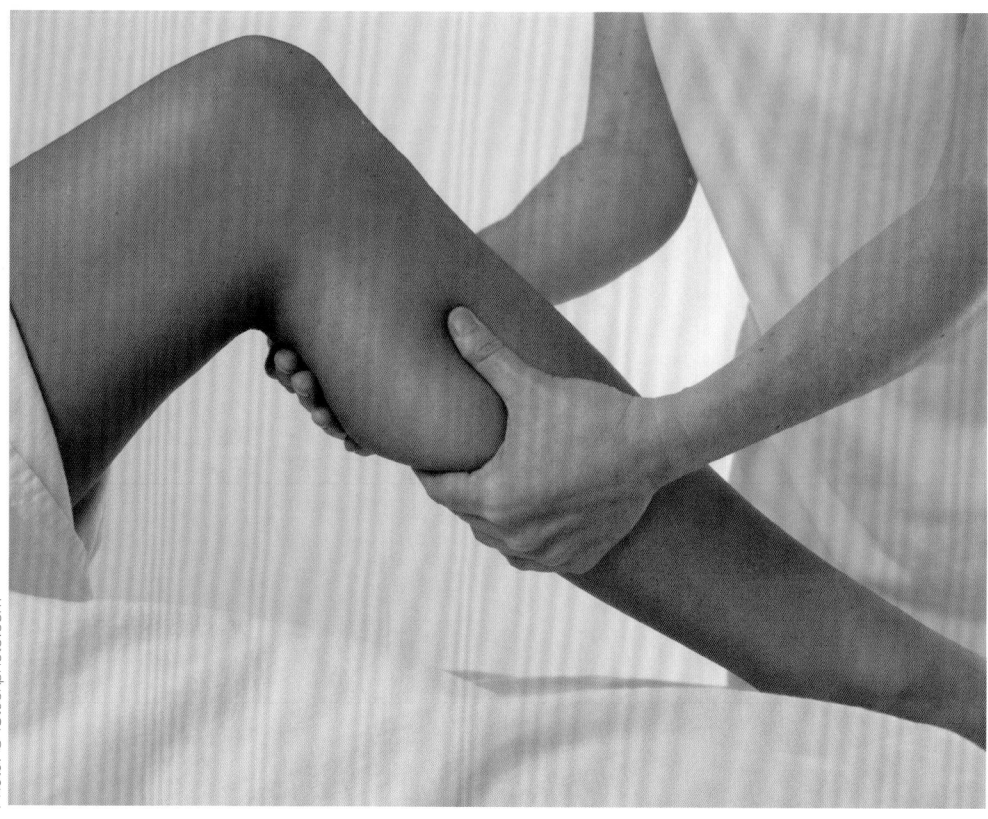

Photo: © iStockphoto.com

PART **9** # Dandruff

## Introduction
Although psoriasis will cause dandruff, the most common cause is seborrhoeic eczema. Both produce flaky white scales but the eczema tends to be slightly waxy. It is a comment on a society that we spend millions of pounds on trying to eradicate something which is completely harmless.

## Symptoms
There may be a slight itch although this is often caused by inflammation from scratching. White flakes of dead skin will fall from the scalp particularly when combing.

## Causes
Psoriasis is an auto immune condition (see *Psoriasis*) while seborrhoeic eczema may be a reaction to chemicals. There is an over production of skin which builds up around the bases of the hair follicles.

## Prevention
Regular washing and brushing will keep the dandruff at bay but at the same time may stimulate its existence.

## Complications
There are no known complications of dandruff. It is now thought unlikely that it causes any hair loss. Too frequent washing and brushing may be bigger factors.

## Self care
Anti-dandruff shampoos do work although they need to be used over a long period. Once they are stopped the dandruff often returns. Avoid strong soaps and over use of hair gels.

## Action
See your pharmacist.

Flaky paintwork can make your car less attractive

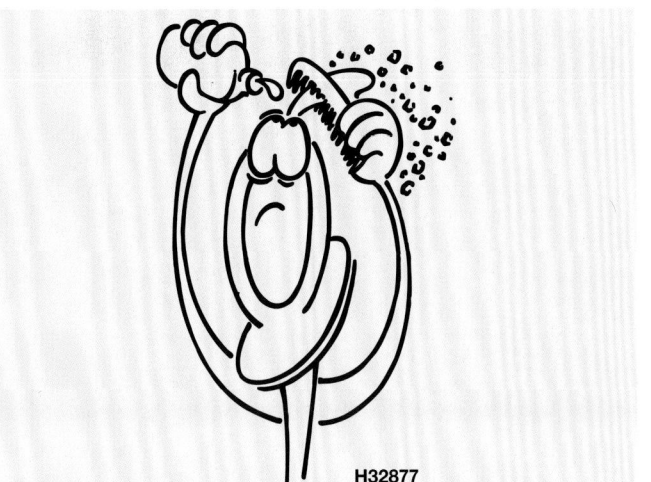

H32877

# PART 9 Fractures

## Introduction

Bones have many functions, not least producing new blood cells, but their obvious job is to support the body. They need to be almost rigid but not to be brittle. Bone is made mainly of a protein called collagen which is stiffened, strengthened and kept fairly rigid by the incorporation of mineral salts, especially calcium salts, and phosphates. Yet it is also a living 'organ' of the body often involved in complex metabolism and blood cell production. Without minerals bones would be quite rubbery, and far too flexible to do their job properly.

There is, of course, always a limit to the stress that a bone can take. And if that limit is exceeded a fracture occurs. Excessive force will fracture any bone, but a bone which has been generally weakened by a disease such as osteoporosis, or locally weakened by a tumour or cyst, will fracture under a smaller force. Such a fracture is called a pathological fracture.

Young bone, subjected to bending stress, often splinters on one side but merely bends on the other. This is called a greenstick fracture.

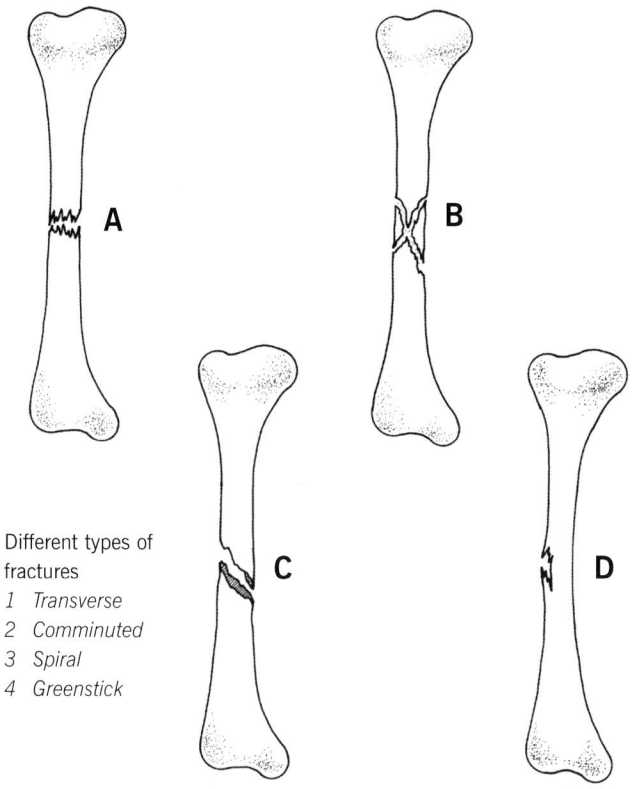

Different types of
fractures
1  *Transverse*
2  *Comminuted*
3  *Spiral*
4  *Greenstick*

H32937

## Symptoms

Signs of a fracture include pain and swelling, abnormal bending of the limb or part, skin discolouration and loss of movement. In the case of a fracture of a large bone, such as the thigh bone, the femur, the swelling may be very considerable, as a large volume of blood may be lost into the muscles and the spaces between them. This may be a cause of important complications.

## Causes

The usual cause of a fracture is a heavy fall or other impact. People with osteoporosis (brittle bones) suffer fractures more easily (See *Osteoporosis*).

## Diagnosis

Most fractures are easily diagnosed on the basis of the history and the symptoms, and are confirmed by X-ray.

## Prevention

Sticks and stones do break our bones. Although fractures may be a part of the risk of living active and healthy lives, this risk can be minimised by taking precautions such as wearing the correct protective clothing.

## Complications

Osteomyelitis is an infection of bone and bone marrow that can also result from an open (compound) fracture. For this reason compound fractures require careful management in hospital by an expert. Intensive antibiotic treatment is necessary if the condition is not to become long-term (chronic).

## Treatment

Fractures must be properly aligned. Once aligned, a fracture must be secured by some form of fixation until the repair is strong enough for weight-bearing. Various forms of fixation are used. These include:
- Plaster casts.
- Cast bracing with a joint to allow joint movement.
- External fixator.
- Sustained traction with weights and pulleys.
- Steel plates and screws.
- Long screws.
- Internal steel rods (intramedullary nail) for long bones.

Plaster casts are, effectively, bandages impregnated with plaster of Paris. Stronger versions now use resins.

An external fixator is a strong steel bar, placed parallel to the fractured bone. It is securely fixed to it by a number of steel pins passed in through the skin and screwed into the bone above and below the fracture site. The pins are attached to the bar by adjustable brackets.

Serious fractures often require internal surgical immobilisation by means of screws, nails or screwed-on steel plates.

Immobilisation may be necessary for a period of a few weeks to a few months, depending on the bone and the fixation involved.

# PART 9 Frozen shoulder

## Introduction

The shoulder is a complex joint with the greatest range of movement. This flexibility comes at a price as there is little stability from the bones of the joint, as with the hip. Instead the shoulder relies on muscles, ligaments and tendons to keep it in place. It is relatively easy therefore to damage a shoulder joint, especially if you play contact sports such as rugby. A frozen shoulder says just exactly what it is; you cannot move it and any forced movement is extremely painful. Sometimes there is pain only when it is moved in one particular direction and then the pain suddenly clears. This is called 'painful arc syndrome'.

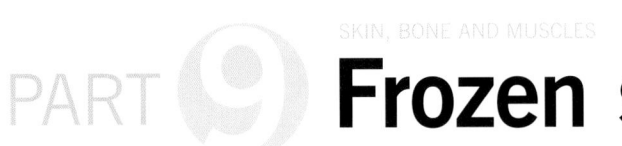

Stiff suspension needs to warm up properly

H32872

## Symptoms

Most frozen shoulders result from an injury which didn't seem too bad at the time. With constant and particularly heavy use afterwards the joint becomes hot, painful and difficult to move. Eventually it is impossible to lift your arm without severe pain. It can also follow tendonitis as seen in repetitive strain injuries (RSI).

## Causes

Most of the problem stems from the tendons which run inside a lubricated sheath not unlike a bicycle brake cable. Following a minor injury or with repetitive movement, the tendon and its sheath becomes inflamed. The point at which the tendon joins to the bone is also affected and may become very tender to touch. As the inflammation gets worse so the tendon is less able to run smoothly in the sheath and eventually it jams or is only possible to move with extreme pain. With painful arc syndrome, one part of the tendon is affected, usually on the muscle which is responsible for lifting the arm straight outwards away from your body. There is intense pain as the arm is lifted then suddenly it disappears once the affected part of the tendon clears the sheath only to return as the arm falls.

## Prevention

All of the ways to reduce the risk from tendonitis apply for avoiding a frozen shoulder (see *Tendonitis*).

## Complications

Untreated, the shoulder may return to normal within a month or so, particularly if the work which produces the RSI is avoided. Unfortunately there can be a permanent effect on shoulder movement so it is best to do something about it when it happens.

## Self care

Anti-inflammatory drugs from your pharmacist will help ease the pain. Massage and warmth also help. Physiotherapy is also useful and many physiotherapists specialise in these types of joint problems. Do not force the joint. This can damage the tendons, muscles and even tear the bone lining where the tendon joins. Avoiding the work which produced the RSI is vital, even if the pain has subsided with treatment.

## Treatment

Steroid injections into the joint can make a miraculous difference. Unfortunately many people then promptly over use the shoulder 'to make up for lost ground', possibly causing permanent damage. Few doctors will inject a shoulder joint more than three times, many will not do so more than once and some refuse to do so at all as there is evidence that it can cause joint damage.

## Action

Make an appointment to see your GP.

# PART 9

# Lice & crabs

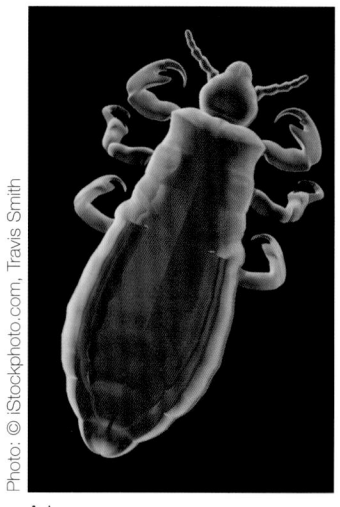

Photo: © iStockphoto.com, Travis Smith

A louse

## Introduction

These tiny parasites live on any hairy bits of the body. Head lice live in scalp hair, body lice will live in the armpits while crab lice prefer the groin but will survive quite happily in your eyebrows. They survive by sucking blood from your skin which is why they are so itchy. Female lice lay eggs every day. The eggs hatch in eight to 10 days. Social status means nothing to lice. They are very common among children, and infestation has nothing to do with dirty living. They are completely harmless, but very irritating.

## Symptoms

Itchiness is a common first symptom. The adults can be seen crawling about in the hair. Nits (eggs) can be seen attached to the hair shafts.

Inflamed areas around the hair shafts are common, usually caused by scratching.

## Causes

There is only one source of lice and crabs: other people and their clothes. You can pick up similar parasites from pets but they don't survive long on people.

It is possible to catch them from second-hand clothes or wearing other people's clothes. Dry cleaning and washing generally gets rid of the adults and their eggs.

## Prevention

- Avoid sharing hats, scarves or combs.
- Act promptly when warned of infection in the child's school.
- Check all the family, lice like to move around and meet people.
- Lice are easily caught from others, so avoid spreading lice by treating the whole family.

## Complications

- Although they are bad neighbours, lice and crabs do not cause any serious harm.
- Scratching may cause secondary infection which may need antibiotic cream.

## Self care

Keep the hair clean. Comb the hair while wet regularly with a fine-toothed comb. Use a conditioner. This helps to prevent the spread of lice.

The most effective treatment is daily combing with a nit comb followed by chemical lotions. Organophosphates are the mainstay of lice treatments, but there is some concern that they may be dangerous if used too often in young children. If in doubt, use only conditioner and nit comb.

As lice can stay alive for two days when they are not on a person, thoroughly clean clothes and hats which have been worn, as well as combs and brushes

## Action

Ask your pharmacist for the most suitable lotion. There will be a local policy on the treatment of head lice.

PART 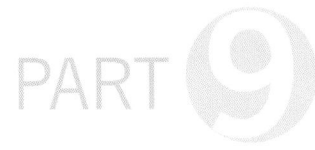 # Multiple myeloma

## Introduction

Multiple myeloma is a cancer of the cells that produce antibodies, called plasma cells. It actually forms in more than one part of the active bone marrow of various bones. These are the regions in the body where blood cells are produced. Antibodies are proteins which attach themselves to bacteria, viruses or sometimes cancer cells. This helps the immune system to destroy them and so protect the body from infection and cancer.

For some reason the abnormal myeloma cells stop making useful antibodies and instead produce large quantities of a useless substance called Bence Jones protein. This has implications for more than simply the immune system, as the large amount of protein produced can block the fine tubes inside the kidneys.

Around one person in 30,000 will develop multiple myeloma, the majority being over the age of 50 years.

## Symptoms

Like some other cancers, myeloma tumour can erode normal bone causing pain and fractures. This bone destruction can lead to high levels of calcium in the blood causing nausea, vomiting, loss of appetite, constipation, dehydration, drowsiness and confusion.

Normal blood cell production is crowded out so anaemia (lack of red blood cells) is often a feature with pallor, weakness, breathlessness on effort and fatigue. The reduction in production of normal antibodies results in increased liability to infection.

## Causes

There may be a genetic element as the disease does seem to run to some extent in families, but it is also commoner after exposure to large doses of radiation.

## Diagnosis

Obvious changes in the bones, most easily seen in the skull, may be visible on X-ray examination. However, the most effective test is to check the blood for anaemia and raised calcium and protein levels. The urine may contain large amounts of Bence Jones protein. One of the oldest tests was to gently heat a sample of urine to show a white jelly like protein appear in a similar way to egg white turning solid.

## Treatment

Anaemia and infections can be treated with blood transfusions and antibiotics. Bone pain can be relieved by radiotherapy and pain-killers mixed with anti-inflammatory drugs. Chemotherapy can significantly prolong life but is aimed really at improving the quality of remaining life. Major progress has come from the use of bisphosphonates (see *Bone metastases*).

# PART 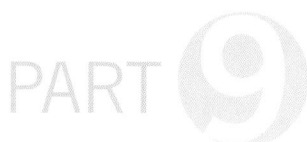 Osteoarthritis

## Introduction

Osteoarthritis is a degenerative joint disorder. Although it is related to age, many younger people show early osteoarthritic changes, and the by the age of 65, about 80% of people have some evidence of the disorder. Osteoarthritis most commonly involves the spine, the knee joints and the hip joints.

## Symptoms

Pain is at first intermittent and then becomes more frequent. Joint movement becomes increasingly limited, at first because of pain and muscle spasm, but later because the joint capsule becomes thickened and less flexible. Movement may cause creaking.

As the condition gradually gets worse stiffness increases and there is progressive reduction in the range through which the affected joints can be moved without pain.

## Causes

The cause of osteoarthritis is unknown. Being overweight makes the symptoms of osteoarthritis significantly worse.

There may be a number of factors which include:
● Injury.
● Excessive pressure from obesity.
● Over-use of certain joints.
● Infection.
● Damage to the joint nerve supply.
● Other joint diseases such as gout or rheumatoid arthritis.

There is also some evidence of a genetic factor in osteoarthritis.

## Diagnosis

The diagnosis depends on things such as:
● The family history of any joint disorder.
● When the symptoms started.
● Where the pain is.
● How severe it is.
● When it is worse.

X-rays can be helpful.

## Prevention

Eat healthy to avoid weight gain. Use gentle exercise to maintain muscle strength around the joint, to reduce problems.

## Treatment

Weight reduction, if necessary, can greatly reduce the severity of symptoms. An exercise program designed to improve the general health and the health of affected joints is also helpful.

Immobilisation on the other hand, is dangerous and can speed the progress and worsen the outlook of the disease.

In osteoarthritis, drug treatment is of relatively minor importance because inflammation is not an important part of the process and infection is not involved. Non-steroidal anti-inflammatory drugs (NSAIDs) are often all that is required to relieve pain. Newer drugs are available which have less effect on the stomach lining.

Surgery to replace the joint is a last resource, usually considered before total loss of function occurs. A large amount of surgical experience of hip and knee replacement for osteoarthritis has now been obtained, and the results are usually remarkably good. Other osteoarthritic joints can also be replaced.

## Action

Make an appointment to see your GP.

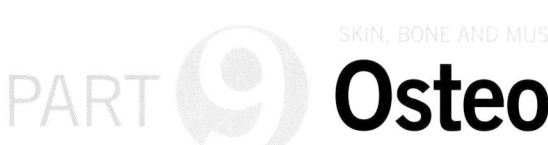

# PART 9 Osteoporosis (thin bones)

## Introduction

Far from simply being scaffolding or girders on to which all the soft living parts of the body are attached, bone is constantly developing and changing its shape to meet the demands set on it. It produces blood cells and actively fights infection while at the same time providing support and protection for vital organs. For various reasons bone can lose its density and become light and easily broken. The constant replacement with new bone is affected by lack of exercise, some drugs and certain illness. It usually affects people in their 60s and older and is unfortunately common in these age groups, with over half affected to some degree. Keeping bones healthy and strong while you are younger pays great dividends later in life.

## Symptoms

Unfortunately there are no real warning signs that your bones are lighter and less dense. A chance X-ray for some other problem will often be the first time a person is aware of the potential problem. Sudden severe back pain may follow a collapsed vertebra from osteoporosis. A simple fall can cause a broken hip.

## Causes

There are a battery of causes of bone thinning. Immobilisation or lack of activity are major factors because the bone density depends on the forces it has to cope with on a regular basis. Long term steroids will also tend to cause bone thinning but the benefits of the treatment for, say, rheumatoid arthritis have to be balanced against the risk of osteoporosis. Osteoporosis is now well recognised in men and the gradual decline in testosterone, or at least in its effect with age, may be a similar factor as with oestrogen decline in women.

## Prevention

Some doctors believe we should be giving men testosterone replacement for the same reason HRT is used for women. There are now drugs intended to prevent osteoporosis in men. This is a developing area; ask your doctor for details if you are concerned.

## Complications

The most serious complication is the increased risk of fractures. Hip fractures are particularly common although with modern surgery this will not mean permanent disablement.

## Self care

Regular activity and a diet rich in calcium and vitamin D are the best forms of prevention. Eating bread, milk, oily fish, fruit and vegetables usually makes supplements unnecessary. Don't wait for osteoporosis to happen before changing your lifestyle as the damage will have been done.

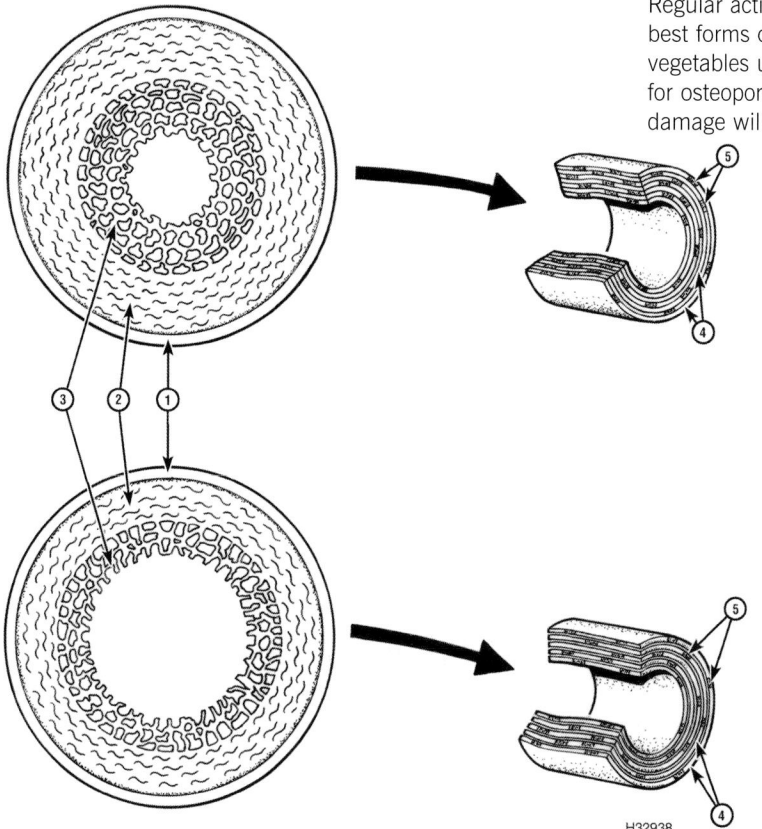

Normal (top) and osteoporitic bone
1  Periosteum
2  Cortical bone
3  Spongy bone
4  Lamellae
5  Bone cell

H32938

# PART 9 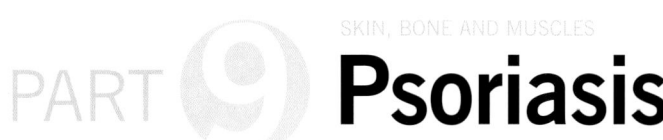 Psoriasis

## Introduction

Contrary to popular myth, psoriasis is not an infection and you cannot catch it from anyone else or their clothes. The silver flaky patches of skin are simply cells which are growing too fast. Around 2.5% (1 in 40) of the population suffer from psoriasis which does tend to run in families.

## Symptoms

Psoriasis is classically found on the elbows and knees and the scalp. It tends to spare the face. In more severe cases it can also affect the soles of the feet, palms of the hands, small of the back and armpits. The oval red patches are often covered with silver flaky scales which come away easily to expose the darker layers underneath. They are not usually itchy unless infected.

## Causes

Psoriasis is an autoimmune condition where for some reason the body attacks itself. It is linked to other similar conditions such as rheumatoid arthritis. We now know there are various triggers which stimulate these areas of skin to start growing too fast. Stress, overwork, changes in climate and even minor infections may be enough to start the process off.

## Prevention

It is difficult to suggest any effective form of protection from psoriasis outbreaks. Dealing effectively with stress through both relaxation and activity instead of resorting to alcohol may be valuable.

## Complications

The rash is not dangerous unless it is very extensive or is infected. When the rash appears on the hands or feet it usually forms fluid filled blisters which resemble pus. There is no infection. A small proportion of psoriasis sufferers, 6-7% (less than one in 10), will experience joint pain resembling that of rheumatoid arthritis.

## Self care

Care and treatment depends on the severity of the condition. Sunlight appears to help some people which is not surprising as ultra violet (UV) treatments have long been used with moderate success. Other advice:
- Avoid strong soaps.
- Avoid overheating by wearing light cotton clothes.
- If the patches itch, use a moisturising cream but do not scratch them.
- Keep your skin moist with special creams called emollients.

Tar-containing products from the pharmacist can be effective, but do unfortunately stain clothes and need to be applied with care only to the affected skin.

## Treatment

Your doctor may refer you to a specialist who can arrange treatment only available in hospital as an out patient.

## Action

See your pharmacist or make an appointment to see your GP.

Psoriasis

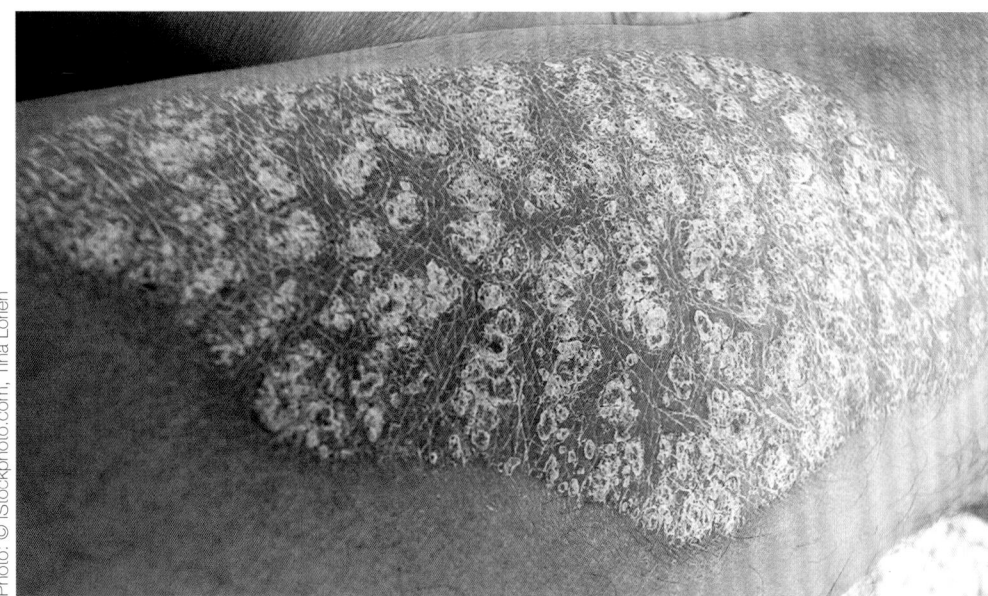

Photo: © iStockphoto.com, Tina Lorien

PART 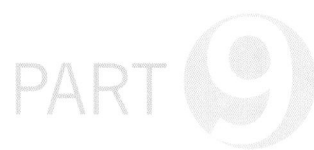 # Ringworm (tinea)

## Introduction

Ringworm (tinea) can affect many parts of the body, particularly the groin and scalp. It is not a worm, simply a fungus.

## Symptoms

It is most noticeable on bare skin when it is referred to as ringworm due to its characteristic appearance as a circular patch of red, itchy skin, which gradually increases in size.

There may also be red itchy areas around the base of hair shafts. With scratching, these areas can bleed and become crusted with blood.

## Prevention

- Keep the area well ventilated and dry.
- Use a separate face cloth and towel – ringworm is infectious.

## Complications

- Bacterial infection from scratching is common.

## Self care

- Keep the area well ventilated and dry.
- Use an antifungal cream or shampoo available from your pharmacist.

## Action

See your pharmacist or make an appointment to see your GP.

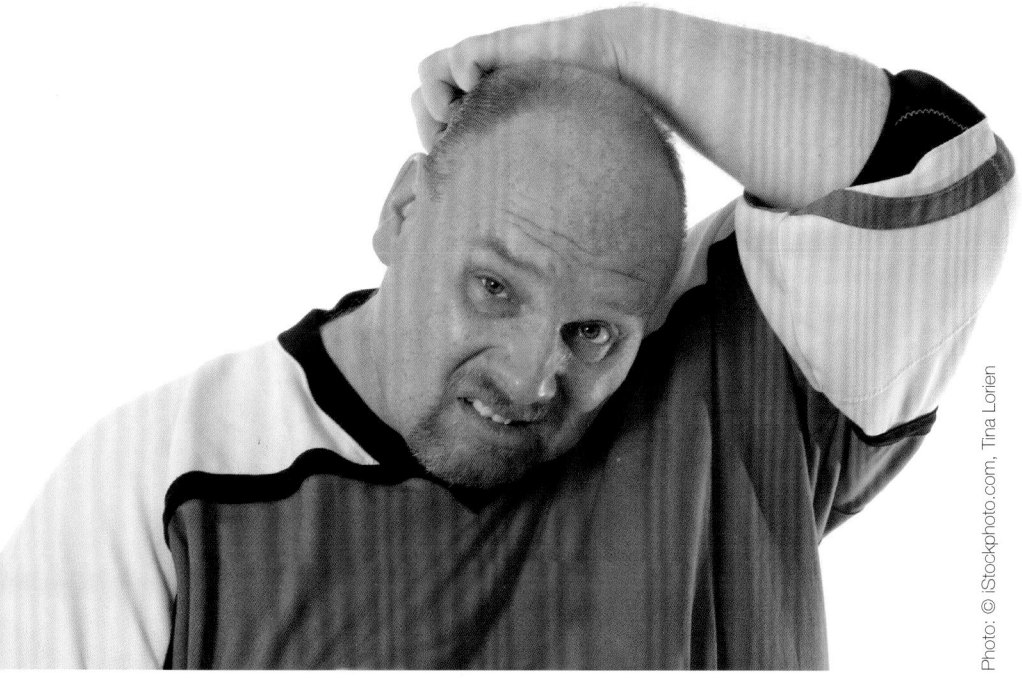

Photo: © iStockphoto.com, Tina Lorien

# PART 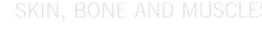 9

# Repetitive strain injuries – RSI (tendonitis)

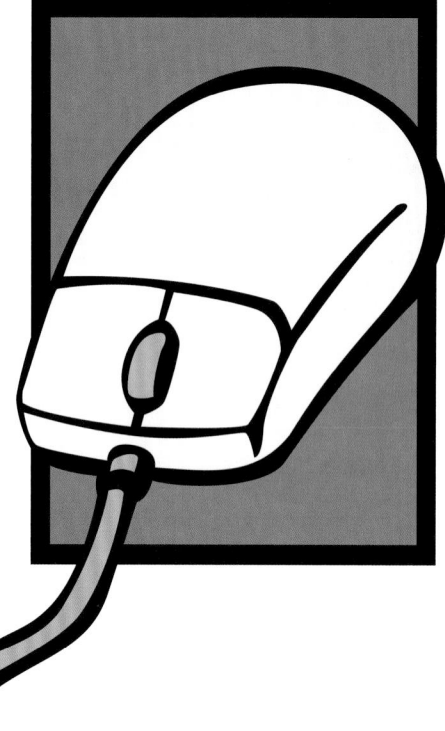

Photo: © iStockphoto.com, Miguel Angel Salinas Salinas

## Introduction

First we had tennis elbow. Now with the explosion in the use of computers, repetitive strain injuries are more commonly associated with the wrists and fingers. In truth there were always a large number of people suffering from this often distressing and even debilitating condition. Musicians, particularly string instrumentalists, were well recognised to be at risk. Other occupations such as carpenters, electricians and nurses can suffer from tendon injury through repetitive movement.

## Symptoms

It's not that difficult to tell if you have RSI. Generally the pain gets steadily worse as the day goes on. During your days off the pain eases only to come back again when you return to work. As the condition progresses you may find it difficult to move a finger, hand or arm.

In severe cases it may progress to tenosynovitis and you will feel a crackling sensation as you move a joint. It may even stick in one place only to suddenly move as you try harder to move it.

## Causes

Tendons move inside a lubricated sheath not unlike an old brake cable. Either from injury or repetitive movement the tendon becomes inflamed and moves as if it were 'rusty' and in need of oil.

Worse still, this movement further inflames the sheath which tightens onto the tendon causing pain. In some severe cases small islands of bone form in the tendon itself which can completely obstruct any movement.

## Prevention

Alternating repetitive movements with others helps reduce the risk. Use exercises which are the 'opposite' of the normal repetitive movement.

Every few minutes lift your hands from the keyboard and flex them downwards (they are normally held in a slightly backwards position, even at rest.

Use a keyboard which keeps your hands in the correct position. Similarly for people using instruments or tools such as screwdrivers. Either spend a few minutes during a job rotating your wrists and elbow in the opposite direction to the repetitive movement.

Consider an electric tool which eliminates the repetitive movement altogether.

## Complications

Most people will find RSI simply a nuisance but for some it can mean the loss of employment and serious disability.

## Self care

As well as the prevention exercises some people find great relief using anti-inflammatory drugs. Gels that you rub in may also provide some relief, but at least some of this comes from the massaging and warmth that it produces.

Applying warm compresses along with gentle massage can ease the pain.

## Treatment

Steroid injection can give almost miraculous pain relief and restore normal function. Most doctors would be reluctant to repeat injections and it can be counterproductive in that the person returns to the work which caused the problem in the first place. Eventually the pain returns and there may be more serious damage.

## Action

See your pharmacist or ring your GP. If the condition is work-related, ask for a work station assessment; if this is unsatisfactory, inform your health and safety representative.

PART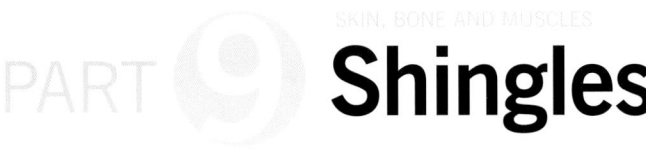

# Shingles

## Introduction

One step up from cold sores, shingles is caused by a closely related virus. It is particularly nasty if the immune system is not working properly, during illness or while on treatment for cancer.

It is rare to develop shingles more than once.

## Symptoms

A tingling itchy feeling precedes a painful rash. It is only found on one side of the body.

It can develop over the next few hours or days into a painful set of blisters. It usually follows a narrow strip of skin, common sites include the chest wall, face and upper legs.

A general flu-like illness often accompanies the rash and may persist after the rash has gone.

## Causes

If you have never had chicken pox you are very unlikely to develop shingles which is caused by the same virus reactivated.

## Prevention

Prevention is difficult, most people will develop the infection without realising where it came from.

## Complications

Although sometimes very painful, shingles is rarely serious.

People who are suffering from any condition or medicine which lowers their resistance to infection can be quite ill.

If it spreads near the ears or eyes, or onto the tip of the nose, immediate attention from your doctor is recommended.

## Self care

- Simple pain killers can help.
- Keep the rash area uncovered as much as possible.
- Try not to scratch the rash. Ask your pharmacist about lotions to ease the itching.
- Pain which follows the disappearance of the rash can be reduced by cooling the area with a bag of ice (don't apply directly to the skin).

## Treatment

Once the tingling sensation begins it is wise to start anti-viral medicine. It is important to start treatment as soon as possible. Once the rash is well developed anti-viral agents are of no great value.

## Action

Make an appointment to see your doctor, especially if:

- The outbreak of blisters occurs near your eye or at the tip of your nose.
- You also have a sore red eye.
- The sores have not healed after 10 days.
- There is also a high temperature.
- You suffer from some other serious illness.

PART 9

# Skin cancer

## Not a lot of people know this

- Skin cancer is the most common cancer in the UK, and not just in women.
- Your risk of growing an extra, unwanted, outside cancerous lump by the age of 74 is one in six.
- Even cloudy days can deliver 9/10ths of the dangerous UV rays.
- Some football shirts are so thin they let almost all the sun's UV radiation shine right through.
- Once the sunburn fades from this year's trip to Majorca it doesn't mean you're in the clear. Damage builds up under the skin just like rust under bodywork paint and can come back to haunt you in later years.
- Virtually all the risk comes from the sun and sun-beds… So cover up and close up!

## Shades of the truth

- Use high factor sun-screens (30+ in sunnier climates). Slap loads on BEFORE you head into the sun and re-apply every 2 hours.
- Cover up, always; and that means when working or holidaying at home too.
- Get ahead and get a hat, a big hat.
- Get out of the midday sun when possible or else look for a nice bit of shade to relax or work in.
- Get those shades on to protect your (next) best assets!
  All men, no matter what colour their skin, need to be sun-smart, but the guys with the following need to be extra careful even when working or playing outside in the UK, as well as abroad:
- Pale or freckled skin that doesn't tan or burns before it tans.

> See that big round yellow thing hanging in the sky? It causes more cancer in the UK than anything else you can shake a pair of sunglasses at. Don't be a mad dog, get out of the midday sun!

Virtually all the risk comes from the sun and sun-beds. . . So cover up and close up!

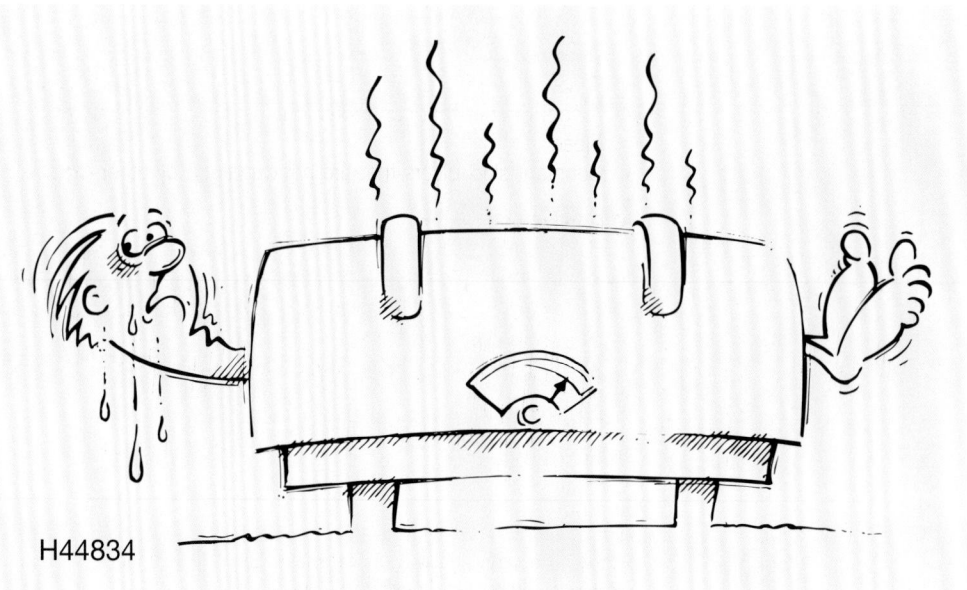

H44834

- Naturally red or fair hair and blue, green or grey eyes.
- A large number of moles (50 or more).
- Easy burnt skin, a history of sunburn or already had skin cancer.

## Sunscreens and smokescreens

People get confused over sunscreens and can damage their skin through a false sense of security, remember:

- The higher the Sun Protection Factor (SPF) number, the greater the protection provided. A SPF above 15 gives high protection.
- Wearing sunscreen does not mean that you can stay out in the sun longer than recommended – it offers some protection, but should be used with cover-up clothing.
- It is very important to apply sunscreen thickly and evenly. Most people get a lot less protection than they think because they do not put enough sunscreen on their skin.
- Those parts of the body that are not usually exposed to the sun will tend to burn more easily. But also take extra care of ears, neck, bald patches, hands and feet.

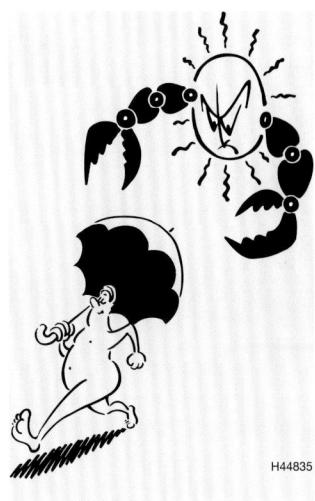

H44835

All men, no matter what colour their skin, need to be sun-smart

## Sun sense

The sun damages your bodywork by its Ultraviolet Radiation (UV) and there are two types:

- UVA. Results in early ageing and skin cancer.
- UVB. Most harmful, causes burning and skin cancer.

Tanned skin is damaged skin. It's a sign that damaged skin is trying to protect itself from the sun's ultraviolet rays. Even when you have a suntan, you can still get sunburn.

There are two main types of skin cancer.

### Non-melanoma skin cancer

Most common form, often seen on the ear tips, nose, forehead and cheeks but is very curable.

Look out for:
- A new growth or sore that does not heal within four weeks.
- A spot or sore that continues to itch, hurt, crust, scab or bleed.
- Constant skin ulcers that are not explained by other causes.

### Malignant melanoma

Most serious form and although relatively rare it is on the increase, especially in men. It most often appears as a changing mole or freckle but the good news is that early diagnosis is likely to produce a cure.

Mole maintenance, watch out for changes such as:
- Size.
- Colour.
- Shape.
- Itchiness.
- Bleeding.

Many skin changes will be harmless, but if you notice anything unusual, you should visit your doctor.

# PART 9 Sports injuries

## Introduction

Muscles, joints and bones are very susceptible to damage when not treated properly. They all have limitations which when exceeded will cause damage, sometimes permanently.

## Symptoms

Some injuries show themselves as a gradual increase in pain on movement. This is typical of a repetitive strain injury or tendonitis.

A snapped Achilles tendon (ankle tendon) can sound like a gun shot, with immediate loss of power to the foot, severe pain and an inability to flex the ankle.

A ruptured meniscus (knee cartilage) invariably causes pain and swelling immediately or soon after it happens. A 'locked' knee is a very obvious sign of internal damage such as a torn cartilage.

Sprains involve damage to tendons and ligaments which stabilise or move a joint. These ligaments can be either stretched or partly torn from the bone. This causes pain and swelling with a restriction on movement.

In all these cases the joint or muscle becomes hot and tender.

H32871

High performance racing increases risk of suspension damage

## Causes

Most sports injuries are caused by a force exceeding that which the joint, muscle or tendon is designed to withstand. It is often the result of a twisting movement under great force (torn knee cartilages) or excessive force to an unprepared or inflexible tendon (torn Achilles tendon). Simply twisting the ankle in a hole can tear ligaments and muscles which surround this highly complex joint.

## Prevention

Warming up is vital. Many men snap their Achilles through sudden activity, especially if they are unused to exercise. Although some injuries are accidental and often unavoidable, the damage is reduced by having the joint kept flexible through regular exercise. It will also heal much quicker because of the improved blood supply.

## Complications

There is controversy over the link between osteoarthritis and sports injuries, but common sense dictates that regular damage to a joint must impair its function eventually.

## Self care

Many injuries do not require anything other than rest and time to sort them out. Physiotherapy may be required to restore normal function. Surgery is common for injuries such as torn knee cartilage or snapped tendons. Many of these treatments do not restore the normal state of the muscle, joint or tendon and there may be reduced movement or power.

The most important part of reducing pain and limiting permanent damage is immediate first aid. RICE is a system used by many first aiders and sports physiotherapists. Following these rules will invariably help immensely:

### R – Rest

Further movement will only make the damage worse. Once the initial inflammation has subsided gentle exercises help restore normal function.

### I – Ice

Cool the joint with bags of ice packed in cloth. This eases the pain and reduces the inflammation. Do not apply ice, bags of frozen peas etc directly to the skin. Remove the pack after 5 minutes maximum. Reapply every hour in the first 48 hours.

### C – Compression

An elastic bandage will help reduce swelling. Make sure it is well above and below the affected joint. Take it off at night.

### E – Elevation

Raise the limb and support it. This helps reduce swelling by draining the fluid away from the joint.

PART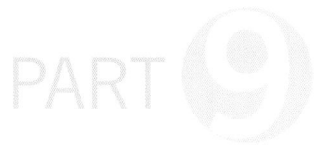

# Sun burn

Although there is some controversy over the danger of exposure to too much sunlight, we do know that it can be harmful. Over the past few decades there has been a dramatic increase in the number of cases of malignant melanoma, a particularly nasty and potentially lethal skin cancer. Once considered rare, it is still increasing possibly due to the desire for sun drenched holidays. Australia has been in the forefront of educating people over the dangers of sunbathing.

## Symptoms
Most people do not realise that they have badly burned themselves until later on in the day. The first sign of a burn is a reddening of the skin caused by blood vessels increasing in size to get rid of as much heat as possible. At this stage damage is already being done to the skin.

## Causes
Ultra violet light (UV) can penetrate the outer layers of skin, especially in fair skinned people. It heats and damages the lower layers causing skin loss. The body responds by increasing the amount of melanin, a black pigment, in the skin which prevents the sun from reaching the delicate lower skin layers. This is the 'sun tan' we crave so much.

## Prevention
It's not too smart to go out in the sun wearing nothing but your union jack shorts. Never mind the crimes against fashion, it's potentially deadly. Use a strong sun block (SPF 15 and over). Cover your body, especially the head, with appropriate clothing. Never leave a baby exposed to the sun, even if the weather is hazy.

## Complications
If the exposure to the sun continues the skin will form blisters just as with a scald. These blisters burst very quickly and the covering skin is then lost exposing red skin beneath. If this is extensive, a large amount of body fluids can be lost; a particular danger to babies and small children who do not have a large body mass.

Like any burn, skin damaged by overexposure to UV can scar.

Long term exposure to the sun causes the collagen network within the skin to become less flexible. This makes the skin lose its elasticity so it droops, folds and wrinkles very easily.

## Self care
A badly burnt baby or small child needs to go to hospital. Treat sun burn like any other burn. There are lotions you can apply which will ease the pain but they cannot prevent the damage which is already done. Take plenty of non alcoholic fluids and stay out of the sun for a few days. Use only tepid baths.

### Note
There is no 'safe' exposure time. The rate at which you burn depends on the colour of your skin. Fair complexions are the easiest to damage with UV. Dark skin is the most resistant but will still be burned with prolonged exposure. Generally after 15 minutes on a first exposure white skin is already damaged.

## Action
See your pharmacist.

PART 9

# Warts & verrucas

## Introduction
Around 5% (1 in 20) school children will suffer from warts or verrucas. Warts and verrucas are less infectious than we once thought. Even so the link with cervical cancer needs to be taken seriously so warts on the penis should be treated as soon as possible.

## Symptoms
Warts can appear anywhere on the body but are most common on the hands and feet. They can also appear at the anus and penis.

## Causes
'Dirty' skin is not a cause. The papilloma virus actually causes the skin to produce warts. There may be a difference between the viruses which cause hand and feet warts to those which cause genital warts.

## Prevention
Wearing protective footwear at public baths may decrease the risk of passing on or picking up the infection.

## Complications
Most warts are not dangerous. Verrucas may cause pain when walking. Warts on the penis should be removed at a GUM (genito-urinary medical) clinic. They are linked to cervical cancer although their link with cancer of the penis is less clear.

## Self care
Warts appear to have a limited lifespan and eventually disappear on their own. It can be a frustrating wait as new warts may appear as the older warts depart. Wart removal creams are available from your pharmacist. It takes great patience as repeated applications for more than a week are often required.

### Note
Do not use wart removal pastes or creams on your face, anus or genitals.

## Treatment
Some GP practices offer wart removal using liquid nitrogen or by burning (diathermy).

## Action
Ask your pharmacist for advice. Ring the local genito-urinary (GUM) clinic if you suspect they are genital or anal warts.

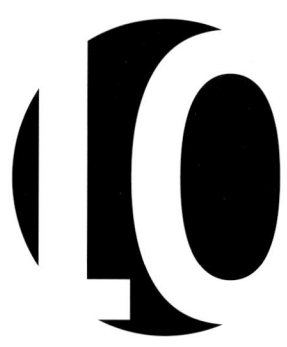

# Endocrine system

The endocrine system
1  Pituitary gland
2  Thyroid gland
3  Parathyroid gland
4  Thymus gland
5  Pancreas
6  Adrenal gland
7  Testes

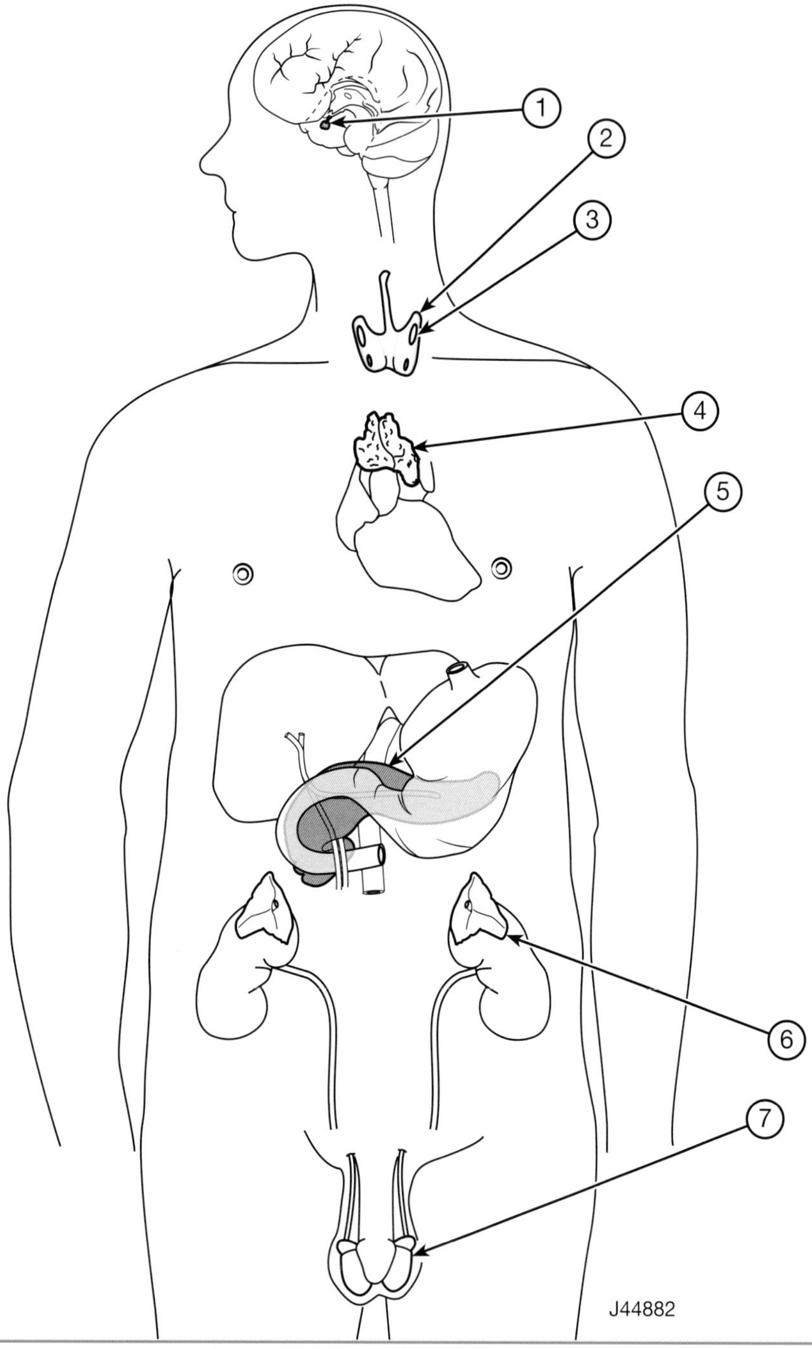

J44882

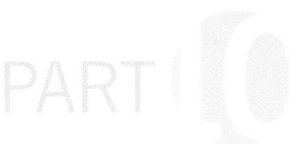

# Breast cancer

## Introduction

Yes, men can get breast cancer, though luckily it is very rare. Only about 1% of all breast cancers occur in men; it is commonest in men over 60. There is a small amount of breast tissue behind each nipple and it is here that the cancer can develop.

## Causes

It is not possible to say with certainty what causes male breast cancer, but there are some factors which are known to increase the likelihood of it occurring. These include:

● Having close relatives (male or female) who have had breast cancer.
● Having close relatives who have had cancer of the ovary or colon.
● Exposure to repeated doses of radiation, especially when young.
  If you think that you fall into one of the above categories, talk to your GP.

## Symptoms

The usual symptom is a lump in the breast, or a change in its shape or size. Other symptoms include changes in the shape of the nipple, a discharge from the nipple and a rash on or around the nipple.

## Diagnosis

An ultrasound scan is used to get a picture of the lump. A sample of cells from the lump will also be taken (by needle aspiration or needle biopsy) for examination. These tests will show whether the lump is cancerous.

## Treatment

Treatment for male and female breast cancer is essentially the same. One or more of the following may be used, depending on the type of cancer and how far it has spread:

● Surgery to remove the affected tissue, and maybe the lymph nodes in the armpit.
● Hormone therapy to reduce the level of oestrogen in the blood. Most breast cancers require oestrogen for their growth.
● Chemotherapy to destroy cancer cells which may be spreading elsewhere in the body.
● Radiotherapy to destroy the cancer cells, either in the original site or (if they have spread) elsewhere.

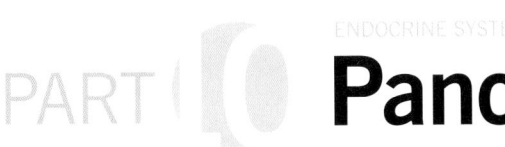

# Pancreatic cancer

## Introduction

The pancreas is a complex organ sitting in the loop of the duodenum (small intestine). It has a number of jobs, not least the controlling of blood sugar levels through the secretion of insulin from discrete 'islands' studded in the pancreas. The surrounding tissue is more concerned with producing digestive enzymes, particularly those for breaking down fat. It is in these parts of the pancreas that cancer is more likely to arise.

Although relatively rare it is unfortunately one of the most dangerous, with a poor survival rate, and is one of the 10 most common causes of cancer death in the UK. Men suffer from it twice as often as women and it is slightly higher in black men.

One of great problems for diagnosis is the lack of any symptoms until late in the development of the condition. There is also a difference in survival depending on where tumour arises in the pancreas.

## Symptoms

These tend to develop over months rather than weeks and include:

- Pain in the upper abdomen under the rib cage which seems to go through to the back as well.
- Weight loss and lack of appetite.
- Jaundice and white motions which tend to float in the toilet can be a sign of later disease.

## Diagnosis

MRI and CT scans are the most useful tools although endoscopy (a long flexible telescope) with the insertion of a small tube (stent) can help release any obstruction which may be causing jaundice. At the same time a small sample (biopsy) can be taken for further tests.

## Treatment

Surgical removal is the only realistic chance of cure, but for most men it will be a matter of relieving the pain. Thankfully this is possible using pain killers and sometimes a nerve block.

## Prevention

There are no hard and fast rules regarding prevention, although moderate alcohol consumption and a low fat diet may reduce your risk.

The pancreas
1 Liver
2 Stomach
3 Pancreas
4 Duodenum

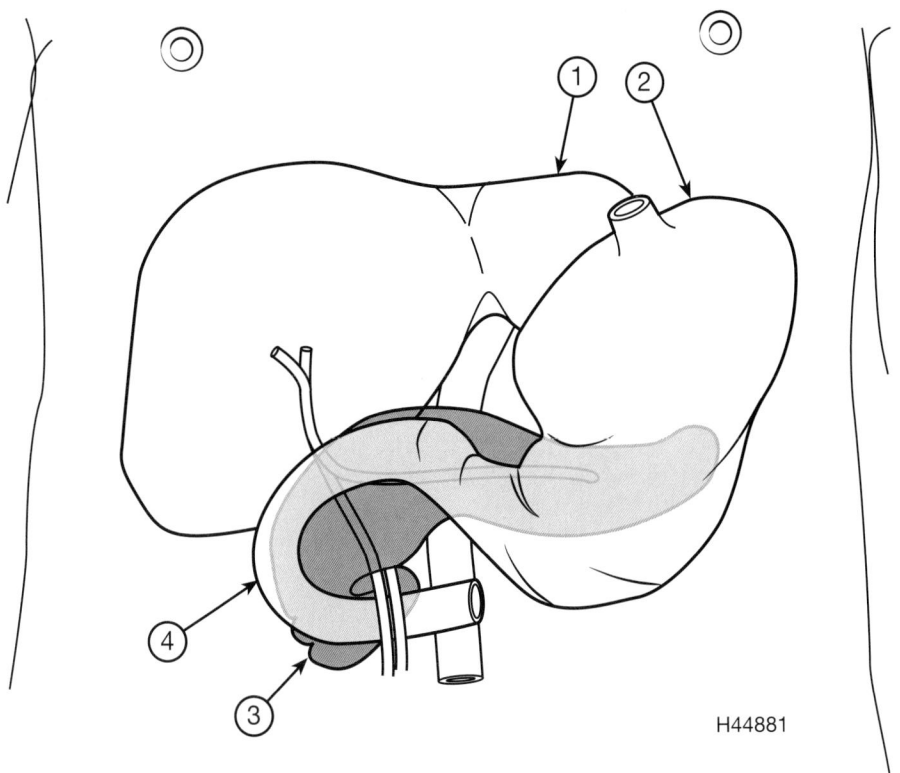

H44881

PART 10 # Cancer of the pituitary gland

## Introduction

Often described as the 'body's orchestral conductor', the pituitary is a complex gland sitting at the base of the brain. It produces a number of hormones which collectively determine to a large extent the way the body functions. Cancer of this important part of the brain is fortunately rare and its treatment is increasingly successful.

The effect of the tumours will depend on whether or not they produce hormones which act on distant parts of the body. Most of these tumours are non-malignant, so spread from the gland is not a problem. Even so, the hormones they produce, or the pressure from the size of the tumour, can cause their own serious problems.

## Symptoms

These will depend on the type of tumour, the hormone it is producing or preventing, and any pressure on surrounding tissues.

- Impotence can result from excess production of the hormone prolactin which suppresses testosterone production from the testes.
- Excess stimulation of the adrenal glands near the kidney can produce a condition called Cushing's Syndrome with characteristic 'moon face' appearance and high blood pressure.
- Visual disturbances can occur from pressure on the optic nerves which run very close to the pituitary.
- Lack of stimulation of the thyroid gland in the neck can lead to hypothyroidism, with symptoms of lethargy, thick skin and weight gain.

## Diagnosis

The warning signs for the doctor will come from what you describe as happening to you. The symptoms can arise gradually over a prolonged period of time so the penny doesn't always drop immediately. Blood tests for abnormally low or high levels of hormones can provide invaluable clues, but MRI or CT scans of the brain can often show the tumour. Although these tumours tend to be slow-growing, early diagnosis makes successful treatment all the more likely.

## Treatment

A great deal depends on the type of tumour. Chemotherapy, radiotherapy and surgery are used often together, and this may require hormone replacement on a regular basis to make up for the loss of tissue that previously produced the essential hormones.

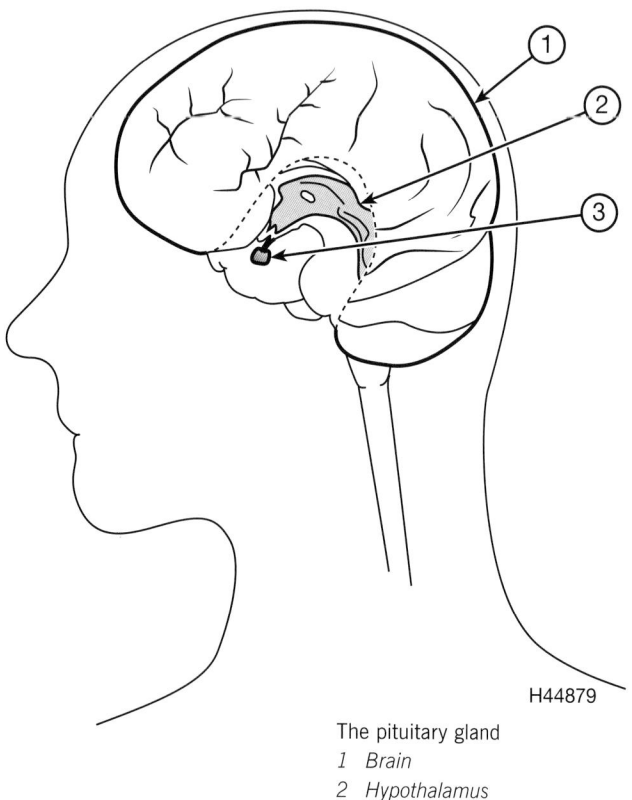

H44879

The pituitary gland
1  Brain
2  Hypothalamus
3  Pituitary

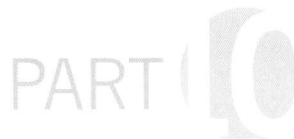

# Cancer of the thyroid

## Introduction
The thyroid gland sits in the throat just below the Adam's Apple (larynx). It has the job of regulating the body's metabolism. Too much thyroxine – its secreted hormone – makes the body work too fast, with the heart beating too quickly. Too little and the body is sluggish with a slow heart rate. A over- or under-active thyroid does not necessarily indicate the presence of cancerous cells.

Cancer of the thyroid is more common in women and previous exposure to radiation may be part of the cause. It is rare, one in 100 of all cancers are of the thyroid. It is more common in people over 40 years old. The good news is that successful treatment for thyroid cancer is amongst the highest for any cancers.

## Symptoms
These depend on the type of thyroid cancer as they can arise in different parts of the gland. The majority tend to spread outside of the gland itself. Symptoms include:
- A painless lump in the throat.
- Difficulty or pain on swallowing.
- Hoarse voice.

## Causes
There are no known causes of thyroid cancer other than the possible effect of direct radiation. Therefore there is little to advise on prevention. Thankfully it is a rare cancer.

## Diagnosis
Examination of your neck and blood tests by your GP will provide most clues to the diagnosis but ultrasound, MRI or CT scanning can give definitive diagnosis particularly after a biopsy (taking a small sample of thyroid tissue).

## Treatment
Surgical removal of the entire gland will often make survival possible. This can be done alongside radioactive iodine, which will only affect the thyroid gland or the metastases. As a result you will need thyroxine replacement, the normal hormone produced by the thyroid gland. Around 95% of people will survive their cancer.

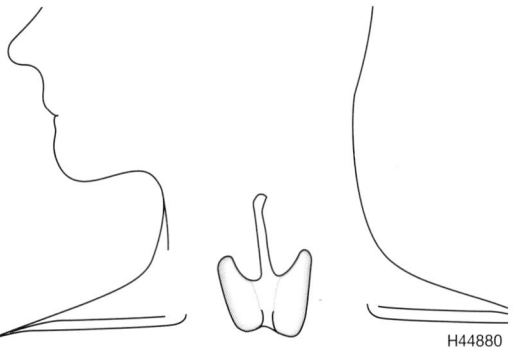

The thyroid gland

H44880

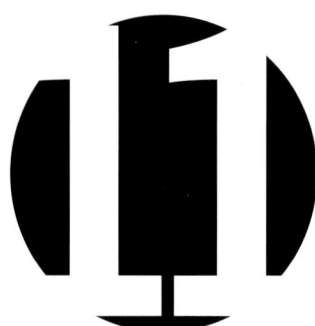

# Ears, eyes, nose & throat

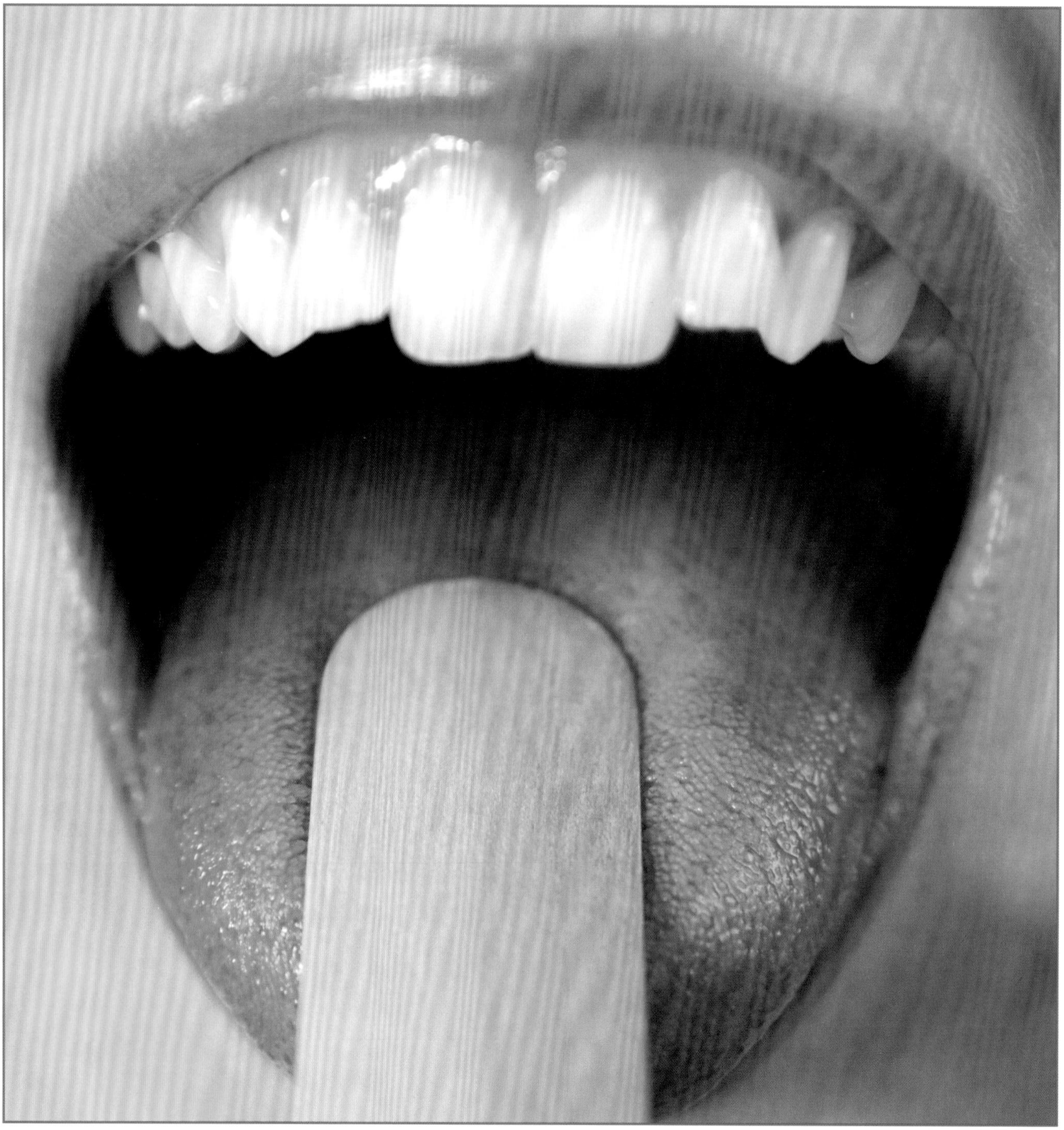

Photo: © iStockphoto.com, Chris Hutchison

PART 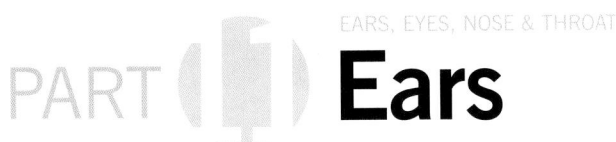 **Ears**

## Ear wax

### Introduction
Ear wax is very common and generally harmless, although It can affect hearing to some degree. Normal soft wax makes its way out of the ear and is removed by washing. Hard, or dried, wax tends to accumulate.

Removal of wax by syringing can give great relief, but this should be done by an expert aware of the risks. It is better to avoid syringing, in case infected material should be carried into the middle ear through an unseen perforation in the ear drum.

### Symptoms
Deafness is not caused by wax until the ear canal is completely obstructed, but this may occur suddenly if water gets into the ears lodging between the wax and the ear drum. Ear wax absorbs water and swells up.

### Causes
The rate of secretion of wax is affected by irritation to the skin, and constant poking of the ears with paper clips. Cotton buds, toothpicks or other objects will tend to produce more wax.

### Self care
The smallest thing you should ever put in your ear is your elbow. Never attempt to physically remove wax. Instead use wax softeners obtainable from your pharmacist. Avoid syringing as much as possible. It tends to stimulate the production of more wax and can pass infection into the middle ear if there is an ear drum perforation.

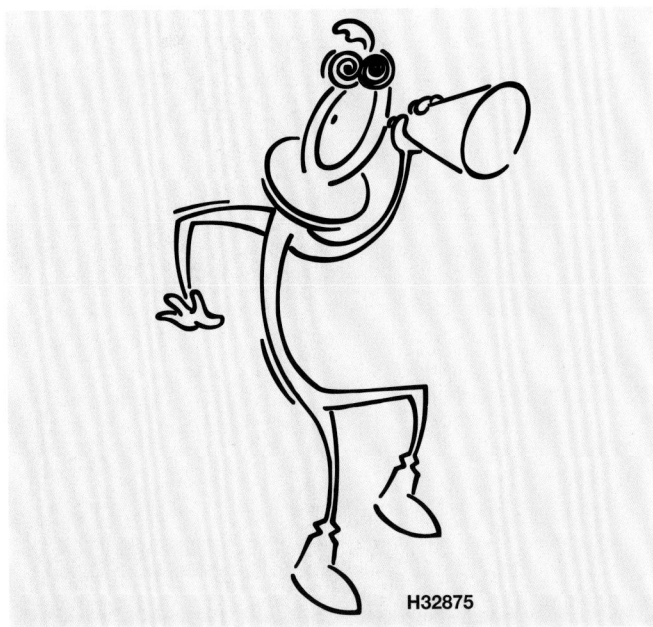

H32875

This sort of thing could affect your balance and roadholding

## Loss of hearing

### Introduction
There are many ways to lose your hearing. Terms like 'Boilermakers Ear' gave way to 'Disco Deafness' and will probably be known as 'Mobile Middle Ear' with the present explosion in mobile phones and personal stereos. Infection is another factor although infection of the middle ear and so called 'glue' ear are no longer thought to be a major cause of permanent hearing loss. Ear wax is a common cause of deafness, made worse by attempts to remove it with a cotton bud. This has about the same degree of success as trying to take a cannon ball out of a cannon with a ramrod.

### Symptoms
Most people do not realise how much they depend upon their hearing until it is impaired or lost. Gradual hearing loss is usually missed or ignored until there is difficulty hearing speech. By this time the damage has invariably been done, particularly if it was caused by prolonged and repeated exposure to loud noise. There may also be a ringing or hissing noise (tinnitus) much worse when in a quiet room or at night. Less often there may also be dizziness (vertigo) although this tends to occur while the damage is taking place.

### Causes
Prolonged exposure to loud noise is a common cause, particularly in industry and farming. Some viral infections may cause deafness and tinnitus. There are basically two types of deafness.
- Conductive deafness involves the poor conduction of sound from the ear drum, along the middle ear bones (ossicles) and on to the sensory structure which converts the sound vibrations into nerve impulses for the brain to understand (cochlea). Diseases which attack the ear drum or middle ear bones reduce their ability to conduct sound.
- Perceptive deafness involves the cochlea or auditory nerve and this permanent damage is commonly caused by loud noise exposure.

### Prevention
Hearing loss is often joked about, and although some hearing loss is inevitable with old age, there is lots you can do, again in earlier life, to prevent going completely deaf. Wearing ear protectors and using sound baffles is relatively easy. More education is needed for young people about the dangers of using personal stereos, head sets and mobile phones with the volume too high.

### Complications
Loss of hearing can cause accidents and potentially dangerous misunderstandings over instructions. It can be a terrible social barrier for some people. Some forms of deafness are accompanied by tinnitus which can be very distressing.

### Action
Make an appointment to see your GP.

# Middle ear infection (acute otitis media)

### Introduction
Infections of the middle ear are common, particularly in children. Various theories attempt to explain this but we do know that the infections are not as serious as once thought. Even so, they are very painful and can cause a temporary loss of hearing. A recent cold or throat infection may have happened before the pain in the ear started.

### Symptoms
Most people complain of a dullness in their hearing as if there was cotton wool blocking their ear. There is also a severe throbbing pain made worse sometimes by coughing. If there is pus behind the ear drum it may leak through a small hole not unlike a boil on the skin. Once the pus escapes the pain rapidly declines. It is difficult not to notice this happening as the pus usually flows out very quickly and has a strong smell. The ear drum repairs itself and there is very rarely any loss of hearing as a result.

### Causes
Infections of the tube which connects the ear to the back of the throat – the Eustachian tube – may help cause middle ear infections. This tends to happen during cold or flu epidemics. Its job is to keep the pressures equal on both sides of the ear drum, pressure builds up in the middle ear which is the main cause of pain.

### Prevention
Some doctors feel that mentholated pastilles sucked during a cold may prevent the Eustachian tube from blocking but there is no hard evidence to support this.

### Complications
It was once thought that middle ear infections caused permanent loss of hearing. This is no longer considered completely true. In the past serious infections of the skull bones next to the middle ear (mastoiditis) were dangerous and often lead to complete deafness in that ear. Thankfully it is now very rare although we do not know why.

### Self care
Pain relief is the main treatment as antibiotics take a long time to take effect. Painkillers will reduce the pain and hard swallowing should be encouraged rather than blowing against a pinched nose to help unblock the Eustachian tube.

### Action
See your pharmacist. If the pain does not subside or respond to painkillers, make an appointment to see your GP.

# Tinnitus

### Introduction
Tinnitus is a constant sound in the ears. About 25% of people with tinnitus experience musical noises, about 75% describe it as hissing, buzzing or ringing.

Nearly everyone has experienced short periods of ringing in the ears. This may be spontaneous or due to a loud noise, a cold or a blow on the head.

In established tinnitus, the sound is continuous, but sufferers are not always aware of it, so that it appears to be intermittent.

Most sufferers say that tinnitus is always worst in bed at night, probably because there is then less background noise. It is, to a variable extent, masked by external background noises that are usually present during the day.

### Causes
Tinnitus is almost always associated with some degree of deafness and is related to damage to the hair cells of the cochlea of the inner ear. These delicate hair cells are the means by which acoustic vibrations are converted into nerve impulses for passage to the brain.

Tinnitus can be caused by any of the factors known to cause deafness, such as:
- Nearby explosions.
- A blow on the ear.
- Prolonged loud noise.
- Fracture of the base of the skull.
- Tumour in the nerve from the ear to the brain (acoustic neuroma).
- Some antibiotics.
- Diuretic drugs.
- Quinine.
- Various ear disorders, such as Menière's disease, otosclerosis, labyrinthitis and presbyacusis.

Explosions, and other nearby loud noises (acoustic trauma) are among the most important causes of tinnitus and deafness. After exposure to noise loud enough to cause temporary deafness, most of the hearing loss is restored, usually in a matter of hours; but some permanent loss occurs.

The causes of non-permanent tinnitus include:
- Ear wax irritating the eardrum.
- Middle ear infection (otitis media).
- Glue ear (serous otitis media).
- Impacted wisdom teeth.

None of these is likely to lead to permanent tinnitus.

# Treatment
Certain drugs, such as local anaesthetics and others which interfere with nerve conduction, have been found to have an effect on tinnitus. Try not to concentrate on your own tinnitus. Distraction is the best strategy. Some people have found it helpful to listen to low-level music on personal headphones. Others have invested in 'white noise' generators (tinnitus maskers). These produce a rival sound on which to concentrate.

# PART 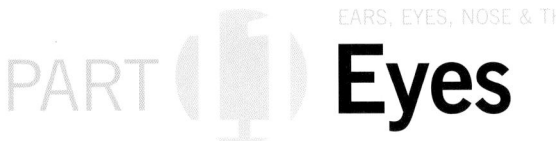 **Eyes**

## Conjunctivitis

### Introduction

Inflammation of the transparent covering over the eye, the conjunctiva, is common. Infection, foreign bodies, constant rubbing or chemical irritation are all causes. People with allergies to plants or certain chemicals may inadvertently cause conjunctivitis by rubbing their eyes after handling the substances. In most cases the inflammation will subside on its own.

### Symptoms

The blood vessels in the conjunctiva enlarge and the eye may appear 'blood shot'. Pus collects during the night under the eyelid and can matt the two eye lids together. Bacterial infections, reactions to chemicals or allergies often affect both eyes whereas viral infections tend only to affect one eye, at least initially. Pus is much less of a feature with allergic or chemical reactions. Instead there can be a quite dramatic swelling of the conjunctiva producing a boggy plastic bag effect around the centre of the eye which remains unaffected. It will settle on its own although it can be treated with anti-inflammatory eye drops.

### Causes

Bacterial from another infected person, often a member of the household or a school child can be passed on through sharing towels or even physical contact. This may also be true for viral infections although they also arise spontaneously. Grass and pollen will irritate the eye, especially if you suffer from hay fever. Wood resin, household chemicals, petrol, and many other common substance will also cause conjunctivitis.

### Prevention

Using separate towels and face clothes while a relation is infected makes good sense. Wear goggles when handling chemicals. Take anti-histamines during high pollen counts if you are a hay fever sufferer.

### Complications

Persistent bacterial infection can cause permanent damage to the front of the eye. Viral infections are more serious if they are on the transparent centre of the eye, not the conjunctiva.

### Treatment

Bacterial infections need antibacterial drops from your doctor. It can take up to a week for the infection to clear but you can make things much better by gently cleaning the crusted pus away from the eyelids with a soft cloth and warm water. Antihistamine drops make a dramatic difference for allergic conjunctivitis and are available from your pharmacist without a prescription.

If there is any change in your vision, whether pus is present or not, you should ring your GP.

### Action

If there is pus, phone your GP, otherwise see your pharmacist.

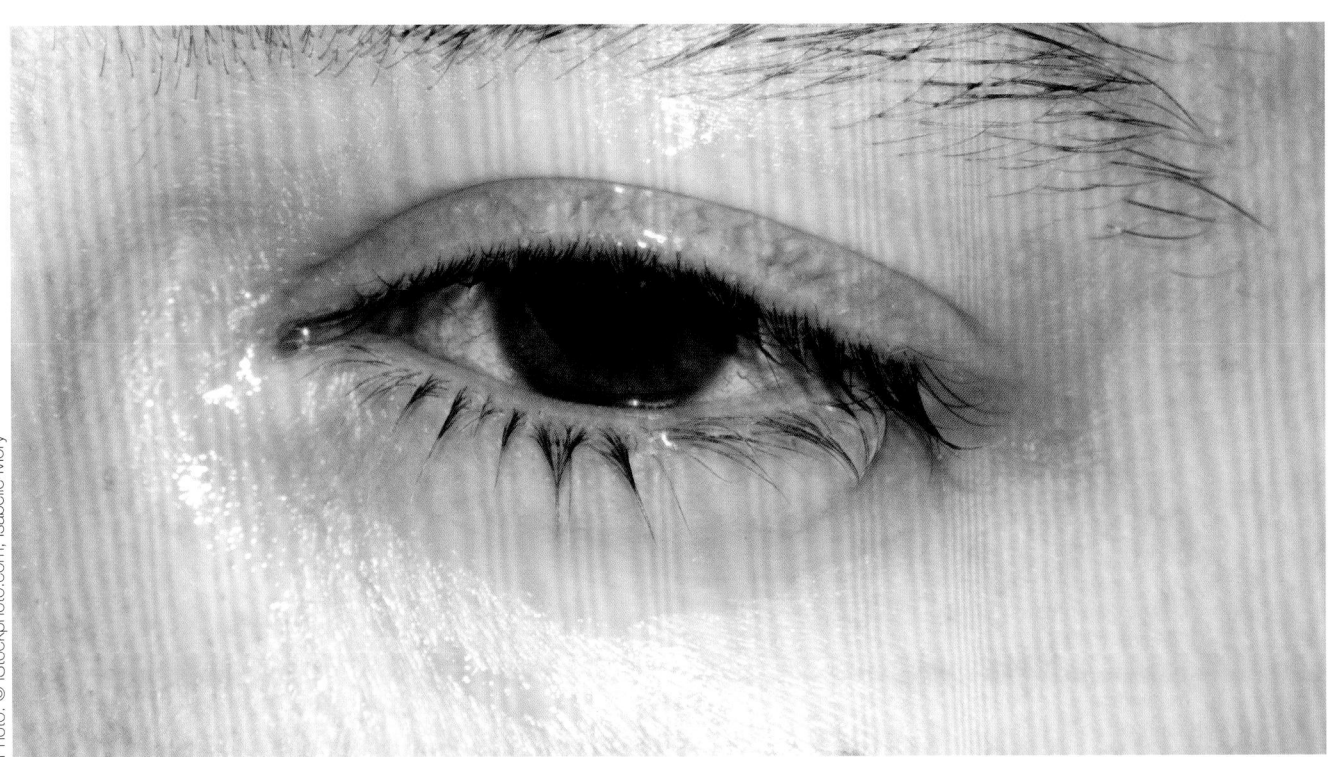

Photo: © iStockphoto.com, Isabelle Mory

# Glaucoma

### Introduction

The outer coat of the eyeball is tough but soft. It needs a steady pressure inside to maintain its shape.

Glaucoma is a group of eye diseases in which the pressure of the fluid (aqueous humour) within the eyeball is too high. This can happen in two ways. Either the tiny openings which allow fluid to leave the eye become partly blocked, or part of the eye moves forwards to block access to the openings.

About one person in 100 has glaucoma at the age of 40, but the incidence rises steeply with increasing age. By the age of 70, about one person in ten has significantly raised eye pressures. Chronic simple glaucoma runs in families and is more likely to occur in relatives of people with the disease. Only in the late stages will there be obvious symptoms. Central vision is usually the last to go and one eye may be completely blinded before it is appreciated that anything is amiss.

In other, less common, forms of glaucoma, the effects may be more obvious, with recognisable symptoms. In the most severe form the symptoms may be dramatic, with great pain and sudden loss of all vision.

### Symptoms

Unfortunately, chronic simple glaucoma produces almost no symptoms until it is at an advanced stage at which much of the outer (peripheral) field of vision has been lost. Surprisingly, very few people notice the loss of peripheral vision despite bumping into furniture.

A less severe and less common form, called sub-acute glaucoma, causes symptoms that should be more easily recognised. These usually occur at night when the pupils are wide. There is a dull aching pain in the eye, some fogginess of vision, and, characteristically, concentric, rainbow-coloured rings are seen around lights. The condition can easily be prevented by the use of eye drops and is curable by a simple operation or outpatient laser procedure.

Acute glaucoma is hard to miss. The affected eye is acutely painful, intensely red and congested, very hard and tender to the touch. The pupil is enlarged and oval and the cornea steamy and partly opaque. The vision is grossly diminished. Urgent treatment is needed to reduce the pressure, so no time must be wasted.

### Effects

If the internal pressure of the eye gets too high it will be higher than the pressure of the blood in the small arteries inside the eye and these will be flattened and closed. This can kill the nerve cells or fibres which detect light.

These fibres are concerned with vision at the extreme outer limits of our fields of vision and it is hard to notice that peripheral vision has been lost. This is because our brains concentrate on a narrow area around the point we are looking at. Many people can lose extensive peripheral vision without being aware of it.

### Diagnosis

The best test is to measure the internal pressure by a technique known as tonometry, using a pressure-measuring device mounted on an eye microscope. This test is routinely performed by opticians when carrying out eye tests. Your eyesight is vital – an eye test costs a lot less than a car MOT.

### Complications

A serious complication of undetected and untreated glaucoma is blindness.

### Treatment

Glaucoma must first be detected, then treated. In most cases the pressures can be kept under control by regular daily use of special eye drops. If eye drops fail, some form of surgery will be necessary.

Laser trabeculoplasty uses a laser to burn several tiny holes in the outflow filter of the eye. This makes it easier for the aqueous humour to flow out and reduce the pressure.

Another option is trabeculectomy, an operation to provide an alternative route for fluid drainage out of the eye.

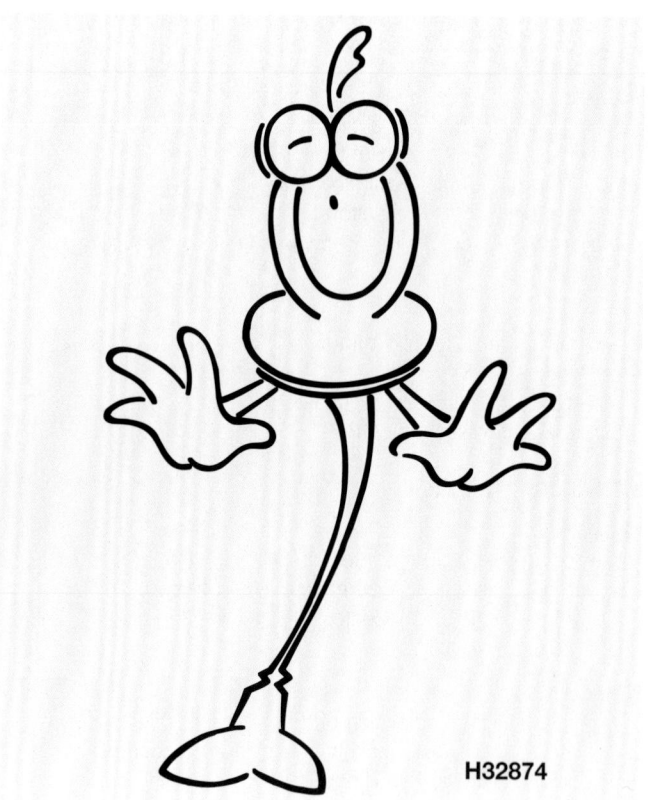

H32874

Make sure your headlights go to full beam. Get them checked regularly

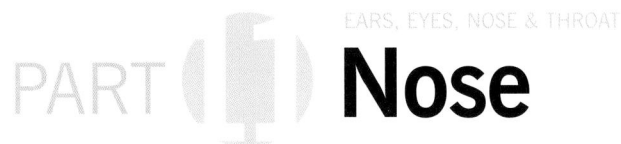

# PART **Nose**

## Nose bleeds

Nose bleeds are common. The vast majority are spontaneous, often following a cold or chest infection. Adults taking anti blood clotting drugs should tell their doctor or clinic as it can mean they may need to reduce the dose slightly.

### Symptoms
Nose bleeds can look quite dramatic but they are rarely serious. They are generally painless and from only one nostril.

### Causes
The blood vessels in the nose are very close to the surface. At one place inside the nose a number of blood vessels meet and bleeding from this area (called Little's area) is common.

In very rare cases it can be caused by a blood disorder.

### Prevention
As there is generally no warning it is difficult to prevent a nose bleed.

### Treatment
Cautery – burning of the blood vessels – by a surgeon does help but if you are prone to them it may well happen again.

### Complications
Avoid swallowing the blood as it irritates the stomach, making you vomit.

### Self care
Tip your head forward over a sink or basin, firmly pinch the soft part of the nose just in front of the bridge and allow the blood to run out of your mouth. It will stop bleeding in around 10–15 minutes. Once it has stopped avoid blowing your nose and cough gently for the next 8–10 hours to avoid starting a fresh bleed.

### Action
● If it fails to stop after 15 minutes, which is rare, you should ring your GP for advice.
● If you are suffering from repeated nose bleeds make an appointment to see your GP.

## Sinusitis (nasal)

### Introduction
Although inflammation and infection of the hollow spaces of the face bones (the sinuses) is extremely painful, it is rarely serious. Some people suffer from repeated sinusitis while others avoid the problem altogether.

### Symptoms
A great deal depends on which of the sinuses is affected. It can feel like severe tooth ache or a headache with tenderness under the eyebrows. Generally your nose feels blocked up and your voice has a nasal sound. It can last for weeks but most will clear up within 7 days.

### Causes
Sinusitis is caused by sinuses which fail to drain though their ducts into the back of the nose. It often follows a cold or an allergic attack.

### Complications
Serious complications such as infection spreading into the bone are now very rare because of antibiotics.

### Self care
Sinusitis really does hurt, so pain relief is important. Use appropriate painkillers. Decongestants may help initially but over use simply makes matters worse, particularly when you stop taking them.

Stop smoking. (You may have heard that before in this manual but it is still good advice.)

Try inhaling steam from a bowl of hot water.

### Treatment
You may be prescribed antibiotics by your doctor but they penetrate the sinuses very slowly and you need to take them in high dose for quite a while.

There are surgical treatments to flush out the sinuses.

See your pharmacist for pain relief.

### Action
If the pain persists make an appointment to see your GP.

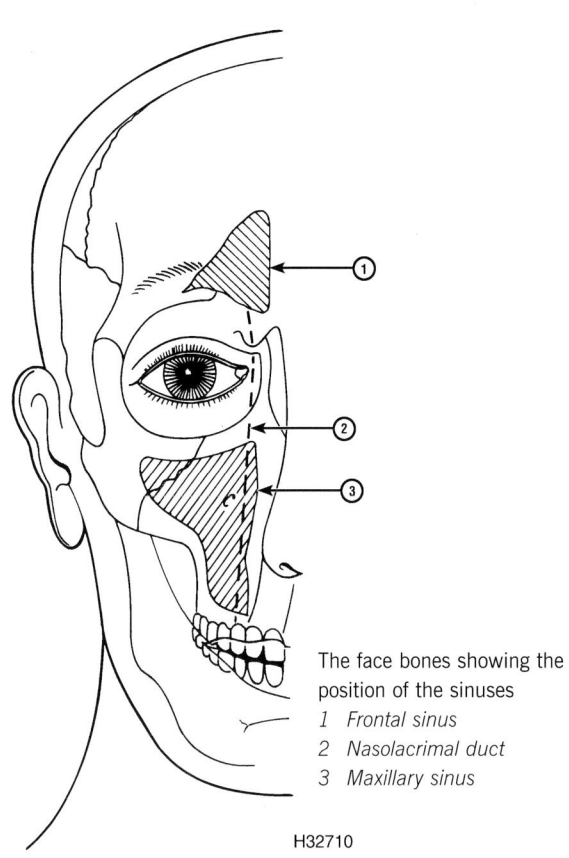

The face bones showing the position of the sinuses
1   *Frontal sinus*
2   *Nasolacrimal duct*
3   *Maxillary sinus*

H32710

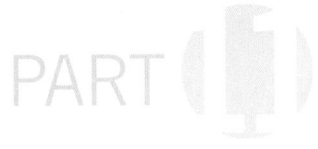

# Throat –
# Cancer of the larynx

## Introduction

Popularly known as the Adam's Apple, the larynx is the box-like structure at the top of the windpipe. Partly composed of gristle (cartilage) it has a prominent front part, especially in men. It has two important jobs: making noise with the vocal cords for the mouth and tongue to turn into speech, and stopping food going down 'the wrong way'. Trying to do both at the same time is one of the tricky bits which can go wrong, especially after a few pints of lager and faced with large chunks of poorly-chewed steak. It has sensitive nerves which make you cough when spaghetti bolognese is boldly going where air should go.

Although relatively rare, cancer of the larynx occurs most often in smokers and heavy drinkers. If the cancer is confined to the vocal cords it causes obvious voice changes and is likely to be diagnosed early. In addition, spread from the vocal cords to other parts is thankfully slow. In this case the outlook is favourable. Unfortunately, cancer elsewhere in the larynx is likely to be well advanced before symptoms of breathing or swallowing difficulty arise, so the prospects of a cure is not so good.

## Symptoms

An obvious symptom of cancer of the larynx is a change in the voice. This is not the usual sore throat of an infection or after speaking for long periods. Singers and actors know this feeling well. With cancer there is a permanent hoarseness. With a longer-standing cancer there can be difficulty in breathing and swallowing.

## Causes

Tobacco smoking is the single greatest cause, but others include alcohol abuse and exposure to asbestos fibres. Obviously stopping smoking, drinking in moderation and using mixers rather than drinking neat spirits makes sense.

## Diagnosis

Any marked change in the voice lasting more than a couple of weeks should be investigated by an expert without delay. It is possible to look at the inside of the larynx using an instrument called a fibre optic laryngoscope and any cancer present is generally readily visible.

## Prevention

As mentioned above, laryngeal cancer is almost totally preventable by stopping smoking, drinking in moderation and avoiding neat spirits.

## Treatment

Early diagnosis is essential as small cancers of the vocal cords can often be cured by local treatment with lasers, or more often with radiotherapy. Larger cancers that have spread to involve the cartilage of the larynx usually require partial or total removal of the larynx (laryngectomy). Obviously this means the vocal cords are no longer there to vibrate and produce the sounds acted on by the mouth for speech. This is where the latest technology steps in with electromechanical devices that mimic their function. Speech therapists can give invaluable support and advice.

# Contacts

**Active places**
Website:
www.activeplaces.com

**Alcoholics Anonymous**
PO Box 1
Stonebow House
Stonebow, York YO1 7NJ
Tel: 01904 644026
Helpline: 0845 769 7555
Website: www.alcoholics-
anonymous.org

**Asthma UK**
Summit House
70 Wilson Street
London EC2A 2DB
Tel: 0845 7 01 02 03
E-mail:
info@asthma.org.uk
Website: www.asthma.org.uk

**Beating Bowel Cancer**
39 Crown Road
St Margarets, Twickenham
Middlesex TW1 3EJ
Tel: 020 8892 5256
E-mail: info@
beatingbowelcancer.org
Website:
www.beatingbowelcancer.org

**British Colostomy
Association**
*Support, reassurance and
practical information for people
with a colostomy.*
Helpline: 0800 328 4257
Tel: 0118 939 1537
Fax: 0118 923 9184
E-mail: sue@bcass.org.uk
Website:
www.bcass.org.uk

**British Heart Foundation**
14 Fitzhardinge Street
London W1H 6DH
Tel: 020 7935 0185
Website: www.bhf.org.uk

**British Infertility Counsellors
Association**
Tel: 0114 263 1448
Website: www.bica.net

**British Lung Foundation**
73-75 Goswell Road
London EC1V 7ER
Tel: 08458 505020
Website: www.lunguk.org

**CHILD: The National
Infertility Support Network**
Tel: 01424 732 361
Website: www.child.org.uk

**Citizens Advice Bureau**
*If money or legal problems are
causing you stress, contact them
for free and confidential advice.
Look in your phone directory to
find your local office.*
Website:
www.citizensadvice.org.uk

**Colostomy Association**
15 Station Road
Reading RG1 1LG
Tel: 0118 939 1537
Helpline: 0800 328 4257
Fax: 0118 956 9095
E-mail: cass@
colostomyassociation.org.uk
Website: www.bcass.org.uk

**Cruse Bereavement Care**
Cruse House, 126 Sheen Road
Richmond, Surrey TW9 1UR
Administration Tel:
020 8939 9530
Fax: 020 8940 7638
General E-mail:
info@cruse.org.uk
Helpline: 0870 167 1677
E-mail: helpline@cruse.org.uk
Website: www.
crusebereavementcare.org.uk

**Diabetes UK**
10 Parkway
London
NW1 7AA
Tel: 020 7424 1030
E-mail: info@diabetes.org.uk

**Digestive Disorders
Foundation**
Tel: 020 7486 0341 (not a
helpline)
E-mail:
ddf@digestivedisorders.org.uk
Website: www.
digestivedisorders.org.uk

**Donor Conception Network**
PO Box. 7471
Nottingham NG3 6ZR
Tel: 0208 245 4369
E-mail:
enquiries@dcnetwork.org
Website: www.dcnetwork.org

**Drinkline**
Tel: 0800 917 8282
Websites: www.downyour
drink.org/drinkline.html and
www.wrecked.co.uk

**Epilepsy Action**
New Anstey House
Gate Way Drive
Yeadon
Leeds
LS19 7XY
Tel: 0808 800 5050
E-mail:
helpline@epilepsy.org.uk
Website: www.epilepsy.org.uk

**Everyday Sport**
Website:
www.everydaysport.com

**Human Fertilisation and
Embryology Authority (HFEA)**
21 Bloomsbury Street
London WC1B 3HF
Tel: 020 7377 5077 (Mon to
Fri 9.30am to 5.30pm)
E-mail: admin@hfea.gov.uk
Website: www.hfea.gov.uk

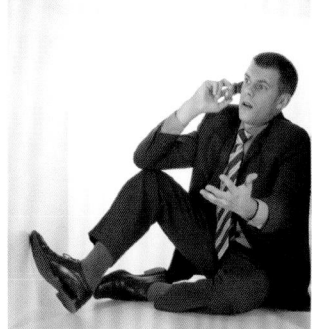
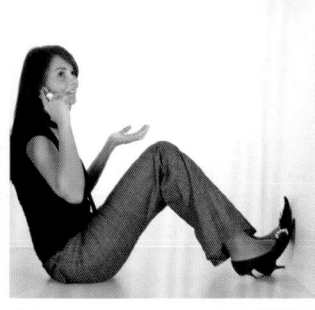
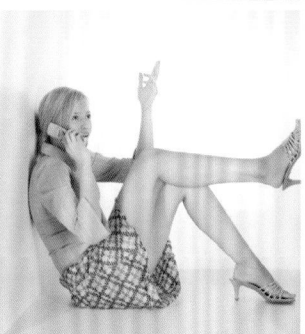
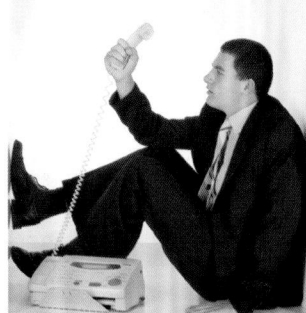

Photo: © iStockphoto.com, Gabriela Trojanowska

**Ileostomy and Internal Pouch Support Group**
Peverill House
1 – 5 Mill Road
Bally Clare
Co. Antrim
BT39 9DR
Tel: 0800 018 4724
E-mail: Ia@
ileostomypouch.demon.co.uk
Website: www.
ileostomypouch.demon.co.uk

**Impotence Association**
PO Box 10296
London
SW17 9WH
Tel: 020 8757 7791
Website:
www.impotence.org.uk

**International Stress Management Association**
The Priory Hospital
Priory Lane
London
SW15 5JJ
Tel: 07000 780 430

**ISSUE: The National Fertility Association**
Tel: 09050 280 300
(25p/min)
Website: www.issue.co.uk

**The Mental Health Foundation**
London Office
9th Floor
Sea Container House
20 Upper Ground
London
SE1 9QB
Website: www.mhf.org.uk

**Men's Health Forum**
Websites:
www.malehealth.co.uk (UK)
www.mhfs.org.uk (Scotland)
www.mhfi.org (Ireland)
www.emhf.org (Europe)

**Mind**
*Mind is the leading mental health charity in England and Wales, and works for a better life for everyone with experience of mental distress.*
PO Box 277
Manchester M60 3XN
Tel: Mindinfo Line
0845 766 0163
E-mail: info@mind.org.uk
Website: www.mind.org.uk

**National Association for Colitis and Crohn's Disease (NACC)**
4 Beaumont House
Sutton Road
St Albans
Herts AL1 5HH
Tel: 0845 130 223
NACC in-Contact Support Line
Tel: 0845 130 3344
E-mail: nacc@nacc.org.uk
Website: www.nacc.org.uk

**National Asthma Campaign**
Providence House
Providence Place
London
N1 0NT
Tel: 0845 7 01 02 03
Website: www.asthma.org.uk

**National Osteoporosis Society**
Tel: 01761 471771
Website: www.nos.org.uk

**NHS Direct** *provides confidential health advice and information 24 hours a day.*
NHS Direct Interactive on digital satellite TV.
Tel: 0845 46 47
(England and Wales)
Website:
www.nhsdirect.nhs.uk
Tel: 08454 24 24 24 (Scotland)
Website: www.nhs.24.com
*Lots of examples of fruit and vegetable portion sizes are on the 5 a day web site.*
Website: www.5aday.nhs.uk

**NHS Stop Smoking Helpline**
*An advisor can put you in touch with your local NHS Stop Smoking Service.*
Tel: 0800 169 0 169
Website: www.
givingupsmoking.co.uk
Websites inspired by hundreds of ex-smokers in the UK
Website: www.ash.org.uk
Website:
www.sickofsmoking.com

**The Orchid Cancer Appeal**
Tel: 020 7601 7808
Website:
www.orchid-cancer.org.uk
*TSE Testicular Self Examination Leaflets from:*
McCormack Ltd
Church House
Church Square
Leighton Buzzard
Beds
LU7 7AE

**The Prostate Cancer Charity**
Helpline Tel: 0845 300 8383
Website:
www.prostate-cancer.org.uk

**QUIT**
Ground Floor
211 Old Street
London
EC1V 9NR
Smokers' Quitline Tel:
0800 00 22 00
E-mail: info@quit.org.uk or
stopsmoking@quit.org.uk
Website: www.quit.org.uk

**Relate**
Website: www.relate.org.uk

**St John Ambulance**
27 St. John's Lane
London
EC1M 4BU
Tel: 0870-010 4950
Website: www.sja.org.uk

**Samaritans**
*Available 24 hours a day to provide confidential emotional support for people who are experiencing feelings of distress or despair.*
General Office
10 The Grove
Slough
Berks
SL1 1QP
Tel: 08457 90 90 90
E-mail: jo@samaritans.org
Website: www.samaritans.org

**Sexual Dysfunction Association**
Tel: 0870 774 3571
Website: www.sda.uk.net

**Sexual Health Direct**
*(Run by the Family Planning Association)*
Tel: 0845 310 1334 (UK)
– Mon to Fri 9am to 7pm
Tel: 0141 576 5088
(Scotland) – Mon to Thurs
9am to 5pm,
Fri 9am to 4.30pm
Website: www.fpa.org.uk

**Sport England**
Website:
www.sportengland.org.uk

**The Stroke Association**
240 City Road
London
EC1V 2PR
Tel: 0845 30 33 100
(Mon to Fri 9am to 5pm)
E-mail: info@stroke.org.uk
Website: www.stroke.org

**Walking the way to Health**
Website: www.whi.org.uk